Body, Breath, & Consciousness

Body, Breath, & Consciousness

A Somatics Anthology

A Collection of Articles on Family Systems, Self-Psychology,
The Bodynamics Model of Somatic Developmental Psychology,
Shock Trauma, and Breathwork

Edited by Ian Macnaughton

Foreword by Peter A. Levine

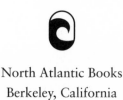

North Atlantic Books
Berkeley, California

Published by
North Atlantic Books
P.O. Box 12327
Berkeley, California 94712

Cover and book design by Brad Greene
Printed in the United States of America
Distributed to the book trade
by Publishers Group West

Body, Breath, and Consciousness: A Somatics Anthology is sponsored by the Society for the Study of Native Arts and Sciences, a nonprofit educational corporation whose goals are to develop an educational and crosscultural perspective linking various scientific, social, and artistic fields; to nurture a holistic view of arts, sciences, humanities, and healing; and to publish and distribute literature on the relationship of mind, body, and nature. This is issue #65 in the Io series.

North Atlantic Books' publications are available through most bookstores. For further information, call 800-337-2665 or visit our website at www.northatlanticbooks.com.

Substantial discounts on bulk quantities are available to corporations, professional associations, and other organizations. For details and discount information, contact our special sales department.

Library of Congress Cataloging-in-Publication Data

Body, breath, and consciousness : a somatics anthology / edited by Ian Macnaughton.
       p. cm.
   ISBN 1-55643-496-0 (pbk.)
   1. Mind and body therapies. 2. Mind and body. 3. Psychotherapy. I. Macnaughton, Ian, 1938–
   RC489.M53C665 2004
   616.89'14—dc22
                                                            2004007818
                                                            CIP

   2 3 4 5 6 7 8 9 DATA 09 08 07 06

Permissions

The following articles are reprinted with the permission of Bodynamic International: *The Body Self in Psychotherapy*; *Ethical Consideration in Somatic Therapies*; *Individuation, Mutual Connection and the Body's Resources*; *The Art of Following Structure—Exploring the Roots of the Bodynamic System*; *Waking the Body Ego, Parts 1 and 2*; *The Body-Knot Model*; *Caring For Yourself While Caring For Others*; *The Therapeutic Power of Peak Experiences*; *Character Structure and Shock*.

Multigenerational Family Therapy is reprinted by permission of the author, David Freeman.

Sensory Functioning in Psychotherapy is reprinted by permission of the author, Erving Polster.

Panic, Biology, and Reason: Giving the Body It's Due is reprinted by permission of the author, Peter Levine.

It Won't Hurt Forever...Guiding Your Child Through Trauma is reprinted with permission of the authors, Peter Levine and Maggie Kline.

Using the Bodynamic Shock Trauma Model in the Everyday Practice of Physiotherapy is reprinted by permission of the author, Barbara Picton.

Acknowledgments

This collection would not have been made without the efforts of a number of people. I am grateful to all the contributors who allowed their work to be re-published here, and to the many colleagues, clients, and friends who have assisted in vital ways, both recently and earlier, to find concepts and methods for understanding and treating the entire person in the full contexts of living. A special appreciation goes to Garry Friesen of designTHIS.net for guiding the development of this book. Richard Grossinger and Brooke Warner of North Atlantic Books have been incredibly helpful in reformatting and with timely advice on how to proceed with the publishing process. Dr. Stuart Miller has been an invaluable "author coach," and Sylvia Sandquist's many hours of word-processing were important. My mother, and my wife, Barbara, have been unfailing sources of encouragement and support. Together with our children, they will find me eternally grateful to rest in such a loving and passionate family.

Table of Contents

Introduction

This book is about Body, Breath, and Consciousness. It presents various pathways to enhance the ease and depth of connection between us all. Within that capacity lays the forging of a sense of personal authenticity, an individuation we recognize as our self. The capacity of such presence allows us to be closely interrelated with others in intimate ways as well as appropriately connected with groups and the world community. To be confident in our ability to maintain a solid sense of self in all those domains of human experience requires a healthy sense of autonomy, a secure self that neither distances nor unduly reacts to the challenges of the range of interpersonal contact.

Our sense of self rests in our history, understanding the legacies, the strengths and losses faced down through our family generations. Here, rather than stories of family dysfunction, are the seeds, the markers, the images that can help recover and honor the losses inherent in every family's stories, and the overt and sometimes subtle heroism of surviving nonetheless. It rests in our personal developmental history, how we individually coped within the family, school, society. From that we developed our character patterns—our defenses; our best friend in times of great challenge; our ways to cope when all else fails us. Learning how to appreciate these limitations as the best we could do in the circumstances—and with a compassionate heart embrace and learn other options—is central to the theme of the various clinicians whose work is presented here. They offer their work as an aid to those travelers who are interested in pursuing a holistic and multi-integrated approach. Each author presents a solid theoretical base for individual exploration; they all address the central unity of the person, whether from a multi-generational systemic perspective or more specifically focusing on the relationship of mind and body in biological, psychological, and spiritual reality.

The understanding of spiritual experience signals an attention to the underdeveloped parts of ourselves. As we live more at ease within ourselves, there is a natural unfolding of the richness of internal experience, without focusing on trying to reach spiritual plateaus. In that way, we come home to ourselves, our nervous systems, our mind body reality. We are essentially biological beings, a part of the cosmos and of all existence. Our task is to grow into the lived experience of that as an increasing emergent consciousness.

The general reader will travel through many perspectives that bridge the themes of body, breath, and consciousness. The material is intended to be useful for the general reader interested in human development. In addition, the present book will be of use by itself to students of family systems—particularly to the many professionals struggling to comprehend the diverse and complex forces, both within and outside the individual, that shape the life of the self: somatic, emotional, mental, interpersonal, social, and spiritual. Somatically oriented therapists will also find the book useful for its discussions of the theory of systems in general and of family systems in particular.

The Bodynamics model of somatic developmental psychology is prominently featured here for its unique contribution to therapeutic theory and practice, as well as to understanding self-development, shock trauma, and spirituality. In the years to come, this profound model will surely make major contributions to our seeing the body-mind as a whole rather than only in its separate parts. The Bodynamics relating of spirituality to psychology is especially helpful in developing an integrative rather than fragmentary view of the human being.

I have divided the book into five parts:

Part One introduces aspects of systems thinking and treats some of its applications to family and body-mind therapy and practice.

Part Two zeroes in on body-mind systems, with specific reference to sensory function, touch, therapeutic touch, and ethical considerations in practice.

Part Three presents the theory and practice of one body-mind approach in greater depth and fullness.

Part Four is about the theory and practice of dealing with trauma from a body-mind perspective.

Part Five explores the current emphasis in body-mind spirituality practices and theory of the bio-energy system.

In order to help readers bridge their understanding of the successive sections of the book, I begin each part with a short preface suggesting how the articles fit together in the section and how the parts relate. In the Afterword, I further explore some of the common threads in the articles and suggest implications for additional theoretical and practical explorations.

I cannot think of a better beginning to the rest of this book than a poem by John Baughan that has always touched me. It sounds the twin notes of exploring and unifying, both so needed in society and psychotherapy and to which this book is dedicated:

What is required of us in our time
is that we go down
into uncertainty
where what is new is old as every morning
and what is well known is not known as well.

That we go down
into the most human
where living men have vanished
and the music of their meaning
has been trapped and sealed.

What is asked of us in our time
is that we break open
our blocked caves
and find each other.

Nothing less will heal the anguished spirit,
nor release the heart to act in love.

—from *The Sound of Silence,* by John Baughan

Foreword

Ian Macnaughton has been a guide and mentor to students of body-oriented psychotherapy for over twenty-five years. Ian's wisdom and warmth have touched those who have had the privilege to study and work with him. During this time, Ian has brought together the knowledge of a select group of innovators who have formed the core of his approach to body psychotherapy. In this volume, he offers a selection of their various works.

For the reader interested in the integration of body, mind, emotions, and spirit, these various perspectives contained here will be a meaningful resource to guide their way. *Body, Breath, and Consciousness* spans the breadth of perspective from the cognitive, behavioral, somatic, and spirit dimensions. The emphasis on speaking to people's underlying health and resources provides a voice toward emergent consciousness versus focusing on psychopathology.

This book has great value as a useful resource for both well-accomplished professionals (such as body psychotherapists, bodyworkers, mental health professionals, educators, medical personnel), as well as those who are just beginning their career exploration.

The integration of these apparently divergent worlds of different approaches is sequenced to present a systemic perspective on the human condition. This writing encourages us to view the whole person and the context within which they reside—their family, understanding the role of cognitive patterns, the family legacies, the driving force of the need for mutual connection, and an appreciation of the uniqueness of an individual's personal journey.

Ian draws from the wisdom of viewing the individual as resting within the field of a dynamic, systemic, interrelated world. In particular, he explores the Reichian, Neo-Reichian, and developmental theorists primarily from Bodynamic Analysis and the trauma therapy of Somatic Experiencing. He also provides a practical article of "trauma first aid" for children, as well as an article of guidance, which delineates the limitations and contraindications of the

Reichian breathing techniques from the vantage point of these other somatic methodologies.

Readers seeking to understand their own personal dynamics and relationships, as well as those in the helping professions, will discover leading-edge perspectives to guide their way. This collection opens up new pathways in the service of greater personal and societal evolution.

I highly recommend Ian Macnaughton's intelligent offering.

—Peter A. Levine, Ph.D., author of *Waking the Tiger: Healing Trauma*

Part One

Family Systems &
the Body-Mind

Systems theory can be a useful way of understanding the incredible complexity we confront in living today. Gregory Bateson, a famous systems philosopher, maintained that ignorance of the context of our lives is the biggest error in our thinking today. He meant that we fail to appreciate our complex and multiple relationships to the world. Our psychological and organizational theories, for example, often ignore the vast social, physical, and other energies and influences within which we live. As our world becomes more socially complex, it becomes more difficult to manage, and our ability even to influence social and political events diminishes. To our peril, we were educated to think mainly in a linear and not a systemic way. Part One, applying systemic thinking to the individual and the family, briefly outlines some principles about how the family is a system with both psychological and somatic influences upon us.

Dr. David Freeman's article, "Multigenerational Family Therapy," outlines the core principles that guide his work, and also the mental health professional training at the Pacific Coast Family Therapy Training Association and PACE, a therapeutic play school for three- to five-year-olds. There we integrate family systems therapy with art and play to help children and their families. As a consultant to PACE, I have also been introducing concepts and interventions relating to early psychomotor development, learned through my studies with the Bodynamic Institute in Copenhagen. Lisbeth Marcher, the founder of this system, and Marianne Bentzen, senior trainer, have generously contributed time to this endeavor. The principles of Dr. Peter Levine's Somatic Experiencing Model have also been helpful. Both Marcher's and Levine's work will be explored further in Part Four.

I am deeply indebted to Dr. David Freeman for the contribution he has made to my view of the family system. As a mentor, friend, and colleague, he has not only expanded my view of the family system, he has also greatly enriched my life.

"Expanding the Field of Family Therapy" is an article that, in fact, reflects on the ideas and practical steps in Dr. Freeman's approach to inviting elders into the therapeutic process—in a way that uses their oral history of the family as an adjunct to therapy.

The final article, "The Narrative of the Body-Mind—Minding the Body," suggests how a broadly systemic perspective can begin to integrate body-mind approaches (in this case Bodynamics) with family-of-origin theories and practices.

Multigenerational Family Therapy

—David Freeman, D.S.W.

Introduction

A multigenerational approach to family therapy honors the family in a special way. The approach recognizes that the family can be both a resource and a problem for its members. One of the goals of the therapeutic process is to maximize the family's positive influences as a way of dealing with the problem areas.

It is critical that the family therapist understand the influence and power the family exerts over its members. Without this understanding, a therapist may unwittingly side with a family member against his or her family. The collusion is subtle but profound. It is common for a client to begin therapy by telling the therapist various stories about how rejecting, critical, and unloving his or her family is. Many therapists assume these stories are generally accurate and focus their efforts on helping the family member deal differently with his or her family. These therapists may have a view of family similar to that of their clients, and may even advise that family contact should be kept at a minimum. Other therapists may encourage their clients to confront family members about the behavior they see as upsetting and destructive. These approaches, although intended to be supportive and helpful to the client, in fact, reinforce the client's preconceived assumptions about family; thereby maintaining distance, a lack of family connection, and a sense of loss.

Multigenerational family therapy emphasizes the importance of family connections in people's lives. Therapists employing this framework encourage their clients to work on family relationships. Ordinarily, people enter therapy feeling quite ambivalent about their families. If the therapist shares this ambivalence, he or she will feel discomfort about involving the family and avoid this potentially positive resource. My model of family therapy views the family as a powerful ongoing influence in its members' lives. My approach may involve seeing aged parents, adult siblings, and other important family members as well as the more traditional parents and children.

This introductory article describes the major family therapy principles that underlie a multigenerational approach to family therapy. When a therapist involves several generations in the therapeutic process, he or she embarks upon a radical approach to problem solving. This article provides a framework for that approach.

Section 1: *Major Principles of Family Therapy*

Principle One: A family member's problem is contributed to and reinforced by the other family members' response to it.

All family therapy models endorse this basic principle. However, there continues to be an active debate about which came first—the problem or the "response." My position is that it does not matter. By the time the family is seen by a therapist, the problem has existed for so long that it has become part of the way in which the family functions.

The family therapist's task is to understand the functional nature of the problem and how the family reinforces it as a way of problem solving. When an individual family member experiences difficulty, either physically, socially, or psychologically, the family system has to respond to him or her in some way. This response will set up certain family behavioral patterns that may influence behavior after the original problem is gone. Family members who define a particular individual as having a problem will do so in relation to their view of themselves as "healthy." Perceived dysfunctional behavior in one family member may contribute to another family member's feelings of adequacy. And so, certain responses, once set in motion, may become part of a permanent behavior pattern.

In a session that I once had with two parents and their three adolescent children, the father told me that his wife usually jumped in to break up any conflict between him and his older adolescent daughters. When I asked him how that affected the way he dealt with his daughters, he answered that he knew he could count on his wife to rescue him if he became too angry. He went on to explain that knowing this allowed him to indulge his anger and, at times, actually get angrier than he felt initially. When I asked his daughters what they had learned about their father from their conflicts, they answered that they had discovered their father was not as safe as their mother because his temper got out of control. In fact, the mother's rescuing the father contributed to the father's unsafe appearance to the daughters, and added to the distance that developed between father and daughters. The family members had not recognized the reciprocal nature of their behaviors.

Whatever the nature of the problem, it is up to the practitioner to take a holistic view of the family and resist zeroing in on the identified problem. The immediate concern of the family is often not the major underlying problem. The important issue is how the problem has affected the relationship network within the family.

Principle Two: Change will not be sustained in a family unless the most powerful members of the family are willing to sustain it.

It is an important systems principle that change occurs from top to bottom. If a child tries to change his or her behavior toward a parent without a corresponding change from the parent, within a short period of time, the child will revert to the old familiar behavior. However, if the parental unit is able to sustain a change in their behavior toward a child, eventually the child will behave differently.

The general principle plays out when one member in the family system changes and remains involved with the entire system, resulting in the other members being unable to maintain their old behavior. The question for the therapist to determine is which members of the family have the greatest potential for change. In many families, the child acts out as a way of connecting with his or her family. It is futile to try to get such a child to change without the cooperation of the parents. A more effective approach is to help the parents understand how their reaction to the child encourages this behavior. The family therapist must analyze the family system to discover the functional nature of the problem and the reciprocal roles the family members play with the problem. The next objective is to determine which unit within the family has the greatest potential for change. In my opinion, the parental unit is the most powerful one in the family. When a therapist helps parents respond to a child's behavior in new ways, the child will modify the behavior, and a new family structure will develop.

A simple experiment will help the reader understand how difficult and risky it is to do something differently in one's family. Think about some traditional behavior that your family counts on you to continue exhibiting. Consider stopping behaving in this manner and think about the reactions. The usual response by family members is anger, hurt, and criticism. In turn, the one who has changed becomes anxious about the reaction that his or her new behavior has brought about. He or she quickly discovers that by resuming the old behavior, his or her own anxiety and the anxiety of family members can be reduced. This example illustrates how difficult it is for a family member to change his or her customary way of taking care of other family members.

Principle Three: Functional families maintain a balance between individual autonomy issues and family solidarity concerns.

When assessing a family, it is important to evaluate how it is able to balance the individual needs and expectations of its members and the solidarity concerns of the group. Often parents enter family therapy with the hope that the therapist will work toward greater solidarity in the family and in effect bring the family members together in a closer, more involved way.

Adolescents and young adult children tend to resist coming into family therapy because they are apprehensive about becoming more involved in family issues. Adolescents are in the process of moving away from the family. Even the term family therapy increases their anxieties about their ability to eventually emancipate from the family. The family therapist, therefore, has a unique balancing act to perform. He or she has to address the parents' concern for greater togetherness while also communicating to the adolescents that their needs for greater autonomy and separateness from the family are understood and supported.

In most functional families, individual autonomy is not a major concern. Family members are able to respect each other's differences, while at the same time feeling connected as a group. When there is a dysfunctional member within the family, whether parent or child, this balance becomes threatened. Some of the family may become over-involved with the dysfunctional member and others may remain on the periphery. Usually, when there is a concern about one family member, the ability of the family to maintain a balance between individual needs and group concerns is lost. The anxiety is too high, and the preoccupation with the dysfunctional member too great to maintain the balance. The involvement of helping professionals usually reinforces the imbalance with its focus on the dysfunctional member. The responsibility of the family therapist is to realign the family boundaries.

The family with an alcoholic parent provides an example of family imbalance. The common pattern is for the non-alcoholic parent to be preoccupied with helping the alcoholic partner give up his alcoholism. During periods of sobriety, the children will tend to feel great anxiety about when the alcoholic parent will start drinking again and throw the family back into chaos. A great deal of thinking, talking, and feeling is directed toward the alcoholic and his drinking.[1] The drinking behavior controls the family. Families function for years maintaining this anxiety. Everyone is cheated because of the preoccupation with the alcoholic. Individual needs of the children are considered secondary concerns and the individual needs of the non-alcoholic parent are seen as less important than taking care of the alcoholic member. When the alcoholic partner ceases to drink, it also creates anxieties within the family because the members have not learned how to function as a family without the familiar preoccupation.

Whenever there is a family problem, it in some way undermines the ability of the family to be able to attend to the individual needs of its members. One of the therapist's tasks is to help the family support the individual growth and development of its members, and in the case of children, to help them leave the family while at the same time feel connected and supported by it.

Principle Four: The family therapy session must be safe for all members and respect individual differences.

Principles three and four are interconnected. One of the ways in which the family therapist operationalizes principle three is by the way he or she relates to the family members in the sessions. It is up to the family therapist to make all the sessions safe for each family member. Family members are worried that they will be scapegoated—held responsible for the problem, focused on excessively, invalidated, etc. It is a great relief to family members to leave the first session feeling respected and understood, and to have had the opportunity to explain their view of the world to the rest of the family. One can understand the anger, ambivalence, and silences of family members as stemming from the anxieties that have been described. The job of the family therapist is to join with each family member around his or her concerns and to help to make it safe for them. I routinely ask family members questions that focus on how they have learned to make it safe for themselves, both in the family and in the work at large.

In addition to providing a safe environment, the therapist must be respectful of the individual differences within the family. The therapist must guard against trying to get family members to perform and/or behave in ways that make the therapist feel comfortable. Some family members may choose to be silent, some may choose to tell their concerns through stories and humor, while others may choose to be angry for a while. All the behaviors that family members exhibit during the early phase of family therapy are representative of the way they cope and make it safe for themselves. When they realize that the family therapist is not going to judge them, control them, and/or evaluate them, they will begin to relax and involve themselves in a positive way in the process.

The therapist plays an active role in keeping the sessions safe. He or she must foresee the reactions by family members that would tend to invalidate what another family member is saying. For example, when a child tells his or her story and describes reality as he or she perceives it, it is essential that the family therapist does not permit the parents to criticize or invalidate the child's story. Allowing parental criticism is a common error of therapists. When a therapist asks a family member to comment on what another member has just said, the member frequently responds with criticism and verbally attacks the other family member. When this happens, the therapist has allowed the session to get out of control. He or she has set up a situation in which one family member has undermined and invalidated what another family member has said. It is essential that the family therapist prevent that from happening. The therapist must give the family members an opportunity to say things through him or her to other family members without the statements stirring up anger, criticism, or hostility. Being heard without being criticized is a powerful experience for a family member. The degree to which the therapist is able to prevent family members from reacting to each other with hurt or anger determines the degree of safety experienced by family members in the session.

Principle Five: The family therapy session must offer the family members an opportunity to experience each other differently.

In the early stages of the family therapy process, the family tries to duplicate their "at home" behaviors in the therapist's office. Family members are both hopeful and anxious about the therapist being wise enough to prevent this duplication of experience. Family members desire change, yet are frightened by it. They will resist it. Behavior that is unpleasant, and makes one sad or unhappy, is nonetheless familiar. Coping mechanisms for dealing with the behavior have been developed. Change that prevents us from reacting in the familiar way will force us to develop a different understanding of ourselves. Many people find this frightening.

When a family therapist offers family members an opportunity to experience each other differently, the members become hopeful that they will be able to achieve something new and more meaningful. Simultaneously, their anxiety levels go up. In the beginning phases of family therapy, the family members will start expressing more of their concerns as they become more comfortable. They will feel relieved and hopeful during the session. However, when they return home and react to each other in the old predictable ways, they begin to feel defeated. They will return to therapy saying that they feel discouraged because they have not been able to react differently with each other outside of the family therapist's office. The challenge to the family therapist at this point is to ask questions that will help the family members identify what the loss for them would be if they were to respond differently to each other. Inexperienced family therapists commonly get discouraged at this point and question their abilities, or think family therapy is not working.

The therapist must continually help the family members understand that their old responses stem from ambivalence and anxiety rather than dysfunction and illness, and that gradually change will occur.

The skilled therapist offers the family members hope that they can connect with each other in a more positive way, and learn about each other while these new connections are occurring. The behavior of the wife in a couple I once worked with illustrates the struggles that we can have about changing. For several months, I had been encouraging the wife to bring her mother into a session. She eventually agreed to do this. However, when the session arrived, she appeared without her mother. When I asked her why her mother was not there, she answered she did not really want her mother to come to the sessions. I then asked her what the loss would be for her if I met her mother. Her answer was that she had spent a lifetime learning how to deal with her mother, and that this allowed her to maintain a comfortable distance from her. If a session with her mother challenged the view she had of her mother, she would lose this comfortable distance. The risk of having to give up her old story about her mother created tremendous anxiety and prevented her, at least at that point, from connecting with her mother differently.

There is no question that it is risky for family members to see each other differently. Once you see someone differently from the old familiar pattern you have to reevaluate your own behavior toward that person. You cannot hold the other person solely responsible for what is going on between the two of you. The ultimate challenge for the family therapist in all this is to shake up old patterns and remain calm in the face of the family's ambivalence when the therapist is successful in doing so.

Principle Six: The family therapist must control the process during the session.

When conducting a therapy session, the experienced therapist is continually focusing on the process and is avoiding becoming caught up in the content. Families will often present a story, and then try to get the therapist to say who is right or wrong. It is, of course, impossible to figure out a story. If you as a therapist can be convinced that one member's view of the story is correct, then you have entered the triangle; and everyone in the family, as well as yourself, becomes the loser.

When looking at the process, therapists should be alert to how individual members within the family use conflict to maintain emotional distance. There are two major types of conflict: (1) non-productive conflict, which maintains relationships the way they are; and (2) functional conflict, which involves the renegotiation and reorganization of relationships.

As discussed earlier, when one family member changes, other members can become uncomfortable and conflict can occur. The way in which the family deals with conflict, rather than the conflict itself, is critical to its functioning. The therapist will want to note which members of the family are most comfortable with change and how they are positioning themselves within the family to deal with that change. The therapist will also want to note what other family members are doing in response to that change. It is not the issue (content) that is important, but how it is dealt with (process).

The family will try with all its might to get the therapist to take a side on content issues. When family members become anxious, they almost always revert to content issues. When a therapist gets hooked into content, it is usually because it has to do with an issue in his or her own life. Later in this text, I will deal with the issue of unfinished business and how it affects the therapeutic process. The success of the therapist in understanding content issues as symbols of struggles and unresolved losses will be determined by the degree to which the therapist has worked through his or her own past losses and struggles.

A popular joke highlights the importance of process over content. A famous rabbi in Russia was well known for his astuteness and ability to resolve marital conflicts. A couple with serious marital conflicts went to see him. When they entered the rabbi's office, they found him there with his rabbinic student. The rabbi asked the husband why he came to see him. The husband responded by telling him many terrible things about his wife. When he finished, the rabbi said, "You're right." Then the rabbi asked the wife why she came to see him. The wife proceeded to tell the rabbi many terrible things about her husband. When she finished, the rabbi said, "You're right." At this point, the rabbinic student was very confused and said, "But Rabbi, how can the husband be right on the one hand, and the wife right on the other hand?" The rabbi reflected for a moment, stroked his beard and said, "You know something, you're right, too."[2]

Principle Seven: The family must own its change and take responsibility for its outcome.

In a family systems approach, the experts are the family members. The goal of the therapist is to help the family develop its own way of discovering how it wants to move from point A to point B. One of the therapist's jobs is to encourage family members to assume the expert role. The initial expectation of the family is that the therapist will provide the answers. This expectation represents one of the first challenges to the therapist. Consequently, there may be an initial struggle between the therapist and the family about who will do what. If the therapist takes responsibility for the solution to the problems, then he or she must also take responsibility for the outcome. If the therapy works, it is because he or she is a great therapist. If it fails, it is because he or she is inadequate. In either case, the family does not assume responsibility for resolving its problems.

One of the most powerful experiences family members can have in therapy is to discover that they have their own effective ideas about how to resolve their dilemmas. The therapist's initial task, then, is to encourage the family to find its own solutions. Typically, when families enter therapy, it is because they have been ineffective in resolving their problems. Often, their view of the picture exacerbates the situation and impedes their finding better solutions. Therefore, one of the first tasks in family therapy is to redefine the problems. In accomplishing this task, the therapist must help the family understand how its problems affect the entire family. This process helps the family members gain a broader, more sophisticated definition of themselves as a system. As this occurs, they will also develop a new set of ideas about how they want to resolve their dilemmas. As the therapist focuses on the family's ideas, the members will begin to see themselves as experts in dealing with their problems.

The course of therapy with the "M" couple illustrates the importance of this dynamic. During the course of therapy, the couple decided to separate. Mrs. M decided to continue in therapy to work on some self-issues. One of her major concerns was doing things alone, which was the basic reason she had remained so long in an unsatisfying relationship. She found it difficult to go to movies alone, go out to dinner alone, travel alone, etc. One day, she came in and announced ecstatically that she had gone to a movie alone and had found it an enjoyable experience. I responded by challenging her as to why she wanted to do this alone. At this point, she became angry and asked if this was not what we had been working toward all this time. I replied I didn't know. I asked if this was something that she thought was good for her, and stated that I was not sure myself. She told me with tremendous energy and conviction that this was the best thing for her, and that she needed to do this. I could not convince her otherwise. I took a rather contrary position with her because I wanted her to "own" the change rather than do something to please me. I did not want her to think about my advice as a way of making it safe for her to go out alone. When she tried to talk me out of my lack of enthusiasm for her activity, it reinforced within her the idea that she was the mistress of her fate. It is important for family members to own their outcome, and not do something to please their therapist.

In addition to the seven general principles described on the preceding pages, there are several specific principles that underlie a multigenerational approach to family therapy. Both sets of principles dovetail, and when taken together form a holistic approach to family therapy.

The following principles represent the most significant themes discussed throughout this text. They are evident in both the basic theory and the practice components of the model.

Principle Eight: The family is a multigenerational emotional system.

Relationship patterns are passed on from generation to generation. One needs to look at multigenerational patterns to understand current family patterns.

Parents will bring lessons from their own families-of-origin and try to put them into practice in their new family-of-procreation. A family has a minimum of three family influences, the husband's family-of-origin, the wife's family-of-origin, and the synthesis of the two families in the nuclear family. The success with which the differences, as well as the similarities, are integrated by the couple will determine the overall balance of the new family unit. Many people assume that when they marry they start with a clean slate and will evolve a unique family unit. The family that the couple develops is indeed unique. However, it has been greatly influenced by the emotional lessons and experiences each person has brought into the family.

It is helpful in understanding how we operate in our families to look back at least three generations. It is not enough to understand just our parents and siblings. The way our parents organized our family and responded to us as children should be understood in terms of their experiences in their own families. Often, a family therapist assesses a family by asking the parents to talk about their experiences in their own families. He or she will ask about what happened between various family members in the extended family: what were the losses, how were emotional needs met, who was the most involved, who was the most distant, etc. This information, though important, does not reach back far enough in helping us understand family structure, function, and development.

Our parents' behavior toward us was, to a significant degree, determined by their parents' behavior toward them. If our parents experienced separation, divorce, or significant loss in their own families, these experiences would have had a profound impact on how they dealt with their family-of-procreation. If we do not understand our parents' experiences in their own families, we will not fully appreciate how their struggles and losses have shaped their behaviors and feelings toward us. A multigenerational approach provides a different framework for understanding why certain reactions, decisions, and positions are taken in a family.

On one occasion, when I was asking a highly conflictual couple about their families-of-origin, the husband told me his father had never really told him much about himself. He grew up seeing his father as being in the background, not really involved in the family, and somewhat unimportant in his life. He described his mother as being more central to the family. He adopted the general notion in the family that his father did not care much about the family. I encouraged the husband to learn more about his father. He discovered that his father was an orphan who had been deserted by his extended family and had raised himself from the age of thirteen. When the husband told me this story, he interrupted himself and said, "You know, I never considered my father an orphan. I never thought of him as a little boy who did not have a family." This new idea about his father led to him viewing his father's separateness from the family differently. He stopped seeing it as a sign of lack of love and caring, and began to understand it as a manifestation of his father's early sense of loss and isolation from his own family.

It is helpful to family members to understand that current concerns have historical significance and, in turn, implications for future generations.

Principle Nine: People's relationships are shaped by their family stories.

One way to change family behavior is to help the family modify its emotional stories about its history. Everyone has stories about his or her experiences with family.[3] Most people think that their stories are accurate accounts of what happened. In truth, many of the stories that we carry in our heads are symbolic of losses and/or important emotional events that have shaped our thinking about ourselves, our family, and the world around us. These stories are often used to maintain safe distance in relationships.[4] If we felt hurt, rejected, abused, misunderstood, or invalidated in our family, we will be cautious about duplicating the experiences underlying these feelings in our adult life. One of our hopes when we marry or form close relationships is that our new partner will either make up for our past losses or replicate the safe, positive experiences we had in our families. When our partner's behaviors remind us in any way of hurtful memories, or when our partner disappoints us by not making us feel okay, we take a defensive stance. This stance is a familiar reaction that allows us to feel emotionally safe.

In order for change to occur in relationships and/or families, we have to rethink the basic stories that we carry in our heads about ourselves and our family. When we feel that our family experiences occurred because we were not lovable, then we will continually look to others to make us feel worthwhile. Paradoxically, we will also be more likely to perceive others' behavior toward us as confirmation of our feelings of inadequacy.

One of the major objectives of a multigenerational approach is to help people rethink their family stories. One must recognize, however, that many of us are not prepared to give up the stories that we have developed about ourselves and our family. These stories allow us to maintain a safe distance in relationships. We know how to function with these stories intact. If we give up these stories, then we have to alter our style and way of relating.

Principle Ten: Significant change in the extended family influences the functioning of the nuclear family.

To understand the family problem, we have to understand the family's developmental history. There is an intimate connection between the nuclear family and the extended family. The nuclear family is commonly described as the family-of-procreation, the biological mother and father raising biological children. One can extend the definition of the nuclear family to include stepparents, stepchildren, and adopted children, but basically the nuclear family is a small unit of parents and children. The extended family includes grandparents, uncles, aunts, in-laws, cousins, etc. Most people are not aware of how they are influenced by extended family changes. The death of a parent, illness of a sibling, the break-up of a marriage within the extended family, the death of a cousin, are all changes that can have a profound impact on the nuclear family.

When one assesses the family on a multigenerational basis and charts all the major events, one begins to perceive a relationship between the timing of problems and developmental shifts within the family. It is not unusual, for example, for the death of a parent to produce marital problems for an adult child. Similarly, the divorce of parents after thirty or forty years of marriage can threaten the sense of family solidarity among the adult children in the family. Not just the behavior, but the response of the extended family to major developmental events in the nuclear family, has a tremendous impact on the nuclear family.

The meaning a family attributes to its problems is often based on its previous experiences with that type of problem. Couples often view a problem as stemming from the husband's side of the family, or the wife's side of the family. It is not unusual for a couple to fight over which side of the family was responsible for producing a particular problem in a child. Our view of a problem and the labels that we give to it are, to a large degree, determined by our previous family experiences of that problem. Professionals, in turn, also contribute to the labeling process. It is a powerful event when the professional definition of a problem coincides with the family member's personal definition of a problem. When this occurs, the label becomes firmly embedded in the family's mythology.

In my practice, I ask numerous questions about the timing and context of family problems. For example, I will ask (1) what losses have occurred in previous generations, (2) have there been any major developmental changes coinciding with the problem, (3) what was going on in the family prior to the problem occurring, (4) what have the family members learned from the family in their attempts to cope with this type of problem, (5) how do the anxiety levels of the two parents compare, and (6) how do the parents understand these differences? When the family addresses these questions, they begin to see how change in a nuclear family may be connected to events in the extended family. They also begin to get a sense of how their previous experiences with a particular problem influences their current perception of the problem.

Principle Eleven: We are never totally free of our family involvements.

Family relationships extend beyond space and time, life and death. By involving members of the extended family in the course of therapy, we bring in new energy and information, which in turn helps broaden and deepen family understanding. We occasionally see people who believe they can escape their family ties. Some individuals on the West Coast feel that the Rocky Mountains have separated and freed them from their family on the East Coast. What they learn, of course, is that family issues and relationships follow us wherever we go.

Some people attempt to suppress any thoughts of their family and avoid seeing them for years at a time. However, they fill the vacuum by looking for replacements. They try to construct a new family based on what was not finished within the old family. When their new relationships begin to feel like and/or remind them of the old issues, they quickly revert to the behavioral patterns that were played out when they were still in contact with their family.

One cannot, by distance, work through old family issues. One must deal with them at the source if one is going to be truly free of difficult issues. During the course of therapy, it is crucial to involve available extended family members. It is always a powerful experience to participate in a session in which aged parents, siblings, or other important relatives tell their stories. The later articles in this text contain general examples of interviews with different family constellations. In various ways, they illustrate that we cannot, by sheer willpower and distance, make peace with our family members. The most solid way for us to accomplish this is to reposition ourselves in the present with family members so that we understand their stories from a new perspective.

It is well known that the more solid the parent/child relationship, the less devastating the parent's death is for the child. Many children who have conflictual relationships with their parents maintain the fantasy that one day their parents will understand and accept them and all will be fair. When that parent dies, the anger, rage, and sense of betrayal increases. They feel that once again the parent has cheated them out of the relationship. Working with adult children prior to a catastrophic loss is a form of prevention. Helping them make peace with these relationships will result in fewer regrets when the parent does die.

Principle Twelve: Children emerge from the family-of-origin with a certain degree of unfinished emotional business.

We all have unfinished business. Unfinished business affects our choice of partners, the type of family structure we create, and the expectations we have of our mates and children. The premise underlying unfinished business is that children take on their parents' anxieties, vulnerabilities, and fears. It is difficult for children to separate their own emotional experiences from those of their parents. When a parent reacts to a child out of anxiety, neediness, or fear the child will, to some degree, act out those feelings for the parent.

One of the most dramatic examples of unfinished business is seen in second-generation survivors of the Holocaust. Numerous studies indicate that the second generation assumes the same fears, anxieties, and phobias of their parents. Many of these children have not been told about their parents' experiences in World War II concentration camps. Nevertheless, they exhibit similar behavioral patterns to those of their parents.[5]

Unfinished business is present in all families. The critical factor is the degree of unfinished business that an individual carries from one generation to the next. There is a certain amount of deprivation built into all family life. The extent of the deprivation one experiences in the family is the main determinant of how much unfinished business one carries into the next generation. Unfinished business does not go away. It is something we need to work on and understand so that part of ourselves does not interfere with our relationships with others.

Principle Thirteen: Relationship problems are a reflection of unfinished business and not an indication of a lack of commitment, caring, or love. One cannot give emotionally to others what one has not received from the family-of-origin.

This principle underscores the importance of reframing relationship problems as family-of-origin issues. One of the more compelling reasons for forming a relationship is to feel special. Most people want to be admired, liked, and needed. Those relationships that produce these feelings are the ones we cherish the most. When someone is asked what he needs from another to make the relationship work, the answer usually focuses either on what the individual did not receive from his or her family or on what he or she wants to duplicate from his or her family.

There are two major issues that get played out in most relationships: One either moves into a relationship as a way of making up for one's losses, or as a way of replicating one's own family experiences.

Relationships based on finding someone to make us feel whole and right are formed out of mutual need. The focus is more on what one needs than on what one can give. There is a high degree of reactivity in these relationships. The parties quickly become disappointed and negative toward each other. Of course, the more a person feels unloved and/or unlovable, the greater the neediness he or she brings into a relationship.

The second major type of relationship is one that is based on the couple's desire to duplicate experiences that they have had in their own families. These types of relationships have their own sets of difficulties. These difficulties come to the fore when one partner is not able to behave in a way that fulfills the other partner's expectations. When one emerges from a family-of-origin feeling special and cared for in a certain way, and has a mate who is not able to reproduce these feelings, disappointment and disillusionment will set in. In summary, most of us look for someone to make up for previous losses or to take care of us in a special way. When we do not find this we feel let down. This feeling leads us to take a defensive, distancing stance in the relationship and relationship problems will occur.

Principle Fourteen: The basic North American family structure is extended.

It is a myth to think that the basic family structure is nuclear. Most people are powerfully involved with their extended family members, although the look of the involvement has changed over time. The current notion of extended family is no longer based on how many people live under the same roof.

Our definition of family structure is significant because it influences who we see as important, and whom we include in family treatment. For many years, North Americans have popularly viewed the family as a two-generational unit. The work of Parsons and Bales[6] has influenced this view. Their studies indicate that the nuclear family is the most viable, flexible family system in an advanced industrial society. Parsons and Bales describe the nuclear family system as a family of parents and children lacking strong ties to extended kin. In a moment's notice, these families can move where the labor market demands its presence. Since Parsons and Bales's work was first published, many articles have appeared reiterating their view that the extended family is dead, and that the nuclear family is the major family structure in North America. This view has become so accepted that family units with close and significant ties to extended families are at times seen as dysfunctional and inappropriate. Although the initial work by Parsons and Bales is over thirty-five years old, the prevailing attitude continues to be that the more functional family structure is a small nuclear family unit. This attitude obscures the importance of the extended family.

The critical question is not whether we call the family nuclear or extended. What we should be looking at are the roles that various family members play in the nuclear and extended family constellation to facilitate and/or handicap the family unit. If we limit our concept of family structure to two generations, we ask fewer or no questions about extended family and can miss discovering the natural resources that are available to family units.

The importance of the extended family is not its physical proximity but rather its emotional impact. A few of the questions that I commonly ask to get a sense of the role extended family members play in the life of a nuclear family are:

1. Who are the most important people in your life?
2. Who can get you upset most quickly?
3. Who do you turn to first for help?
4. Which family members do you spend the most time talking about?
5. Who has had the strongest impact on your own development?
6. What relationship in the family do you have the most regrets about?
7. If changing one relationship in your life would help you feel better about yourself, what would that be?

Section 2: *Values Underlying the Family Therapy Process*

It is important that the family therapy model be guided by clearly articulated values. Values are the "oughts" or "shoulds" of behavior. They set the parameters of acceptability, and prevent us from experimenting with families in harmful or unethical ways. The therapist's intervention must always honor the family's sense of itself as a positive unit. Therapy should never undermine the solidarity of the family. As previously discussed, one of the major tasks of the family is to help its individual members grow, develop, and leave, while at the same time fostering the need for continuity, connection, and belonging. When a family therapist enters the family, his or her challenge is to address both of these opposing developmental goals. On the one hand, the parents will want the therapist to support their needs for family solidarity. On the other hand, the adolescent children will want permission to begin to move away from the family, their concerns being with issues of autonomy.

The therapist must be aware of his or her own values and refrain from superimposing them on the family. The therapist's job is to learn about the family culture—its values, its goals, and its vision. The therapeutic strategies and expectations must be based on that knowledge. Each family has a unique value system based on the values that each parent has brought into the relationship, as well as the values of the children. The children's values are, in turn, influenced by school and peers and may be in conflict with the parental value system. In actuality, a family has several value systems, which may be competing with each other. The fact that issues arise from a conflict in values is not always addressed. Often value differences are not even discussed, yet these differences get acted out around incidents and problems. Understanding the family's values will allow the therapist to see when conflict arises from different belief systems. The skilled therapist will ask questions that allow each family member to articulate his or her value system, and how he or she developed it over time.

Honoring the family's value system allows the family to own its outcome. The therapist should not impose solutions on the family or assume that he or she knows best how the family should function. There is no hard data about what makes a family functional. We are guided by our hunches, hypotheses, myths, and values. This makes it all the more prudent to take a research stance concerning families and to allow the family members to teach each other and the therapist about how they have learned to get the job of living done.

The value system of the family therapist should be open enough to allow the family a greater range of differences. The therapist must guard against preconceived ideas about what does or does not work for the family. At the same time, the therapist must have a bottom line about what is permissible, or basically unacceptable, in terms of family behavior. Families cannot change or risk talking about important matters when there is a threat to the members' safety.

The family therapist has the responsibility of making it clear to families that when there is any suspicion of violence or abuse, that the family members' safety must be guaranteed or the family therapy process cannot proceed.

To be effective, the family therapist must not be involved in secrets, nor should he or she collude with or align with certain family members against other family members. The family therapist must honor his or her commitment to all the members of the family—those present as well as those in the background. The underlying goal of the family therapist is to help family members at all levels connect in a deeper way. It is important that the family therapist be a positive force in a family's life. The therapist accomplishes this by serving as an impetus to the family as it re-discovers its basic wisdom.

A school counselor raised an interesting value dilemma during one of my recent consultations. It covered a family that consisted of a biological mother, her lesbian lover, and two adolescent children. One of the children was acting out at school, which initiated referral to the school counselor. The counselor was in a quandary about whether he should invite the mother's lesbian partner into the family sessions. He was not sure if the partner was truly a member of the family. Clearly, our own attitudes about what constitutes a family will determine whom we invite into the sessions. As it developed, the children in this family saw the mother's partner as an important caretaker and family member. It is critical that the therapist honor the family's definition about who is family. When we block the family's definition, then we become part of the problem.

Other value dilemmas commonly experienced by therapists arise from their views of "proper" lifestyle and "appropriate" parents. An example of a value stand that is presented as fact can be seen in the following quote:

> *There are also three-generation families, which are more typical of lower social economic groups and lower middle-income groups. In such multigenerational families, where there are grandparents and parents, parents and children—the question many times becomes: Who is parenting what child?*[7]

The inference here is that families that use extended family members for childcare exhibit more confusion about parenting. This value bias would interfere with an open-minded approach to assessing the family and the way it uses its natural resources.

Section 3: *Goals and Objectives of the Family Therapy Process*

The therapist must have clear, concise goals and objectives for the family therapy process. Goal-setting for a system like the family is complex and involves four major levels. Each individual has personal goals and hopes; the family unit has its expectations as well. The community at large has goals, particularly when a family member is having difficulties outside the home, at school, or at work. The therapist's goals and expectations comprise the fourth level.

To facilitate goal setting at the various levels, it is helpful for the therapist to communicate his interest in helping the whole family as well as its individual members.

As mentioned previously, the *two major developmental goals of the family* are:

1. to help its individual members be competent and independent, and

2. to maintain and foster commitments to the family as a whole.

One of the major successes of family living is to learn how to be part of a group, while at the same time be separate from that group. Many families have difficulty achieving this balance. They may emphasize family solidarity to the point that individual members must relinquish their autonomy. Alternatively, they may emphasize autonomy to the point that there is no family commitment whatsoever. Difficulties in balancing the two poles of individual autonomy and family solidarity underlie many of the problems experienced by families.

When a family first enters therapy, symptom relief is one of its major goals. Symptom relief is the elimination or alleviation of a problem that has been attributed to one of the family members.

It is unusual for a family to begin therapy with the understanding that family change is desirable. The usual complaint centers on one member.

For example, Johnny is misbehaving and the family cannot control him or dad is drinking and is disruptive to the family. The task of the family therapist is to help the family develop broader goals. The therapist must help the family expand its perception of the problem from an individual focus to a group interactional level. It is enlightening for the therapist to ask each family member to explain how he or she sees the problem. This process quickly illustrates how subjective our perceptions are. It also provides an opportunity for each member to express related difficulties and to thereby bring additional goals into focus.

Another aspect of goal setting is developing short-term and long-term goals. The therapist should be setting goals for each session as well as long-term goals. For example, one of the major goals for the initial session is to create a safe environment for the family, in which no one feels solely responsible for the family experience. Simultaneously, the therapist is developing goals for the long-range therapeutic endeavor. The long-term goals will encompass significant behavioral change within the family. However, if the therapist is unable to accomplish the initial short-term goal of providing a non-threatening environment, the achievement of long-term goals will be severely limited.

The major long-term goals of family therapy are to help the family to:

1. Reframe the problem from an individual concern to a family focus.

2. Improve the ability to deal with and accept differences.

3. Improve individual and family problem-solving abilities.

4. Decrease the need to use scapegoats.

5. Develop an intra-observational capacity of its own internal function.

6. Improve autonomy and individuation.

7. Develop a balance between individual autonomy and family solidarity.

8. Expand the boundary of the family to include important extended family members as resources for the family.

9. Work through its unfinished business.

10. Become its own resident expert.

References

[1] Stanton, Duncan, & Thomas Todd & Associates. *The Family Therapy of Drug Abuse and Addiction* (New York: Guilford Press, 1982).

[2] Freeman, David. *Techniques of Family Therapy* (New York: Aronson, 1981), 99.

[3] Stone, Elizabeth. *Black Sheep and Kissing Cousins* (New York: Penguin Books, 1989).

[4] Ibid., 21–24.

[5] Bergmann, Martin, & Milton Jucovy, Eds. *Generations of the Holocaust* (New York: Basic Books, 1982).

[6] Parsons, T., & R.F. Bales. *Family Socialization and Interaction Process* (Glencoe, IL: Free Press, 1955).

[7] Pillari, Vimala. *Human Behavior in the Social Environment* (Pacific Grove, CA: Brooks/Cole Publishing Company, 1988), 252.

Expanding the Field of Family Therapy

—Ian Macnaughton, Ph.D.

This article deals with utilizing interviews of the parents of adult children (clients) as an intervention in the therapeutic process. In describing this approach, it is crucial to understand that this model is not presented as a "technique" to be administered, but rather as a general framework in which certain principles of family systems theory and practice can be utilized.

This approach is not about confronting parents or involving them in therapy. It is about creating a safe atmosphere for the parents to tell their own story, to honor their truth and wisdom, and to assist in the development of appropriate boundaries between the adult children and their parents. Used appropriately, this approach can be of great assistance in facilitating healing in the family. The discussion that follows describes the model in terms of four themes: the pitfalls to avoid, safety considerations, post-session work, and the ongoing repositioning of the adult child.

Pitfalls

The most crucial issue is to provide a safe environment for the parents to tell their story—the story of their lives. They really have three generations to describe: the families from which each spouse came from, the family they made by deciding to be a couple, and lastly, the family they created. The counselor must continually be alerted to the possibility that the parents' story may stir up reactivity in the counselor or the adult child. If the counselor is being critical or judgmental, wanting to distance, or otherwise feeling anxious, it is likely that something in the parents' story is echoed in the counselor's own unfinished business. It is not safe for the parents to tell their story if the counselor becomes reactive rather than maintaining a proactive curious stance.

In this model, the parents have not come in for therapy, per se, but have been invited by their adult child to tell their story about their life and experiences of the family. It is considered an error if the counselor attempts to change the contract by offering therapy, rather than utilizing the presence of the parents as a way of honoring their truth about how they have experienced the family over the years.

It is important that the counselor does not buy into the content of the parents' story, deciding whether it is "right" or "wrong," or editing it. In this way, the story can be heard as a metaphor, with the counselor listening for the way parents relate their life stories and the themes that have run through their lives, and those of different generations. These important themes will include the losses that the family has sustained, and how the family has coped with those losses.

Encouraging interaction between the adult child and the parents can lead to reactivity and a repeat of the old relating patterns. In this approach, it is important that the adult child take an observational position, witnessing the counselor interview the parents about their life story. The parents are speaking directly to the counselor, leaving the adult child free to hear the story in a new way.

A lack of preparation can lead to difficulty in the session, and increase the risk that the session will serve as a reinforcement of the old story about the parents. The interview should be structured, and the role of the adult child clarified, in order to create a safe environment. The counselor should ensure that the adult child is at a stage of therapy where it is possible to sit in on this kind of interview relatively unencumbered.

Safety

The adult child must be in the middle phase of therapy to be able to sustain a proactive curious stance in the interview. At this stage, the therapist has shifted to more of a coach or consultant, encouraging curiosity about family, guiding thinking about conducting research about family stories and how they are constructed. If this approach is used prematurely when the adult child is still in the beginning phase, it will be difficult to maintain an independent sense of self, and may begin framing thoughts in terms of blame, criticism, and distancing. It takes a considerable degree of emotional maturity for the adult child to take responsibility for personal reactions and to not project them out in a reactive way.

If the client is not able to maintain a proactive attitude, the safety of the session will be impaired, and there is a danger of further solidifying the old perceptions about parents. Clients must be fairly secure within themselves in order to risk a shift in their perceptions about their parents and family.

Ideally, the interviews would cover three sessions. In the first session, the stories of the parents' families-of-origin would be heard; during the second session, the story about how they came together and created their own family. The last session would afford an opportunity for the adult child to ask the parents any questions about which there is still curiosity. The interviews would usually be 1½ hours long and spaced out over a few months, allowing time for therapy to proceed with the material that arises for the adult child from the interviews.

The interviews are highly structured, with the counselor conducting the interview and the adult child listening. This arrangement should be very clear before the parents come in, and it should be restated at the outset of the interview.

Parents come in afraid that they will be further blamed, or feel guilty for what they "didn't do" for the adult child. It is crucial that their fears in this regard be allayed by the conduct of the counselor and the framework for the process. It is useful to ask them what they were told by their adult child about the session. The counselor should restate that the interview is about learning the history of the family. By videotaping these stories, the family will have a record for future generations. Explaining that the counselor will conduct the interview, and that the role of their adult child is just to listen as they tell their story, can relieve any fears that they will be confronted. The counselor's own ability to maintain a curious proactive stance can model for the adult child a new way to be with the parents.

The use of the genogram (Jackman, 1991) can be a safe and systemic framework for guiding the process of generating stories about family. Learning about the family by discussing significant events in their family, such as births, deaths, marriages, and geographical moves, will elicit stories surrounding these events and ease the parents into a natural flow.

Post-Session Work

Following each interview, the adult child (client) is instructed to view the video during the next week. This viewing should be done alone in order to avoid the possibility of anyone else commenting on the interview and perhaps influencing the client's perceptions.

Shortly thereafter, the counselor and the client should meet to discuss the client's perceptions of the session and reactions to viewing the video. The crucial point here is to determine where the client has made a shift in thinking, and where old stories about parents and family have been reactivated.

The intent is to support clients in understanding that the way they were parented and the reason for deprivation or withdrawal was not about some lack in them. It is about the losses that the parents sustained in their own families-of-origin. You can't pass along what you didn't get. To hear about the parents' losses, to let go of the old sense of criticism, blame, and distancing on the part of the client, produces a profound shift in relationship with self and a movement to true self-differentiation.

The next step in the process can be to have the client view the tape with a significant other. Concerns that might be raised can be discussed in future sessions. Supporting the client to take a research perspective can aid in fostering curiosity. This can extend to considering interviewing aunts, uncles, grandparents, and other family members.

Ongoing Repositioning

The movement into the family, to a position of an increasing sense of a self that can sustain the anxiety of being different in family, will foster further self-definition. This evolving self no longer retreats into safety by distancing, blaming, or criticizing the family, but is curious about how the family is the way it is. At this point, the client becomes the healer in the family, no longer defined by others' reactions. When family members become controlling, angry, or upset, the client begins to understand that his reaction is not about him/her, and so does not have to respond in a "knee jerk" way. Over time, the client can react less and recover sooner, learning to hear that the others' reactivity (and his/her own) are attempts to create safety and to buffer any further loss.

This process can be facilitated by the client making family visits to different members of the family. These visits should include time alone with the family member, utilizing the curious stance of a researcher about family. Attending significant family events such as births, deaths, marriages, reunions, and holidays can generate many opportunities for connecting with family differently.

Conclusion

In my work with clients and my own family-of-origin, I believe that to truly foster a strong sense of self, we need to develop a curiosity concerning the reactivity in our family, and develop the capacity to shift from reactivity in our family to a proactive curious perspective. The reactivity is protecting losses experienced by family members who are isolated and hurting. Often we hope that family members will assist us or accept the changes that we want to make. The true test of whether those changes are well integrated is in what we do when others become reactive toward us. If we can sustain our changes in the midst of that reactivity, then we are emotionally more solid. True change occurs without the cooperation of others to shore us up. It is important to support our clients and ourselves, to sustain new behavior under old or increased reactivity from family members, without becoming counter-reactive in return. Then the reactivity of family members becomes a further impetus to self-definition, freeing our clients and ourselves to react not with criticism, blame, and distancing, but to respond with curiosity and compassion.

If, as therapists, we have not done our own work with our own family-of-origin and come to terms with our own reactivity, we will run the risk of colluding with our clients' stories about their family and "how impossible" it is for them to be different in their family.

The model described above can be helpful in assisting clients to shift their perceptions about their parents, their family and themselves. Parents in turn can feel respected for what they tried to do, and begin to connect differently with their adult child.

Reference

[1]   Jackman, M. (1991). "The use of the genogram," *The Clinical Counselor* 1 & 2:42–49.

The Narrative of the Body-Mind—Minding the Body

—Ian Macnaughton, Ph.D.

The rain was coming down in sheets as if a dam had burst far above the dark clouds. It was a dreary November afternoon, buffered only by the warm glow of my office lamps and the soft gold upholstery of the chairs, as Ethel and Bob enter. They had started therapy two sessions before because their sixteen-year-old son, Tom, was refusing to go to school and seemed to rebel at almost every reasonable act of parenting.

The two parents presented very different physical appearances. Ethel, I noticed, looked depleted—a slender pale woman with a slightly sunken chest. She had entered the room like a delicate, timid bird, greeting me with a certain deference. I had been struck by the softness and tentativeness of her hand-shake and her general demeanor. Bill, by contrast, entered in a positive, even determined way, as if he and the ground were somehow over-connected. His eyes were penetrating and he greeted me with a sturdy handshake.

During that first and the succeeding session we had begun an initial explo-ration of their own intergenerational histories and the differences in their indi-vidual family-of-origin parenting styles. Among other important facts, I learned that Bill's father had largely been absent; Ethel's had been present in a very strong way. Now was the moment to explore some of the concrete results of those differences by bringing the treatment into the present and its problems.

I was glad when Bill began the session by jumping into the moment: "I don't think we are getting anywhere here. We still haven't found out what we need to do with Tom. Ethel just won't support me in laying the law down to him."

As he was speaking, I saw Bill's jaw tighten, his shoulders tense, and his eyes hardened into a near glare as he turned to face Ethel. To my "mind-body" perspective, these signs, the silent language of his body, spoke his message louder than the words he used.

"So Bill, when you say Ethel won't back you up and lay down the law, what is that like for you?"

"Terrible. I feel I'm stuck either way. If I go ahead with my sense of what to do, Tom won't pay much attention to me, because his mother disagrees. She will undermine my efforts. And if I go along with her, then I think I'm doing the wrong thing."

I had explained to both Bill and Ethel at their initial interview how, in addition to a multigenerational approach to family therapy, I utilized a somatic perspective. In fact, they had come to work with me because of that reason, having been referred by a couple I had worked with previously. Because they both had expressed an interest in the mind-body connection, I felt free to address Bill's awareness of his somatic reality.

"Bill, what else happens? What do you sense in your body, right now, as you speak about this?"

"Well I feel all bound up, like I'm stuck."

"Bound up how? How do you know that—in your body?"

"Well, I feel tight, and like I have all this need to do something and she is stopping me. She won't cooperate!"

"Tight where? Where in your body are you tight?"

"In my shoulders and back, my arms." At this point Bill leaned forward slightly, lifting his arms as if he was reaching out in a futile gesture. Then they dropped down in his lap, seemingly disconnected from the rest of him.

"Bill, I'd like to come back to you in a minute. Right now I'd like to check in with Ethel about her experience before we go further working with you. Is that okay for now?" Looking slightly relieved to be out of the center of attention, Bill nodded and leaned back in his chair.

"Ethel, how do you see the situation? What happens for you when you hear of Bill's frustration?"

"Actually, I become scared when Bill is so intense that I should do things his way. I'm not sure his ideas about 'shape up or ship out' are the way to go with Tom. I think he'll just drive Tom out of the home." As Ethel spoke, the color began to come back in her face as if blood was returning.

"What is it like, here, now, as you listen to Bill?"

"Scary. I just feel I'm torn between my son and my husband. I don't agree with either of them, but they seem to be locked into this contest—'who's going to win.'"

"Ethel what are you aware of in your body, as you speak about this?"

"Well, my hands are cold, I don't feel very strong and I'm trembling inside."

"Trembling where?"

"In my torso, inside."

"Would you be willing just to focus your awareness on the trembling that you experience for a few moments?" She nods.

"Just be aware of the experience of the trembling." As I observe Ethel, she begins to tremble and shake, her torso, neck, and head are shuddering, and then her feet rhythmically begin to twitch. At this point I ask her to stand up and sense her feet on the ground—because I know that without her grounding the intense sensations of the trembling, she may be more overwhelmed than ever.

"What do you notice as you do this, Ethel?"

"My legs. I realize I was not feeling them—as if they were not there."

"And what is it like to have them there now?"

"I feel so much different." (Her trembling begins to slow down noticeably.)

"How?"

"As if I am connected to the floor." (Her voice becomes deeper and her head, which had been leaning forward, now begins to come up.)

"What would you be willing to say to Bill from this sense of support, from your grounding and support in your legs?"

(She looks at Bill.) "I love you both and I don't think dealing with Tom this way will work. I want you to listen to my ideas also."

"Will you say that again and reach out to Bill with your arms?" (This movement is a typical somatic expression of "reaching out" to another. We learned it as a part of our natural development as a child and it is, therefore, a usual way of expressing ourselves when we are ready to receive, to be open to take in. In somatic developmental psychology, such a typical human movement is known as a "psychomotor movement.")

She reaches out to him and then brings her arms down to her sides.

"What is your experience now?"

"I feel more solid, as if I'm inviting him in, into working it out together."

"What do you sense in your body now?"

"My legs are tighter. They have more energy, more sensation, as does my back."

"Would that be enough for now?"

"Yes."

"I would like to turn to Bill now. Is that all right?" (Nods.)

"Bill, what happened when Ethel reached out to you in this way?"

"Well, I don't know, I have not really heard her say 'let's work it out' before."

"What did you sense in your body?"

"I don't know." (I had noticed that Bill's shoulders went up and tightened, his breathing was held, and his facial color had become slightly red when she spoke to him.)

"What happens now in your shoulders and the back of your arms?" (Bill's posture, movement, and build had alerted me to the possibility that he might be operating from some held anger and judgment, a position of *you're wrong, I'm right!* Now I want to test my assessment.)

"Now that I notice them, I can feel they are tight."

"Will you extend your arms for a moment as if pushing something away, pushing away what you don't want, and notice how your arms and back of your shoulder muscles feel as you do that?"

Bill nods, pushes, and then brings his arms back in.

"Okay, now will you do that again, and if you had words for what this action means, what would they be?"

"Back off, don't push me!" (Face gets red, voice elevated.)

"What happens to your shoulders and arms?"

"They are more relaxed." (This movement is intended to establish a better sense of boundary for Bill—activating the posterior deltoids and triceps is a movement joining the words so as to bring body and mind together, allowing Bill a further expression of his felt meaning. The results of such mind-body dramatizing nearly always include a sense of relief, deriving from a closed gestalt, a sense that both parts of the organism have been joined, and there-fore, the expression of self is more complete.)

"How are you?"

"I'm more relaxed!"

"Where? How do you know that?"

"Well, I mean that I'm more relaxed in my shoulders and the back of my arms, but also I'm feeling that my torso, I mean I'm noticing my torso more."

"What happens now when you think about what Ethel said, and how she reached out to you?"

"I want to try and hear her more. I don't think I will agree with her, but we do need to find a way to work this out together!"

"What happens when you think of not working it out together?"

"I tighten up in my shoulders and arms and back, and I think I'm on my own again. Alone!"

"Ethel, what happens when you hear that?"

"I just want to reach out to him," (She turns to Bill.) "—to you. I know you had that alone and threatened feeling growing up, and I don't want to be a part of reinforcing that. At the same time, I need to have you hear that I have some other ideas about how to be with Tom."

Ethel had grown up with a father who was a hard-driving, self-made man with strong opinions. She found it difficult to express her opinions and hold her ground with her father. This pattern, of not being able to have enough impact with her father, someone close to her existence in childhood, has been replayed in her relationship with Bill, and dramatized in her body.

"Bill, what is it like to hear this?"

"A little cautious, but maybe it will work. It's worth a try."

Some Theory Behind What's Been Done So Far

This excerpt of Bill and Ethel's third session illustrates in a small way how utilizing the story the body tells can assist a person's ability to generate new insights, and also become more resourceful dealing with current issues in the family. Bowen family systems theory teaches us how to use a multigenerational perspective to direct our attention and curiosity to how the family is a system of interrelated patterns. Therapy includes examining these patterns, and particularly how they condition or affect individuals' sense of connection in their relationship. Of particular interest is how connection was dealt with in their original family, the legacy of the family's emotional field, and its continuing impact on them as individuals in relationship. As is well known to professionals in the field, a partial list of themes usefully explored include how the family-of-origin handled loss, grief, and abandonment, as well as boundary and triangle issues. In such explorations, clients look at their own "stories," their family-shaped personal realities that continue to be theirs both in regard to themselves and their present world. But if clients are to move beyond their own story to embrace a larger understanding and better functioning, they must experience a perceptual shift about themselves and the world. To achieve this, they need sufficient personal and professional resources to be open to creating respectful doubt about their initial version of self and world, including other people. For the most part, these shifts are usually supported by family therapists utilizing only cognitive interventions.

Therapists, however, can also assist clients to access increased personal resources by using another language—the silent language of body-mind awareness. In the first place, thinking can only go so far without expanding consciousness to include the data of the functioning body-mind. Body awareness, and especially awareness of body sensations, bridges thought, action, and emotion, and assists ego functioning. Furthermore, it enables a client to contain them and digest many levels of stimulation and activation of the nervous system.

At the point where we left Bill and Ethel, I have these three phased outcomes in mind: increased awareness of their body sensations and experience; bridging between thought, action, and emotion; and utilizing that awareness to increase their sense of personal resourcefulness.

In Bill and Ethel's case, after helping them to increase their body awareness, including calling up the abilities inherent in using a psychomotor developmental movement (Ethel's standing on her own two feet, standing up for herself, and reaching out), I expect that both will be a little bit better able to reflect accurately and more flexibly on their experience in life. They are beginning to know themselves, to *be* themselves in a more "embodied" way. This embodied sense of self, as it develops, will increase their possibilities for being able to stay connected with each other, even when their opinions may differ. All too often, one person reacts unconsciously to maintain the stability of the "old" system, during family therapy or real-life changes. With the new resources they discover in their body-mind—the greater totality of themselves, their ability is enhanced to stand firm, to feel safe in their solidity in order to listen, to experience, and appropriately contain whatever troubling feelings, thoughts, or images that become stirred up by change and confrontation. With these new abilities, spouses can become genuinely curious about and attentive to the other person's story.

This sort of body-mind work goes far beyond the body-language manuals, which define the meaning of this or that gesture and posture. What is involved is becoming aware of the body-mind continuum in its full presence and temporal dimension. A person, therapist, or client, is the embodied result of a lifetime's development. Early developmental resignations or holding patterns can be tragically important in limiting personal adaptation and resourcefulness, thereby causing much of the pain with which patients come to us. Learning to see these can help the therapist, not only in assessment, but also in intervention choices. One must learn, for instance, how to differentiate between shock trauma and developmental trauma in choosing an intervention. Muscle tonicity responsiveness, movement patterns, knowing one's way around the nervous system, and attention from a somatic perspective to how particular clients explain their worlds can be immensely useful.

When Bill comes in, he is stuck in his own story—that Ethel (and Tom) are "the problem." My own view is that Ethel and Bill are not connecting in regard to the issue with Tom. My hypothesis—not unusual for a family therapist—is that their pattern of non-connecting has a lot to do with each of their family-of-origin themes and the intimacy, personal space, and comfort level each of them has individually about connectedness in general. But how can such themes and issues be approached most fully without attention to their embodiment, past and present, in each party? How they exist in relationship depends not only on their thoughts, values, and beliefs, but also their body awareness and their embodied character structure, who they have become over time, for better or worse, for quicker or slower, for full or empty, and so on. The fundamentals of this approach include body awareness (sensations—hot, cold, tight, loose, gravity, spatial awareness) and body-based associated experiences (emotions, memory, fantasy, images, thoughts). Clients and therapists need to learn how to observe and utilize these elements of the whole person. Each major aspect of that embodied self can serve as a powerful aid or a severe hindrance in helping the client resolve his problems by making new choices.

Bill and Ethel's Ninth Session

Over the next five sessions, we continued to work with body awareness related to their issues between each other, family-of-origin themes, and their attempts to reach some common agreement of what to do concerning Tom. During this time, we explored their views of what they each had (or had not) learned in their families-of-origin about connecting, despite differences, and how that might be affecting their own relationship, parenting style, and their relationship with Tom. Ethel talked about how it had been difficult to assert herself in her family. Instead, she had learned just to quietly resist doing what did not seem fair or right to her. Bill became more aware of how his deep concerns were so often expressed in anger and judgments, and how Ethel would then lose her sense of centeredness and grounding. Eventually, he discussed how his parents had broken up when he was only fourteen, and, when his father moved away to a distant city, he felt he had to be responsible for his mother's household, and somehow had to take charge. As the therapist, I wondered how I could assist Bill to share the depth of this early loss with Ethel, in order to create some emotional common ground. He still spoke of his loss in the most hard-boiled and big-brave-boy manner. "That's just how it was— life can be hard sometimes!" Before the ninth session, I decided to explore this theme once again.

When Bill and Ethel came into the room that day, I found myself vividly recalling earlier times when Bill looked more angry, and Ethel more collapsed. Though Bill still seemed over-contained to me, there was more lightness in his movements crossing the room, Ethel's fragile-ness seemed to be fading away, and she also seemed more connected to herself and to the ground. After the usual greetings, I inquired about what had transpired since the last session. Ethel spoke first:

"We are doing better together and somehow, Tom is doing better too. He even went to a movie with us the other day. I'm not so frightened of Bill's frustration, and know I'm stronger than I thought. I said to Bill the other day, 'You have got to do something about your anger—what's this all about?' It came out of my mouth before I knew it!"

"What was that like for you, Ethel?"

"Surprising, but the most surprising thing is Bill just looked at me and said, 'I don't really know, this is just all too much!' Then he walked out of the room. I didn't know what to do after that. So I thought I'd like to talk about that here."

"What do you think it was about?"

"Confusion, giving up, or something."

"Bill, what was all that like for you?"

"Well she's right—confusing. I just get frustrated and angry. I know we have talked about my sense of loss in my family and taking responsibly very early, but still this reaction all happens so fast—I don't know exactly how to do anything differently."

"What's it's like for you then that this happens?"

"Not good!"

"Want to explore it?"

"Yes!"

At this point, many schools of mind-body psychotherapy would work toward expression of the anger or, at the other polarity, encourage exploration of "mindfulness," i.e., of Bill's experience, his ability to be "non-attached" to his ongoing experience. In the approach I practice, that of Bodynamic Analysis, there is a third option. While at some time in the future it may be useful for Bill to experience his anger and cathart it, a couple's session tends easily to an exaggeration of both emotional contents, and reaction to them. One can easily create more problems than one resolves. My assessment was that Bill had now developed sufficient cognitive and somatic consciousness to be able to reflect by himself, and make his own judgment of whether he is over-containing some of his emotions. In short, he is ready to explore this kind of material. Furthermore, he is beginning to wonder about how his present anger connects to his early losses. His story, his narrative about the reality around loss, hurt, and anger, is beginning to soften, and so, subtle body-mind awareness and trying on psychomotor patterns can be used. On the other hand, his resources to investigate body sensations and experience are still limited. He is not yet equipped for the best use of cathartic interventions, which include their attachment, in guided regression, to the original imprinting experiences. On the basis of Bill's movement, body posture, and shape, as well as his perceptual framework and his anger, my characterlogical assessment is that he remains somewhat "stuck" in the will stage (2 to 4 years old). His concern with having to do everything on his own, distancing himself from help, implies even younger roots in autonomy issues (8 months to 2½ years). This kind of person, especially after only eight previous sessions, is hardly ready for such a deep plunge.

The use of anger as a defense against underlying feelings of helplessness and sadness, however, *can* be addressed now, in a powerful way, at the fourteen-year-old level—the level that Bill's consciousness is already aware of.

"Bill, what happens when you think back about that time when you were fourteen—what particularly comes to mind?"

"Watching my dad packing and not knowing what to do—or say."

"What happens in your body when you remember this?"

"My chest gets tight and I feel numb, like I don't have any emotion. I'm stuck again."

"What happens in your heart?"

"I can't feel—it's like I'm living on the surface of my body all over."

"What's that like for you?"

"Dead."

"What would a dead heart say right now?"

"I'm dead—I won't feel any more."

With that, Bill's chest takes a heave and his eyes fill with tears, then his shoulders seem to tighten.

"Bill, as an adult man now, what do you wish you could have said then to your dad?" (Bill's chest begins to move in deeper spontaneous breaths.)

"Don't leave me, don't go away." (Sobs come up and tears run down his cheeks.)

With that, Bill reaches out with his other hand, to hold on to Ethel, and his sadness emerges in hard, then soft bursts. By this time, Ethel is softly crying and my own eyes become quite wet as well!

Bill speaks: "Sometimes it's just too hard to let you help, to feel I can hold on to you for strength. It's hard to even know when I need help. In some ways you are much stronger than me." (Ethel quietly responds by slightly nodding.)

"Bill, what does help look like?"

"Like this, just like this."

"What happens in your body when 'this' happens?"

"I feel full inside and softer, my shoulders and back relax."

"And your heart?"

"I can feel it, it's not dead anymore."

"What's 'it' Bill?"

"My heart, my—my feelings—I can feel myself more, like I'm whole."

"Ethel, what's this like for you?"

"I guess I had still been thinking when we came in—that Bill didn't need me in quite this way. Actually I feel more connected to myself and Bill right now. I feel like I'm in a precious state right now, seeing clearly into what it can be like for Bill underneath, rather than wondering if I'm a full partner in this relationship."

"What happens in your body, right now?"

"I, too, feel softer and more connected in my whole body, and I wonder how we will not lose what we have discovered here. "

The session progressed with further movement toward connecting Bill's sadness and his inability to ask for help, not knowing he needed help, and his prickly reactivity around his son's acting out. In this and later sessions, he moved toward appreciating that at least his son was still "in there fighting" (even if it came out in resistance against him!), and that pushing on Tom would not help. Ethel came to understand that Bill's anger had caused her to dig in her heels and distance herself from contact, which only aggravated both her and Bill's sense of isolation. In ensuing sessions, they found new paths to revisit and explored many issues in their relationship where they had "lost their way." They uncovered the sources of the early patterns in their families-of-origin, and the mind-body awareness (or lack of it) that was contributing to not understanding and connecting with each other. A central movement in the therapy process was visiting with their own parents and families, researching the family stories—their multigenerational histories. Patients who share this information with each other usually come to a new understanding of their heritage, and of their parents' lives. As they found the edges of their own reactivity around these stories, we utilized both cognitive and somatic approaches to work through those impasses. This shift in thinking and felt reactivity helped them each understand themselves as well, and connect better with each other and other family members. Over time, they discovered that, even through the ups and downs of life, they could stay connected to themselves, and become less reactive and more able to listen and connect to one another's struggles. Tom slowly settled down, and we did a couple of sessions with Bill, Ethel, and Tom together, mostly hearing from Tom about what his needs were in the family. Therapy ended when Tom managed to move to a school where he felt supported in "catching up" on the schooling he had missed. The whole process extended another twenty sessions.

Theoretical Considerations and the New Somatic Psychotherapies

In the past, practitioners of many body-mind approaches believed that therapy was a process of reducing or breaking down defenses—in somatic psychotherapy terms—"armor." Some theory held that people are "armored" through their character structure from experiencing the deeper, more authentic *self*, the sense of vegetative (autonomic) flow, and their sensations of well-being. In the early mind-body theories of psychotherapy, character was originally defined as a fixed pattern of behavior, the way an individual typically handles his or her striving for pleasure. It is structured in the form of chronic and generally unconscious muscular tensions that block or limit impulses to reach out. Character was also thought to be a psychic attitude, buttressed by a system of denials, rationalizations, and projections, and geared to an ego ideal that affirms its value. The functional identity of psychic character and body structure (or muscular attitude) was then conceived to be the key to understanding personality, for it enables the therapist to read the character from the body, and to explain a bodily attitude by its psychic representations—and vice versa. In holding the premise that people *only* need to be released from the tensions of their character armor, however, earlier theory fell into an overly simplistic trap. Many contemporary somatic practitioners now believe the need to rethink this older theory, since the reduction or dissolution of an individual's armor can disorganize a person's whole system of adaptation and coping. When we, as therapists, intervene to remove some of this defensive armor, it is essential that other, more functional resources be found for the individual. In the instance of this case, our earlier work developing body awareness, maintaining an adult perspective in the intervention, and monitoring Bill's connection with Ethel and myself as therapist, enabled him to maintain and improve the stability he needed to remain functional in the world.

When Wilhelm Reich, one of the founders of mind-body psychotherapy, developed this de-armoring process in pre-World War II Germany, people's defenses were particularly strong. Today, our intent should be to help create better organization in a person's psycho-physiological functioning, so that the person's resources are developed and integratable over the long-term.

Properly worked with, body-mind approaches can facilitate very clear and functional connection with the person's own wisdom, the inner knowing of how to manifest, in behavior, one's very best intentions. It is very useful in that regard to understand early childhood developmental patterns, and the relationship between motor development and psychological development. A fine example of newer and more sophisticated approaches is the Bodynamics Analysis method, mentioned previously and developed by Lisbeth Marcher and her colleagues in Denmark over the last fifteen years, and now being taught internationally. This model is based on these psychomotor patterns and the work of Stern and Mahler, among others. It achieves its power through integrating new research on the psychomotor development of children with the knowledge of depth psychotherapy systems. This developmental approach allows for direct activation of undeveloped motor (body) skills and psychological (mind) resources.

Marcher took Reich's idea that children frustrated in an activity may tense their muscles to hold back that activity. She realized that when the frustration of developmental activity is early or severe, the child may become resigned, and the corresponding muscles will be flaccid (under-responsive). When, on the other hand, response to the environment is appropriate, the muscles will have a neutral responsiveness tone, and the child will exhibit healthy actions to future situations. Since each developmental stage is comprised of specific sets of developmental psychomotor tasks, and since these tasks all have associated muscles, there can be any one of three overall outcomes for each stage: **resigned** (early frustration), **held back or rigid** (later frustration), or **healthy** (appropriate response). This information is then applied to the family-of-origin history and any "shock" trauma the person may have experienced, and used to explore various areas of ego functioning; i.e., grounding, centering, balance, boundaries, habits of interpersonal connection, and the like.

Typical of the new body-mind psychotherapies is a more sophisticated attitude toward touching the patient. The interventions with Ethel and Bill were made without my touching them. Much useful work can be accomplished without using touch, just by asking questions and directing the client's attention. In the helping professions, there are many ethical and legal prohibitions against touch, and it goes without saying that the whole business of touch is a very sensitive topic, and appropriately so: "Fools rush in where angels fear to tread." In my opinion, however, what the professions have done (due to unethical practitioners being justly confronted about their behavior) is taken too "safe" a route: no touch—no matter what the circumstances. Though touching is an exceedingly complex subject, requiring the greatest sensitivity, the highest moral standards, the deepest theoretical and practical psychotherapeutic training, and ethical professional supervision, many mind-body therapists, including myself, do utilize touch some of the time in their therapeutic interventions. The whole subject merits, again, our collective professional attention. A useful review of some of the research in this area has been made by Kertay and Reviere of Georgia State University[1] and also by T. M. Field of the Touch Research Institute, University of Miami Medical School.[2] In a less academic way, a wonderful caption about touch and connection was included in *Life* magazine,[3] illustrating that lack of appropriate touch and connection can have profound implications for well-being.

Conclusion

In this short article, I have taken a single case to illustrate one mind-body approach, emphasizing somatic developmental psychology. By calling attention to some somatic principles, theory, and practice interventions as an aid to the family systems approach, I hope to stimulate some curiosity about mind-body modalities and lead some family therapist readers to explore reference materials and training in this area.

References

1. Kertay, L., & S.L. Reviere. "The Use of Touch In Psychotherapy: Theoretical and Ethical Considerations," p. 47.

2. Field, T. M. Touch Research Institute, University of Miami's Medical School.

3. *Life* Magazine, June 1996, featured a story regarding two premature sisters and the importance of touch and contact in sustaining health for one of them.

See also: Bernhardt, P., M. Bentzen, & J. Isaacs. (1996). "Waking the Body Ego, Bodynamic Analysis, and Lisbeth Marcher's Somatic Developmental Psychology." *Energy & Character* 27(1).

Part Two

Body-Mind Approaches & Self-Psychology

Theory and Implications for Practice

"The Body Self in Psychotherapy" places the psychology of the body self in an historical perspective, and outlines some of the basic guiding principles of practice. It continues exploring the integration of family systems theory and practice with body-mind approaches (as exemplified by Bodynamics) begun in the last paper of Part One.

Dr. Erving Polster's "Sensory Functioning in Psychotherapy" is a fundamental article about human experience. Erv is co-director of the Gestalt Therapy Training Institute in San Diego along with his wife Miriam. He is surely one of the most profound therapists and teachers with whom I have been able to study. Body awareness, particularly of sensation, is a fundamental building block of the Bodynamics and many other somatic approaches. Erv places body sensation in terms of ordinary life experience, even though many spiritual meditative systems also address sensation from a mystical framework. He often chided me for working to make experience more complicated and mystical than it needed to be. This article is pivotal, both in itself and certainly in understanding the material to follow in this and other Parts.

The article "Ethical Considerations in Somatic Therapies" discusses some overall guidelines important to consider in approaching somatic (body-mind) training and practice.

The Body Self in Psychotherapy: A Psychomotoric Approach to Developmental Psychology

—Marianne Bentzen, M.A., Erik Jarlnaes, M.A., & Peter Levine, Ph.D.

"The mind has forgotten, but the body has not—thankfully."
—S. Freud

"When psychologists speak of the unconscious, it is the body that they are talking about."—F. M. Alexander

Abstract

In this article, the role of body consciousness in the developing self will be explored, both as a conceptual underpinning of developmental psychology, and as a vehicle for therapeutic change. Views will be related from the neurosciences, from developmental motor theory, from ego psychology, and from the experiences of therapists developing and practising body oriented psychotherapy. A Scandinavian tradition of psychomotoric therapy will be described as representing a new direction in the emergence of a body-oriented psychotherapy and somatic education that can enhance object relations and self psychologies by giving direct access to vital developmental material. The psychomotoric approach attempts to assess the progression and completeness of each stage of the individual's childhood psychomotoric development. This assessment offers the possibility of using psychotherapy to renegotiate maladapted or lacking stages—and associated personality patterns.

The role of body-oriented therapy tools such as empathic mirroring, nonverbal regression, body sensing, affective expression, and somatic identification will be described briefly, and cases will be given to illustrate their use in establishing the clients' body awareness, authentic sense of self, and feelings of mutual connection.

Introduction

In speaking of the ego initially forged as a body ego, Freud formulated a basic developmental theme of maturational evolution—that bodily processes are an indispensable foundation for the nascent self and developing ego. The integration of body and psyche as a developmental process is also a basic tenant in Piaget's theory of representation, where all later learning processes develop from early sensory motor phases of exploration. This premise is also supported by current research in infant development (see Stern 1985). In this article, the body-mind as a developmental unit will be explored.

As Krueger (1989) points out, an emerging view of developmental theorists is that of a "body-self," which encompasses a wide range of kinesthetic experiences on the body surface and in its interior. It is out of early experiences in this formative self that the psychological self emerges. The body-self, according to Lichtenberg (1978, 1985) is made up of body sensations, body functions, psychic experience, and body image. He argues that the integration of body-self into the (larger) *self* occurs through reality testing in a definite developmental sequence. Since body experience is the first reality of the infant, later psychological development will be dependent on his perception of body experiences.

Movement, Perception, and Psyche

Sperry (1952), a pioneering neurophysiologist, from a very different perspective, also makes the point that the fundamental basis of perception derives from motoric potentiality:

"If there be any objectively demonstrable fact about perception that indicates the nature of the neural process involved, it is the following: In so far as an organism perceives a given object, it is prepared to respond with reference to it. This preparation-to-respond is absent in an organism that has failed to

perceive.... The presence or absence of adaptive reaction potentialities of this sort, ready to discharge into motor patterns, makes the difference between perceiving and not perceiving."

In experiments stimulated by the Sperry Principle, Held and Hein (1963) had their subjects—human adults—wear special prism goggles that made everything appear to be upside down. After some time (usually a week or two) the brain could adapt so that the environment appeared to be normal (right side up) again. This occurred, however, only if the subjects were free to move about actively, touching and manipulating their environments. The subjects who were not allowed to move around and explore did not experience visual normalization.

Held (1965) also carried out experiments that illustrate the developmental significance of motor responses. Newborn kittens were put on a movable apparatus and placed within a circular enclosure. One group of kittens walked and pulled the apparatus around the enclosure with them while the other kittens were pulled along passively. Both groups had exactly the same visual experiences moving around the enclosure. The kittens that were moved around passively—in a way that did not actively explore their environment—could not then use sight to guide their movements. They could not place their paws properly or move away from a place where they could fall. This deficit was swiftly reversed when they could actively (motorically) explore their environments.

On a more personal level, the authors unwittingly created a similar experiment. One author, competently used to finding her way in strange countries and cities on foot and bicycle, had consistently allowed herself to be driven from place to place in a car while visiting in another author's home town. Even after numerous stays she had no sense of the lay of the city, and would certainly not be able to find her way to most of the places she had been taken to. During later visits, however, she began to move around the city on her own, and quickly learned to orient herself.

These experiments, both intentional and unintentional, demonstrate how dependent perceptual adaptational learning is on motoric experience. In the following pages we consider the linkage of motor activity, perception, and psychological states.

The Thinking Body

Of course, we all think we know that the body doesn't think. The mind thinks. And we think that the mind lives in the brain, or in that general vicinity. So thinking about the thoughts of the body is nearly unthinkable. The separation of mind and body, however, is a theoretical construct—well represented in our daily language and thought patterns, but quite unsubstantiated in fact. Are we unwittingly still bound by the cultural spell of Cartesian dualism and seventeenth-century scientific positivism? In contrast to the cogito, ergo sum: "I think, therefore I am," the functional-developmental view sees body and mind as representing an undifferentiated field of formative experience. In the body/mind view: "I sense, I perceive, I feel, I respond, I act, I evaluate, I am . . . and therefore I am able to reflect on my being." In short, "I am, therefore I think!"

In mapping and interacting with an increasingly rich and complex environment, the body/mind unit must register and model its interactions with it. This means that the organism carries with it experiences and action patterns from past situations as a basis for future responses. These registered experiences are what shape the child's interaction with his or her environment.

The dramatic psychological effects from deficits in sensory-motoric interaction with the environment have been described in restrained children and adults. Levy (1944) studied hospitalized children restrained for medical reasons and found pronounced deficits in psychological development. In roughly the same time period, Spitz (1946) made his landmark studies on sensory-motor and contact-deprived children in orphanages, describing the resulting anaclitic depression. Zubek and his colleagues (1963), in an interesting series of experiments, immobilized the necks of a group of university faculty members with halters. They found that restriction of neck movement alone resulted in "intellectual inefficiency, bizarre thoughts, anxiety, exaggerated emotional reactions, and unusual bodily sensations."

Obviously, mechanical movement restriction causes emotional symptoms in both children and adults. What then about self-sustained functional movement restriction?

Control and Resignation

The interlinking of neurosis and muscular restriction (armoring) was proposed by Wilhelm Reich (1949), who established techniques for dissolving "muscular defenses" as an integral part of his psychoanalytic practice. Alexander Lowen (1976) has extended and popularized this work in the form of Bioenergetic analysis. Also inspired by Reich's findings, Wilimar Johnsen (1975), a Norwegian therapist in clinical practice since the mid-1930s, established that the body-mind responds to its environment not only with tension—muscular armoring—but also with weakness of response, hypotension. Both of these tension patterns restrict movement; hypertension in an active restraint similar to that of the unfortunate faculty members above, hypotension rather by an inner relinquishing of the option of movement. In Johnsen's therapeutic practice, an exciting shift occurred. The psychotherapeutic focus moved from the neurotic defense systems to the unrealized potential in the client—the unfolding of those growth patterns from childhood that are still dormant in the adult. In formulating her therapeutic method, "IRT," Johnsen notes the differential transmission of a "respiration wave" through the hypertonic and hypotonic muscles. When the hypotonic muscles are sensitively perceived and manually contacted by the therapist, "lost" emotional and physical resources emerge in the client's perception, sometimes in the form of repressed memories.

In Denmark in 1968, one group of Relaxation Educators (physical therapists, nurses, psychologists, and others in the healing professions concerned with body education, relaxation, and the impact of body states on psychological functioning—see Bulow-Hansen, 1982), led by Lisbeth Marcher, began developing a similar line of investigation. The descriptive testing of Kendall and McCreary (1949, 1983) formed the anatomical basis for Marcher's interpretation of psychological functioning (studied by Ollars, 1980). Trained in the Danish tradition of relaxation therapy, and acquainted with Johnsen's work during her further studies, Marcher developed the concept of muscular defense and resignation into a describable, palpable, and observable muscular activity. The term "muscular response" was used to describe emotional control or resignation reflected in the motor system—*control* being described as hyper-

and *resignation* as hypo-response. To physical palpation, hypo-response is often perceived as a special kind of "flabbiness" or viscosity, and just as hyper-response expresses the feeling state, "I need to hold on to this, to keep control of it," the hypo-response reflects a resignation that says, "attempting to do this is too exhausting; I give up." These interpretations opened the possibility of doing accurate body readings of the personality, both of general character traits and of presently active issues. The Bodymap, a pictorial display of the palpatory findings, rapidly became a valuable research and clinical tool in assessing developmental completeness and emotional health (Rothschild, 1989).

Functional Analysis

One hypothesis currently being developed by Marcher and her colleagues at the Bodynamic Institute is that of psychological functional analysis. To their way of thinking, every part of the body may be said to be part of the mind—with a clearly defined psychological activity growing out of the physical function. In the muscular system, the muscle's "feeling" about its function is observable from its response: does it express resignation, showing hypo-response, or is its action rigidly controlled with hyper-responses? These feeling responses may be mild or severe in degree. There is also a third possibility—neutral response. This corresponds to a full but non-inflected feeling about the function involved, joyful and simple. It seems quite possible that we will find the same triad of possibilities—over-activity, under-activity, or neutrality in other structures of the body (Levine, 1977, 1986). Present empirical findings indicate that these physical states generally correspond to psychological ones (Hammer, 1990; Barral, 1991).

Research and validation in the field of correlating psychological and physiological function is as yet largely confined to clinical findings of practitioners spanning the two fields. The most extensive of these findings concern the muscular system, and the anatomical function of muscles is to move—to act. Marcher and her colleagues observed that children in their journey through the well-charted world of developmental movement use specific muscles at each stage. The young child will respond with the appropriate movement to a touch of an age-active muscle, while another muscle, situated next to it, will evoke no response (it is important to note that biological and individual differences must be taken into consideration when using this information for diagnostic purposes). The Bodynamic group then used this discovery to correlate age levels and initiatory activity in muscles. In older children with better motor control, touch on an age-active muscle no longer evoked overt movement, but a vibrating activity in the muscle tissue, manually discernible to the trained therapist.

Psychological content has been found to relate to these initiatory activities. In psychotherapy, children as well as adults will reliably associate issues related to the developmentally indexed motor action during sensitive touch or specific activation of a muscle (Jørgensen, 1978; Hvid, 1990; Marcher, 1992). This is the foundation of Bodynamic Analysis.

Psychomotor Development

Joints give us our range of movement, of possible action, and muscles affect that movement. However, a muscle's activity is defined by its placement in relationship to the joint(s) it acts upon. Take an example. Grip the back of your upper arm, between the shoulder and the elbow. You are now holding the triceps muscle. One of the three heads moves the upper arm backwards (as in jabbing your elbow into something behind you), and all of them stretch the elbow joint. If you then stretch your elbow, you will feel the whole muscle contract and harden under your hand. The question asked in the psychological function analysis of the triceps is: What personal or interpersonal activities involve stretching the elbow? Throwing, hitting, pushing, stretching out, getting elbow space—all movements associated with expanding personal territory—are all likely to be socialized out of the young child in favor of more acceptable ways of expressing his or her impulses and feelings. These movements indicate a developmental spectrum of psychological function, of creating personal space by being able to push objects and other people away, an important aspect of boundary formation.

From Held and Hein's experiments, we must expect it to be essential to the adequate adult formation of boundaries that the child has come to grips with the feelings and developmental potential expressed by these movements—and that he, from this fullness of experience, has learned to clarify his boundaries as competently in more contained ways.

To return to the triceps: each of its three heads has a separate physical and psychological subfunction, since they act on the joint in slightly different ways and become functionally active at different ages. In addition, the triceps as whole is part of a larger pattern of muscles throughout the body, all expressing different aspects of boundary formation. In similar fashion, the whole motor system is involved in expressing aspects of existential issues, which may be read from movement, posture, extension, and flexion. Muscle responses are charted to become a virtual map of the body self (Rothschild, 1989). Thoughts, feelings, and images that emerge when a muscle is activated (touched or used) arise out of the person's experience correlated with that muscle's overt or derived function. The triceps participates in "thinking" of getting personal space. Similarly, other muscles are involved in feelings connected to actions in which they are, or have been, activated. From the point of view of Nina Bull's attitude theory of emotion (Bull, 1945; Pasquerelli and Bull, 1951), feeling is actually the perception of motor attitude, and is essentially a consciousness of preparation or readiness for action.

How the triceps "feels" about pushing away can be seen in its response— by the degree of holding or resignation in it. If it is hyper-responsive, the person will seem somewhat unapproachable—have "automatic push"—and easily tends to set limits to the contact, whether consciously or unconsciously. If, on the other hand, the triceps were hypo-responsive, this would be consistent with that person's resignation about protecting her personal space—allowing other people to overstep her boundaries as a matter of course, and getting enmeshed in contacts she really doesn't want. Through analysis of the muscular responsiveness, it is possible to construct a hypothesis of both extraordinary complexity and great simplicity from the understanding of the physical-emotional structure of the body.

Britta Holle (1976), a Danish physical therapist, has worked extensively with children characterized as slow or slightly retarded. She has achieved consistent results in improved learning capacity by meticulously diagnosing their motoric standard and helping them learn the next motor stages—the ones, often from infancy, they never quite mastered or which never unfolded with ease. Observers of her work, however, mention a fact that she does not explicitly discuss; that she responds to the children's psychological needs as well as their motoric ones. Her diagnostic test, which essentially consists of checking normal perceptual and motor learning patterns up to the six year level, has been applied to adults and uncovers the same age deficiency patterns that the Bodynamic visual reading or Bodymap will show (Bente Kjaer, 1989).

In the psychomotor developmental view of both Johnsen and Marcher, parallel to Holle's work, psychological disturbances are seen to be arrested rather than faulty. What the Bodymap then uncovers is the living "inner child"—at different age levels—unable to complete its mastery of the crucial age-appropriate issue without support. In adults, as well as in children of any age, these issues show in the Bodymap as well as in the habitual patterns of posture, behavior, and speech.

Returning to the example of the triceps, its three heads are activated at three different ages. The medial head comes into use when the child, at about six months old, pushes his upper body away from the floor or from the body of his mother to orient himself in his explorations of the environment. Many other muscles are activated at the same age as he learns to coordinate his body in rolling and creeping movements, as he grasps and manipulates objects in new ways and refines his differentiation of desired stimuli. In the Bodymap, the pattern of response in these muscles indicates the relative success in negotiating the developmental stage. The psychological function of the medial triceps is interpreted as the subject's feelings about holding his support system (parents and others) at the distance relevant to his need for personal space and orientation; clearly a motor function of early (oral) boundary formation. The other two heads of the triceps are activated at later ages; in the throwing and pushing movements of the rapprochement and practicing stages at eight to twenty-four months, and in the hitting and pushing of the two- to four-year-old exploring his personal power in his dealings with peers and elders. The different ages of activation give the three triceps heads slightly different feeling contents, concurrent with the context of age-relevant issues and activities and the individual's experiences with them.

The Nascent Self

Psychotherapists treat patients whose body-self experiences are disrupted by mirroring insufficiency in the object relationships, and by trauma. Cohesion and orientation are recognizably disordered in these individuals. Krueger (1989) points out that empathic parental mirroring forms body sensations into the distinct and coherent functions of the self. He further adds that prolonged absence or deficit in care-giving leads to distortions in the body self and to subsequent ego development. Also, physical boundaries are not clear, resulting in a failure to develop a functional and coherent recognition and distinction of internal states. Krueger cites a rare case of a congenital neurologically based absence of sensation, studied by Dubovsky and Grogan (1975). The subject, adult at the time of the study, had been unable to develop a reliable sense of self; he was unable to maintain the simplest of personal boundaries, to know where he ended and others began. Generally, in the process of human development, the boundaries of the body become specific and differentiable from the "out-there" world. In the traumatized or developmentally deprived child, however, this discrimination does not develop coherently.

In formulating this developmental self model, a view consistent with the Sperry principle of neurological organization, Krueger (1989) states:

"The first reality is the reality of the body. Motor activity is the first mechanism with which reality is tested: whatever can be touched in the external world is real. Reality is persistently influenced by the present, past conscious, and unconscious images of one's body self. The body is the primary instrument through which we perceive and organize the world. We regularly return to the body as a frame of reference throughout development. Subsequent learning and experiences are referred to what has already been sensorially experienced for confirmation and authentication. The first symbols and metaphors refer simultaneously to the body and to the outside (non-body) world."

It is here, in directly affecting the body-self, that the psychomotoric approach offers exciting possibilities for psychotherapeutic intervention. It recognizes that each stage of (self) development is associated with particular motoric patterns. Each of these movement patterns provides the mold in which the major developmental tasks will be accomplished. It is the child's experience of these ontogenetic transitions which form the basis of his emerging body-self. This process begins in the womb and extends into adolescence and adulthood. It also merges the earliest preverbal developmental processes with phylogenetic history.

For about 280 million years, animals have had to move in relation to terrestrial physical space. They have had to master gravity and other vectors of nature. For humans, the physical environment begins in the womb. Here, gravity receptors provide a reference coordinate, while vestibular stimulation, through maternal movement, gives the early sense of direction and speed. From this information, the fetal brain begins to "infer" and "map out" the world outside the womb and gradually prepares the organism for extra-uterine life. Such prescience for the next is implied within each stage of development. Appropriate sensory and motoric patterns come into play that are necessary for that stage of life and for following ones. Associated with each of these motoric patterns are specific modes of perception and expectation of the needs of the next stage.

The rhythmic movements in the womb, for example, later provide the match between mother and neonate (Gidoni et al., 1988). At birth, the infant seems to relate with an early (pre-)sense of self-experience through rhythmic proprioceptive sensations within his body (see Stern, 1985). During the first weeks after birth, the developing awareness of body surface resonates with the primitive, proprioceptive in utero mapping. Through touch, definition, and delineation the infant's vague, relatively boundless proprioceptive sense is enhanced. The infant begins to develop an interconnection (though rudimentary) between internal and surface (tactile) representation. In normal development, these experiences achieve an increasing coherence where the need for greater intensity gradually evolves into finer differentiation and clarity of affect and intention. In abnormal development, this process becomes discontinuous. Derailed, it leads to disorientation and to gaps in the nascent self and later personality.

The Bodynamic Institute's studies of childhood psychomotor development define their theory of adult character structure. They have traced maturational development through seven periods from birth to adolescence and describe the basic tasks of each period in terms of motor development, perception, affect, and cognition (Bentzen et al., 1989; Hvid, 1990). Each stage is considered to be organized around a specific need or "right" of the developing child linked to the age-specific activities. These rights, in chronological order, are the right:

1. to exist, linked to fetal stretching movements and avoidance responses;

2. to have needs met, experienced through suckling, grasping, and biting;

3. to be autonomous, founded while crawling, walking, and practicing;

4. to be intentional, directed, and willful, explored in powerful controlled gross motor movement;

5. to express loving and sexual feelings, discovering gender-role posturing and movement;

6. to have personal opinions, while learning fine control of balance and other gross motor activity;

7. to feel accepted and respected as a member of a peer group, whether performing well or poorly, while fine-tuning motor skills in single and group activities.

All of these various theories and experimental findings describe different aspects of the interface of the body/psyche developmental patterns. How then does this apply to the therapeutic relationship?

Psychotherapeutic Strategies

The psychomotoric approach attempts to define precisely the individual's childhood motoric progression and to assess relative completeness and incompleteness at each stage of development. It then offers a means to renegotiate (within the transference-counter-transference relationship) those stages that are lacking and/or maladapted. Body awareness (tracking and correlating sensory and kinesthetic experience with images, memories and emotional states) and regression to early verbal as well as nonverbal states are commonly used in this renegotiation process. When failures in empathic mirroring are restructured, feelings of mutual connection with other human beings and illumination of the "real self" can gradually be restored (Bernhardt, 1992). Some primary tools, in addition to the therapist's empathic attunement, are the specialized (subtle) skills of motoric-postural observation and directed touch, used toward the client's own emerging sense of body awareness and body experience (Levine, 1990, 1991, 1992; Marcher, 1992).

In the therapeutic process, resolution of issues is attempted in a specific order. More current age issues are first dealt with—building, as it were, a bridge of health from the present into the disturbed areas of childhood experience. This ensures that the client in therapeutic regression always has areas of resource in later stages of development.

Generally, this makes growth toward mature functioning more attractive. In dealing with an issue in the client's present or past, the therapist emphasizes the factual perceptions of the client in as detailed a fashion as possible. Since meaning is intimately interwoven with perception, this brings out the original depth of the meaning he found in the actual situation, aiding his insight in the actions of himself and others. During this process, forgotten experiences often emerge, offering the subject the possibility of a new interpretation growing spontaneously out of his explorations of kinesthetic and perceptual (body) experiences. When the subject's relationship to the issue addressed is mainly characterized by hyper-responses (signifying control) catharsis may be encouraged. Catharsis occurring unrelated to a specific perceptually evoked situation, however, is strongly discouraged. In the view of Boadella (1987), Nichols and Efran (1985), Levine (1990, 1991, 1992), and Marcher (1992), the destructuring process of catharsis should be directed selectively at the thwarting forces giving rise to the frustration and over-control of the subject, rather than be allowed outlet in a more general way, to the possible detriment of the personality.

The authors have found a common problem in clients with extensive unfocused cathartic therapy experience. They tend to have a relatively weak capacity for containment, perceptual experiences are often chaotic, and they are easily caught in repetitive patterns of unrelated emotive expression. They may be said to have learned cathartic expression as a general remedy against any occurring stress or deepening of feeling, making it difficult for them to deal appropriately with the common fluctuations of ordinary living and relationships. In general, much work in containment and body awareness should determine the shape and structure of their therapy.

One example that comes to mind is of a woman in therapy regressing suddenly and cathartically into an experience of being extremely ill and about six months old. The combination of her observable visceral contraction and her almost expulsive verbal flow prompted the therapist to ask whether she had been treated with purgatives. This proved to be the case: ill and crying for several weeks at the age of six months, she had had numerous laxatives applied before finally being hospitalized in a comatose state (information given by family) and treated for malnutrition and hunger. This experience, besides giving her hysterical-depressive symptoms, seems to have given her an unusual proficiency in previous catharsis-oriented therapy. Her basic imprint was that all inner sensation was bad, and she valiantly attempted to expel it by any means available, lending a great deal of force to her abreaction. The subsequent therapeutic work concentrated on the disturbed developmental issue: her ability to sense the incorporation of physical and emotional nourishment, and to perceive its containment and integration in the body.

In the case of clients with hypo-response (resignation) toward the problem issue, catharsis seems useless or worse. Since there is no charge to release, abreactive work easily leads to further depletion of an already weakened energy system, often compounded by the client's distress about the insufficiency of his "performance." The job of the therapist is rather to provide encouragement, support, and perceptual stimuli that allow the dormant motor impulses to awaken, helping the client to claim his long unused potential of sensation, feeling, choice, and action.

For example, the Bodymap of a forty-year-old woman overwhelmed by legal problems showed significant and long-standing hypo-responses in the triceps and in specific muscles in both legs—showing that her relationship to setting limits and claiming her own power (issues activated at two to four years of age) were quite resigned. Exploring the possibilities of using her arms to push in different ways, she discovered that the right arm wanted to push straight ahead in a confrontative way, while the left took pleasure in pushing sideways. The appropriate quality (determined by the client's feeling of "rightness" after experimenting with different possibilities) of both movements was firm and definite. Her experience was of being able to defend herself with her right arm and get "elbow room" (to not concern herself with the legal problems) with her left. This significantly changed the impact that the pending lawsuit had on her. Subsequent sessions focused on character analysis, but the basic shift in perspective was already well under way. This woman's perceptual image of herself— her "imprint" of who she was—had not included the possibility of pushing, i.e., of being able to establish her boundaries. This basic imprint caused her to perceive many things as potentially threatening. Discovering her arm's ability to protect her was a "re-imprint," a new interpretation or negotiation of her possibilities, and in observably better accordance with reality.

This re-imprinting, the making of new inner experiential maps, is a factor stressed by several systems of body psychotherapy and education, notably Boadella's *Biosynthesis* (1987), Levine's *Somatic Experiencing* (1990, 1991, 1992), Marcher's *Bodynamics* (1992), and Pesso's *Psychomotor Therapy* (1969). All of these consider insight and catharsis in psychotherapy to be useful only in so far as they aid the perceptual re-imprint.

In working with clients whose basic sense of self is weak or disturbed, the body-self approach offers significant new avenues of intervention. When emphasis in the therapeutic interaction is placed on sensory and kinesthetic experience as the context of thought and feeling, working with adults whose personalities have been shaped by physical and sexual abuse, or by disruptive experiences from the first three or four years of life (including the so-called borderline and narcissistic personalities) becomes easier. For these people, life experiences have been so deeply traumatizing that they have dissociated from the deep sense of life flow inherent in the inner perception of the body-self, giving rise to feelings of devastating worthlessness, loneliness, and fragmentation. This inner self-perception is more or less hidden to other people, and occasionally to the person himself, behind a role with which the person is often identified.

In the search for the true inner self, the main difficulties facing both client and therapist are the client's understandable fear of dismantling his known, everyday self-experience and his difficulty in trusting the new images, perceptions, and memories emerging in an often chaotic and disjointed fashion. Traditionally, the therapist can offer little help in this process; he should not become the client's new outer authority on what reality is. This is where attendance to somatic perceptions becomes an invaluable tool. Faced with the confusion of who he really is, and which experiences to believe, the client can learn to use his body sense as a reliable guide. This is possible because experiences and memories are stored perceptions, and will always carry a different feeling tone and kinesthetic "map" than created images, however dearly held.

A brief excerpt from a session with a thirty-eight-year-old man, beginning to access terrifying images of being sexually violated by his father at the age of five, may serve to illustrate this point. As the shadowy images of being beaten and raped once again started flitting through his mind, the client appealed to his therapist: "But how do I know if it really happened? Couldn't I just be making it up?" The therapist admitted that he did not know, but offered the means to find out. He directed the client to make statements that were false, as well as ones that were true but painful and frightening, while paying attention to the subtle sensations that create the inner reality sense and "flavor" of such statements. After some time spent comparing these different sensations, the client had established a clear feeling of his inner "truth sense." Slowly and painfully, he then sorted through his images of abuse and perceived most of them to be true. During this process, he relied on the therapist for emotional support and validation of what he himself felt to be true rather than for outer definitions of reality. This method allowed the client to find the beginnings of his own knowledge about what was and not true, as well as deepening his relationship to the therapist in terms of the trust and support necessary to his growth.

In body-oriented psychotherapy, somatic identification (the nonverbal transmission of body sensation or affective states between people) has been found a useful tool in the course of working with clients with a weak or immature sense of self.

The authors have found that the client is occasionally involved in what seems to be a direct absorption of information perceived from the body-self of the therapist. This appears to be an ordinary, if poorly understood, way of learning—especially in children. Also, adults with character structures dominated by disruptive experiences from the first three or four years of life (including the so called borderline and narcissistic personalities) exhibit this kind of identification learning procedure. In the therapeutic process, it is often considered to be part of the projective identification received by the therapist, and useful mainly as a diagnostic guideline. In the following example, we describe a client discovering the growth potential in learning by somatic identification.

Toward the end of a session, a thirty-five-year-old woman, after regression to early infancy, having experienced her mother's postpartum psychosis and her own deprivation, was lying curled up in the arms of the therapist. The therapist was relaxed, looking at a tree outside the window, enjoying the warmth of the contact and the play of the wind in the branches outside. Suddenly the client exclaimed: "You enjoy living!" "Yes," the therapist replied, mildly surprised. "I can sense it in you right now. My mother couldn't do that, couldn't enjoy living. It's as if I never learned from the inside how that's supposed to feel!" Through subtle shifts in the body posture and breathing of the therapist, the client was perceiving the therapist's body-self feeling at that moment, using it as a role model for her own emerging joy in life.

It seems that the existence of this mode of imprinting alone could offer a whole new set of therapeutic methods to be explored—methods equally useful in verbal and body psychotherapy. As with many other avenues of development in the psychomotoric understanding of human development, however, the bulk of this work is still in the future.

Conclusion

The conceptual framework and tools presented in this article represent an important direction in the formative field of body psychotherapy. It encourages the reader to look more closely into the developmental, motoric, and physiological realms as they are experienced and perceived (rather than as they are measured and described) for further depth and nuance in the understanding of personality development and psychotherapeutic practice. Observing the mutable patterns of the body-self interacting with other body-selves seem to reveal processes similar to those described in chaos theory, a system of understanding developed mainly in biology, meteorology, physics, and mathematics (Bleick, 1988; Briggs & Peat, 1989). More recently, this theory has also been applied in medicine and the neurosciences.

In the computer film, "Valley of the Seahorses," Mandelbrot's fractal pictures of incredible beauty open into new astounding shapes of loveliness as the viewer enters into yet another magnification of the fractal shape, ending in the final movement into the unknown, with a perfect representation of the original Mandelbrot form. The formation of these fractal images, and their relatives in the realm of chaos theory, have revolutionised multiple sciences—allowing new depths to be plumbed and the validity of new hypotheses to be explored.

In the same way, the equation of the body-self sensitively opens itself to expose, to the attentive viewer (or therapist), the colored and shifting information of psychological function, development, and interaction. It is the firm belief of the authors that the process of psychotherapy has its roots in the comprehension of the body-self—its physiological symphony of perception, psychological functions, psychomotoric developmental stages, and the sensitive interaction between it and others.

References

Alexander, G. *Eutonie* (Germany: Koesel, 1981).

Barral, Jean-Pierre. Personal communications with Peter Levine, 1991.

Bentzen, M., S. Jørgensen, & L. Marcher. (1989). "Bodynamic Character Structure." *Energy & Character* 20(1).

Bernhardt, P. (1991). "Individuation, Mutual Connection and the Body's Resources: An Interview with Lisbeth Marcher." *Energy & Character* 23(1). See also p. 66.

Boadella, D. *Lifestreams: An Introduction to Biosynthesis* (England: Routledge & Kegan Paul Ltd., 1987).

Briggs, J., & D.F. Peat. *Turbulent Mirror* (New York: Harper & Row, 1989).

Brooks, C., & C. Selver. *Sensory Awareness* (New York: Viking Press, 1974).

Bull, Nina. (1945). "Toward a clarification of the concept of emotion." *Psychosom Med* 7:210.

Bulow-Hansen, E. *Aadel Psykomotorisk Behandling* (Norway: Universitetsforlaget, 1982).

Dubovsky, S., & S. Grogan. (1975). "Congenital absence of Sensation." *Psychoanalytic Study of the Child* 30:49–74.

Gleick. *Chaos* (England: Cardinal Publishers, 1988).

Gidoni, A., M. Casonato, & N. Landi. (1988). "A further contribution to a functional interpretation of functional movement." *Prenatal and Perinatal Psychology and Medicine.*

Hammer, Leon. "Dragon Rises Red Bird Flies." In *Psychology and Chinese Medicine* (New York: Station Hill Press, 1990).

Haxthausen, M., & R. Lema. *Body Sense* (New York: Pantheon, 1987).

Held, Richard. (1965). "Plasticity in sensory-motor systems." *Scientific American* 213:84–94.

Held, R., & A. Hein. (1963). "Movement-produced stimulation in the development of visually guided behavior." *Comparative and Physiological Psychology* 56:872–876.

Holle, B. *Motor Development in Children; Normal and Retarded* (England: Blackwell Scientific Publishing, 1976).

Hvid, T. *Kroppens fortaellinger* (Denmark: Modtryk, 1990).

Johnsen, L. *Integrert Respiration Terapi* (Denmark: Borgen, 1976).

Jørgensen, Sten. *Kropsorienteret gruppeterapi* (dissertation) (Denmark: University of Copenhagen, 1978).

Kendall, F.P., & F.K. McCreary. *Muscles, Testing and Function, 3rd Ed.* (Maryland: Williams & Wilkins, 1983).

Kjaer, Bente. Personal communications with Marianne Bentzen.

Krueger, D.W. *Body Self and Psychological Self: A Developmental and Clinical Integration of Disorders of the Self* (New York: Brunner Mazel, 1989).

Levine, Peter. "Stress, Psychophysiology." In M.G.H. Coles, E. Donchin, & S.W. Porges (Eds.) *Psychophysiology: Systems, Processes, and Appliations* (New York: Gilford Press, 1986).

Levine, Peter. *Accumulated stress, reserve capacity and disease* (doctoral dissertation, University of California, Berkeley, 1976).

Levine, Peter. "The Body as Healer: A Revisioning of Anxiety and Trauma." *Somatics* VIII(1)(1990).

Levine, Peter. "Transforming Trauma, Giving the Body Its Due." In Maxine Sheets-Johnstone (Ed.) *Giving the Body Its Due (Suny Series)* (New York: State University of New York Press, 1992).

Levine, Peter (1992). *The Body as Healer, Transforming Trauma.* Book under preparation.

Levy, D.M. (1944). "On the problem of movement restraint." *American Journal of Orthopsychiatry* 14:644.

Lichtenberg, J. (1978). "The Testing of Reality from the Standpoint of the Body Self." *Journal of the American Psychoanalytic Association* 26:357–385.

Lichtenberg, J. *Psychoanalysis and Infant Research* (Hillsdale, NJ: The Analytic Press, 1985).

Lowen, A. *Bioenergetics* (New York: Coward, McCann, and Geoghegan, Inc., 1975).

Marcher, L. *Den Kropslige Erkendelse* (Denmark: Kreatik, 1992).

Nichols, M., & J. Efran. (1985). "Catharsis in Psychotherapy: A New Perspective." *Psychotherapy* 22(1).

Ollars, L. *Muskel Palpationstestens Palidelighed* (Denmark: Copenhagen University Print, 1980).

Pasquerelli, B., & N. Bull. (1951). "Experimental investigation of the body-mind continuum in affective states." *Journal of Nervous and Mental Disease* 113:512–521.

Pesso, A. *Movement in Psychotherapy* (New York: University Press, 1969).

Reich, W. *Character Analysis, 3rd Ed.* (New York: Vision Press, 1949).

Rothschild, B. (1989). "Filling one of psychology's gaps." *Journal of Biosynthesis* 20(1).

Sperry, R.W. (1951). "Neurology and the Mind-Brain Problem." *American Scientist* 40:291–312.

Spitz, R. (1946). "Hospitalism: A Follow Up Report." *The Psychoanalytical Study of the Child* 2:118–133.

Stern, D. *The Interpersonal World of the Infant* (New York: Basic Books, 1985).

Zubek, J.P., M. Aftanas, K. Kovach, L. Wilgash, & G. Winocur. (1963). "Effect of severe immobilization of the body on intellectual and perceptual processes." *Canadian Journal of Psychology* 17:118–133.

Sensory Functioning in Psychotherapy

—*Erving Polster, Ph.D.*

I would like to show how psychotherapy can help close the gap between a person's basic sensations and the higher experiences derived from these sensations. Identifying these basic sensations has become difficult for people because of the complexities of our society. A person may eat not only because he is hungry but also because certain tastes delight him, because it is mealtime, because he likes the company, or because he doesn't want to feel depressed or angry. His sensations are often only obscurely related to each other. What he does about the resulting muddle contributes to our current, frequently described crisis of identity because in order to know who we are, we must at least know we feel. For example, knowing the difference between being hungry, angry, or sexually aroused surely is a lengthy step toward knowing what to do. In this interplay between feeling and doing lies the crux of our search for good living.

As conceptual background for identifying and activating sensation, I would like to introduce the concept of *synaptic experience*. The synaptic experience is an experience of union between awareness and expression. You may feel this union if you become aware, for example, of breathing while talking, of the flexibility of your body while dancing, or your excitement while painting. At times of union between intensified awareness and expression, profound feelings of presence, clarity of perception, vibrancy of inner experience, and wholeness of personality are common.

The term *synapse* is derived from the Greek word meaning conjunction or union. Physiologically, the synapse is the area of conjunction between nerve fibers, where they form a union with one another. The synaptic arc facilitates union between sensory and motor nerves, bridging the gap between these neural structures by special, though not altogether understood, energy transmissions. The metaphoric use of the synapse focuses our attention on united sensory-motor function as represented by awareness and expression.

Various therapies differ as to their methods for bringing expression and awareness together, but most, if not all, do share in calling attention to the individual's inner processes, sometimes including sensation as well as expression. Some therapies do not acknowledge any concern with inner process (the operant-conditioning people are among them), yet they repeatedly inquire about how the patient experiences anxiety. Most therapists would agree that if a patient were, for example, to tell about his feelings of love when his mother sang him to sleep, his story would have a greater effect both for him and his listener if he were aware of his feeling. The patient, if given timely direction, may become aware of many sensory phenomena as he speaks. His body may be moist, warm, flexible, tingly, etc. The emergence of these sensations increases the restorative powers of the story because through the resulting unity of feelings and words it becomes a more nearly incontrovertible confirmation of a past love experience.

Exploring sensations is, of course, not new to psychology. Wilhelm Wundt foresaw sensory experience as the root support from which all higher feeling emerged, but his research and that of many others never had the humanistic flavor that attracts the psychotherapist. However, there are many recent humanistic views that do herald a new recognition of the power of sensation. Schachtel (1959), for one, has shown the commonality of the infant and the adult in their experience of primitive, primary, and raw sensation. He says, "If the adult does not make use of his capacity to distinguish ... the pleasurable feeling of warmth ... [from] perceiving that his is the warmth of air or the warmth of water ... but instead gives himself over to the pure sensation itself, then he experiences a fusion of pleasure and sensory quality which probably approximates the infantile experience ... the emphasis is not on any object but entirely on feeling or sensation."

The child's sensation tone is the paradigm for the purity of sensory experience. Although sensations do become cluttered over the years, early experiences need not be merely infantile. In our quest for fulfillment, many of our energies are directed toward the recovery of early existential possibilities. The early innocence of sensation has been neutralized by social forces that dichotomize the child and the adult into altogether separate creatures. However, the adult is not merely a replacement of the child. Rather, he is the result of accretions, which need not make the character of childhood irrelevant. A childlike sense may orient and vitalize us even in the face of newly developing realities. As Perls, Hefferline, and Goodman (1951) have said about the recovery of past memories, "The content of the recovered scene is unimportant but the childish feeling and attitude that lived that scene are of the utmost importance. The childish feelings are important not as a past that must be undone, but as some of the most beautiful powers of adult life that must be recovered: spontaneity, imagination, directness of awareness, and manipulation."

Reports of LSD users also extol the primacy of sensation. Alan Watts (1964) says that while on LSD, he is aware of changes in his perception of such ordinary things as "sunlight on the floor, the grain in wood, the texture of linen, or the sound of voices across the street. My own experience," he adds, "has never been of a distortion of those perceptions as in looking at one's self in a concave mirror. It is rather that every perception becomes—to use a metaphor— more resonant. The chemical seems to provide consciousness with a sounding box . . . for all the senses, so that sight, touch, taste, smell, and imagination are intensified like the voice of someone singing in the bathtub." In our own way, we psychotherapists may also provide a sounding box for resonance, as I shall now describe.

We may start by dividing the whole range of human experience into *culminative experiences* and *ingredient experiences*. The culminative experience exists in a composite form. It is a total and united event of primary relevance to the individual. As I write these words, for example, the act of writing is the culmination of a lifetime of experiences leading to this moment and forming a part of the composite structure of writing. Furthermore, each movement of my finger, each breath I take, each tangential thought, each variation in attention, confidence, zest, and clarity join together to form the composite experience *I-am-writing*. As elements in the composite unit, however, each of these is an ingredient experience. These ingredient experiences frequently go unattended, but when one does explore their existence and discovers their relationship to the culminative event, one may develop a heightened experience. The gourmet does this as he tastes a sauce. Hopefully, he encounters the quality of that taste in totality, as an integrated experience. However, he also examines his experience more pointedly so that he may identify certain herbs, a familiar wine, proportions of butter, etc. This awareness enriches him, leading him to a new dimension of taste experience. That analysis and resynthesis create a rhythm between destruction of the composite taste and re-creation of it. This reverberation between destruction and re-creation occurs over and over, helping to intensify the vibrant taste. So also, when we explore our inner sensations, we may identify the ingredients of the everyday experiences, which form the substance of our lives. Enrichment occurs when there is maximal possibility for the emergence of underlying or component parts into the foreground of our knowledge. The adventure of unlimited accessibility of experience and the fluctuations between a synthesized experience and the elemental parts of our existence provides a dynamic and continually self-renewing excitement.

The recovery of his dynamic process frequently requires close attention, much as relearning to walk after an illness. Concentration is one technique for the recovery of sensation. It is well known that one must concentrate to do good work, but instructions to do so usually sound vague, moralistic, and general. Yet, concentration can be a specific mode of operation that involves giving close regard to the specific object of one's interest. It must be pointed and single-minded. When these conditions are satisfied and one's concentration is brought to bear on internal sensations, events may occur that are remarkably comparable to events arising out of hypnosis, drugs, sensory deprivation, heroic eruptions, and other conditions that take the individual out of his accustomed frame of reference. Although not usually as potent as these other conditions, a great advantage of concentration for heightening experience is that one may readily return to ordinary events and ordinary communications. Thus, one may move in and out of other modes of interaction such as talking, role-playing, fantasy, dream work, etc., which makes it easier to accept the experience as relevant to everyday consciousness.

Moving now to the therapeutic situation itself, I shall describe the role of sensations with three therapeutic purposes in mind. They are: (1) the accentuation of fulfillment, (2) the facilitation of the working-through process, and (3) the recovery of old experiences.

First, with respect to fulfillment, there seem to be two kinds of people, the action-oriented and the awareness-oriented. Both can live rich lives if one orientation does not exclude the other. The action-oriented person who has no deep barrier to the awareness of experience will, through his actions, arouse his experience of self. The swimmer, for example, may discover many powerful inner sensations, as may the business executive who won leadership of a new company. The individual who is oriented toward awareness will find that so long as he does not exclude action, his awarenesses will direct him to action. The psychologist may write a book or create an organization, the restless person may move to another city, and the sexually aroused person may have intercourse. Psychological troubles result when the rhythm between awareness and expression is faulty.

To illustrate, an action-oriented person—a successful businessman—came to therapy because he was not experiencing fulfillment in life. Unusually vital and active, he needed to make every second count and became impatient with any moment of nonproductivity. He could not accept the accumulation of sensation either through action or through planning action. Consequently, he was having great difficulty knowing "who I am." During the first ten sessions, we talked a great deal and made some introductory explorations into his inner experience. These included certain awareness experiments and breathing exercises. Then, one day when I asked him to close his eyes and concentrate on his inner experience, he began to feel a quietness in himself and to experience a feeling of union with the birds singing outside the window. Many other sensations followed. He kept them to himself, as he told me later, because to describe them would have meant interrupting himself, a wise but atypical appreciation for feeling rather than productivity. At one point, seeing that his abdomen was not integrated into his breathing, I asked him to use his abdomen more fully, which he was readily able to do. When he did, he began to feel a new ease of breathing, accompanied by an easy strength as distinct from the impatient strength with which he was familiar. He could really tell the difference between the two kinds of strength. He said he felt like a car that had been perfectly tuned. He then left, saying he was recovering a missing link in his life. He felt as though he had *experienced* time rather than having *wasted* it.

We may illustrate our second therapeutic purpose, the facilitation of the working-through process, by the story of a woman who recently became an executive in a toy factory. Her secretary had been in her department for years, but was a disorganized and controlling person. My patient became aware that this secretary was the root of many of the previous departmental troubles and confronted her with certain departmental requirements. This was a great blow to the secretary, who suddenly looked "like a waif." My patient felt as though she were now sitting face-to-face with another part of herself. She and her brother had grown up in an impoverished section of New York and had indeed been waifs. However, since she had always nurtured her younger brother, she only saw him as a waif, not herself. In her life, she had alternately supported waifs and played the waif herself.

In our talk, she realized she didn't want to be a waif anymore and knew that in this confrontation with her secretary, she had accepted the chance to get rid of the waif in herself, and become a woman in her own right. As she told me about his, a new look came over her face, a mixture of absorption, alert introspection, and yielding to puzzlement. When I asked her what she felt, she said in surprise that she felt a tightness in her breathing and in her legs. She concentrated on these sensations, and, after a few moments of silence, looked surprised again and said she felt a tightness in her vagina. I asked her to attend to this sensation, which she did. Again, after a few moments of concentration a brightness arose in her face, and she said the tightness was leaving. Then she seemed startled and suddenly had a deep sensation that she didn't describe but instead burst into paroxysms of crying, calling out the name of a man she loves and with whom she has for the first time had a relationship of mutuality and strength. When she looked up, there was great beauty and wholeness apparent in her. As we spoke further, she realized the importance of her confrontation with her secretary, whom she subsequently fired, and the rediscovery of her feelings about waifs. But she knew that her deepest breakthrough came with the discovery of the sensation in her vagina. The subsequent awakening of her palpable feelings of womanhood gave substance and therefore primal resolution to problems which might otherwise only be verbalized.

Finally, a third purpose served by the recovery of sensation is the recovery of old events. The unfinished situation moves naturally into completion when barriers are dissolved and when new inner stimulation propels one toward completing the unfinished business. Psychoanalysis, although differing from Gestalt therapy in many details of conceptualization and technique, has made the return of the old and forgotten a familiar expectation in psychotherapy. Although many words about the past have been spoken in therapy, these are frequently without the accompaniment of deep sensations. The next situation illustrates how sensations, rather than mere words, may lead the way to an old event.

A woman whose husband had died about ten years previously had spoken about her relationship with him but had never gotten across a sense of the profundity of their experience together. In one session, a series of awarenesses evolved, including the experience of her tongue tingling, a burning feeling around her eyes, tenseness in her back and shoulders, and then dampness around her eyes. Following a lengthy sequence of these experiences, she caught a deep breath and realized that she felt like crying. There was a sense of tears in her eyes and a sensation in her throat that she could not describe. After a very long pause, she felt an itch, which she concentrated on at some length. It should be said that with each new sensation, the silence and inner concentration was lengthy, frequently lasting for minutes. Silence when joined with focused concentration has the effect of building up the intensity of feeling. Soon she began to feel itchy in many places. She found it difficult to stay with these sensations without scratching, but she did. She was feeling somewhat amused about the surprising spread of her itching sensation, but she also began to feel frustrated and sad again, as though she might cry. She talked about an irritating experience she had had the night before at the home of her parents where she had not been able to show her irritation. Then she felt a lump in her throat, and after a period of concentrating on the lump, a palpitation appeared in her chest. Her heart started beating rapidly and this made her quite anxious. She verbalized the *pump, pump, pump* sounds, then became aware of a sharp pain in her upper back, then said under considerable stress, "Now I remember that horrible night that my first husband had a heart attack." Another lengthy pause followed where she appeared under great tension and absorption. Then she said in a hushed tone that she was aware again of the pain, the anxiety, and the whole experience of that night. At this point she gave in to deep, heartfelt crying, which lasted about a minute. When she finished she looked up and said, "I guess I still miss him." Now the vagueness was gone and I could experience the reality and wholeness of her relationship with her husband. The clear transformation from superficiality to depth was apparently brought on by the build-up in sensation through self-awareness and concentration, letting her own sensations lead the way rather than her ideas or explanations.

To summarize, the concept of synaptic experience provides a background for the relevance of sensation for good living and accentuates the importance of the rhythm between one's awareness and one's expression. Although it represents only part of the total therapeutic methodology, the individual's discovery of his sensations, where it becomes relevant, may lead him to an experience of fulfillment, may help complete the working-through process, and may stimulate the recovery of old events.

References

Perls, F., R. Hefferline, & P. Goodman. *Gestalt Therapy* (New York: Dell, 1951).

Schachtel, E. *Metamorphosis* (New York: Basic Books, 1963).

Watts, A. "A Psychedelic Experience: Fact or Fantasy." In D. Solomon (Ed.) *LSD: The Consciousness Expanding Drug* (New York: Putnam, 1964).

Ethical Consideration in Somatic Therapies

—Ian Macnaughton, Ph.D., Marianne Bentzen, M.A., & Eric Jarlnaes, M.A.

Introduction

This article addresses the need to develop ethical standards in the field of body psychotherapy. It is directed to those counselors and psychotherapists who utilize somatic approaches in their practice as well as those in the larger psychotherapeutic community. The authors' intent is to expand the information available in the field, hopefully leading to increased awareness of ethical concerns and the development of appropriate ethical standards of practice.

Somatic approaches in counseling and psychotherapy are becoming more prevalent. In North America and Europe, there are now some fifty-two teaching institutes with training programs extending as long as five years.

The inclusion of the body in understanding the psychological development of the person is relatively new in the Western world. Some research is being done in the different aspects of this approach, but as with any emerging field, more is necessary. This paper points out some useful directions for the development of ethical practice consideration.

Somatic approaches need additional and more extensive ethical standards than those for conventional counseling and psychotherapy because of (a) the nature of touch and personal boundaries, and (b) the ability of somatically oriented approaches to bypass a client's "usual" defenses and coping abilities and by doing so, often activate more powerful and dramatic reactions.

This paper will analyze areas of specific concern, explore alternatives to address these concerns, and recommend specific ethical guidelines for those involved in somatic approaches. The development of an actual code of ethics is beyond the scope of this paper. These guidelines are intended to enhance and expand ethical considerations found in professional counseling and psychological organizations.

Nature and Scope of the Issue

A major focus of somatic ethical considerations is the issue of boundaries. Body psychotherapy brings to consciousness aspects of unconscious subtle processes between the client and therapist that are not discernable or are difficult to detect in verbal therapies.

It is possible to engage in body psychotherapy without involving actual touch. In this instance, the ethical considerations are simpler to formulate and contend with. Where a therapist asks a client to direct their awareness to their breathing, body sensations, or experiences, it is not necessary to engage in touch. Nor is touch necessary if a client is asked to merely exaggerate a tension pattern or relax some particular area of their body.

In the case of body psychotherapy where touching is used, the situation is more complex, and a greater degree of care is necessary to ensure that ethical issues are fully addressed. This paper is directed to the ethical considerations of body psychotherapy in the broadest sense. The European Association of Body Psychotherapists (EABP) have developed standards of practice, a code of ethics, a definition of body psychotherapy, and competency criteria for therapists. Their definition and criteria are included here to provide a sense of what body psychotherapy is, and what areas of competency EABP deem appropriate.

Directly and indirectly, the psychotherapist works with the person as an essential embodiment of mental, emotional, social, and spiritual life. She/he encourages both internal self-regulative processes and the accurate perception of external reality.

Through his/her work, the body psychotherapist makes it possible for alienated aspects of the person to become conscious, acknowledged and integrated parts of the self.

In order to facilitate this transition from alienation to wholeness, the body psychotherapist should have the following qualities:

1. Intuitive awareness and a reflective understanding of healthy human development.
2. Knowledge of different patterns of unresolved conflicts from childhood and their chronic splits in mind and body.
3. The ability to maintain a consistent frame of reference and a differentiated sensitivity to the interrelatedness of:
    a. signs in the organism indicating vegetative flow, muscular hypertension and hypotension, energetic blockage, energetic integration, pulsation, and stages of increasing natural self-regulative functioning.
    b. the phenomena of psychodynamic processes of transference, countertransference projection, defensive regression, creative regression, and various kinds of resistance.

Introducing the body more directly into the therapeutic process, especially with touching, can generate transference with need fulfillment, sexual, and boundary issues.

The types of touch, as well as the issues of how, where, and when to touch, will be the subject of a later article. All of these areas will result in different outcomes for the client. For the purposes of this article a short introduction to the issue of touch will assist the reader to understand the complexity of touch.

Boundaried touch means that the therapist's hand is well boundaried—that their touch is firm and definite. In merging touch this sense of boundary is lacking. This type of touch can be simulated by putting two hands together, palm to palm, for an extended period of time. The difference between the two surfaces as separate entities disappears as time goes on. The sense of the two hands has dissolved; they are now one. If the therapist touches with the intention to join in this way, the touch is termed a merging touch.

Erotic touch involves a sexualized wish that is expressed through the fine motor movement of the therapist's hand. The neutral touch carries with it a lack of these latter messages; rather, the information does not evoke a meaning other than "being touched."

The issue of transference can be somewhat different in body psychotherapy. The following describes some concerns:

1. **Need fulfillment:** In giving need fulfillment, Bernhardt and Bentzen (1991) have found it is necessary to give the clients some resources in the form of touch but also in the form of enabling primary ego formation, which is largely based on the body ego.

   The use of touch can be very powerful in the therapeutic process. The type of touch, its location, and the timing involved may elicit very different responses; i.e., a person that has yearned for physical comforting may be quite stirred by a soft and nurturing touch. This could generate a powerful positive transference response. If the person has a deprived history with little connection with family and social network, the transference generated may make it difficult for the client to maintain their sense of balance. In some cases, the therapist may also not be ready to deal with the degree of attachment that is created, and avoid it by touching mechanically, hence counter-transference reactions may occur.

2. **Sexual connotations:** The issue of where to touch and the type of touch are of course very important with any person where there has been or there is any suspicion of a history of inappropriate sexual behavior. It is quite obvious that touching any areas of the body that are directly involved in sexuality is an inappropriate event. In addition, great care should be exercised in any touching of the inner thigh muscles. Not so obvious but equally important is the type of touch involved, i.e., whether it is a boundaried or a merging touch, a touch with erotic intent, or a neutral touch.

3. **Boundaries:** When touch is involved in the therapeutic process, the client's sense of personal space is being entered. This is a different experience for each person, depending on the setting, the agreement around touch, the type, depth, and duration of the touch, and the sensitivity of the therapist. This speaks to the obvious need for the client's consent for touching.

The issue of boundaries is extremely important. The interaction between client and therapist can reach a deep intimacy, i.e., the therapist being able to perceive and mirror inner body sensations may allow the client to surrender into a dependency, which may reflect early dysfunction, and give a strong transference onto the therapist's perceived magical abilities.

The therapist requires a high degree of skill in sensing his/her and the client's boundaries. When touching, it is necessary to know when a touch is boundaried or merging, erotic or neutral. It is also important for the therapist to be aware of what is happening in their own and the client's energy fields. The following discussion serves to describe some of the differences in their boundary issues.

The Physical Boundary

There are various types of boundaries that come into play in body psychotherapy. The first boundary we tend to think of is in the concrete sense, that of physical boundaries. An example of this would be thinking of the skin as a physical boundary, the place where the physical person contacts their environment, and where the body psychotherapist may touch the client.

The Energetic Boundary

The second boundary to be addressed is the energetic boundary, that is a boundary that extends beyond the person's physical body. This sometimes is thought of as a person's "energy field" that exists around the person's physical presence. There are different theories of what this field consists of in scientific terms. Some therapists speak of the electromagnetic or electrostatic field around the body; others utilize the models of the oriental philosophies and religions referring to the energy envelope that is postulated to exist around every person. This is often referred to as the person's aura, consisting of some seven different aspects of "subtle" bodies around the physical body. Suffice for this discussion is the authors' experience that often people have reported very accurate awareness of the distance the therapist's hand is from their body even though their eyes are closed and no noise or breeze is generated in the movement of the hand. This simply means that even though you have not touched the client, they can have a subjective awareness of how close the therapist is with their eyes closed. Thus a client can feel invaded or comforted by your energetic "touch" even though you have not physically touched them.

In the case of a client with poor boundaries, a merging type of touch may precipitate an experience of the client "losing" themselves, while a too firm touch may be experienced as invasive and violation.

The Interpersonal Boundary

The third boundary to be considered is the interpersonal boundary. The concept of individual variation in what constitutes closeness and distance has been researched by Hall (1966). Hall explored the different norms that various cultures have of what generates safety, respect, and anxiety. We would add that the attention to body awareness, experience, and expression in the therapy process adds a dimension that is rather novel in our culture. This can often result in clients becoming conscious of a sensitivity to their interpersonal boundaries that is new and sometimes disturbing. The necessity to conduct the process in such a way that the client has a therapeutic environment of safety is extremely important.

Safety

The nature of body psychotherapy is quite intimate, and intimate in a rather unfamiliar way, certainly in a therapeutic setting. Clients may be used to massage, chiropractic, or physiotherapy. Attention to the body in psychological healing may not be familiar to them. To develop an appropriate therapeutic rapport, it usually is necessary to educate the client in more of the actual process—the theory and principles of practice, than in some other therapy approaches.

It is necessary to pay attention to the matters discussed previously, and not to engage in any violation of the client's norms in terms of their body awareness; for this, experience is needed. The impact on transference from this approach should be observed carefully. Then the type of transference elicited must be assessed by the therapist for its impact on the client.

Nothing will replace the commitment of the therapist to the development of his/her skill in the practice of body psychotherapy. Treating that matter with due respect is paramount. In the field of what has come to be known as body-work, there are many well-meaning practitioners with a variety of intuitive approaches. Some of these practitioners do excellent work. When we speak of developing broad guidelines for the protection of the public we need to move beyond these exceptions and address the need for solid grounding in theory and practice. In verbal therapies, the physical boundary and interpersonal boundaries are reasonably focused on, but there is little or no consideration of energetic boundaries. The authors have found that body psychotherapists and verbal psychotherapies alike often engage in energetically merging contact, without being aware of it.

The therapist must have the ethical responsibility and experience to address these considerations. Without a thorough and well-developed supervised background in this field the therapist can unwittingly engage in unethical behavior even though she/he is well intended.

Practice Considerations

The intent of this section is to provide a more complete picture of practice issues that have theoretical, practice, and ethical implications. These practice considerations will be the subject of a forthcoming paper by the authors.

To practice effectively, the therapist must develop the ability to intervene in an appropriate manner. This section illustrates two patterns of intervention that can cause distress: *too much too soon,* and *not enough too late,* within the context of timing. The examples here are intended to serve as a partial reminder to practising body psychotherapists of some of the theory and practice dilemmas in this type of therapy. It is also directed to those professionals who do not now use a somatic approach and who are interested in more concrete examples of what practice concerns could arise in body psychotherapy.

Too Much Too Soon

It is all too easy for the therapist to overwhelm the client with a body-oriented approach. Clients are not used to what will happen if they breathe differently, allow certain muscles to be palpated, or stand in certain stress positions. They are much more familiar with the effect of thinking, visualizing, or speaking. When we engage in an approach that is relatively unfamiliar to clients, they do not have the usual sense of appropriate and healthy defense. It is possible for them to slip into unfamiliar states of consciousness, access post-traumatic shock experiences, or collapse into regression toward early wounds without adequate internal support to resolve these issues. If the client does not have the same access to resources while exploring the therapeutic process, then it behooves the therapist to be even more aware of the possible negative implications of any intervention in the client's sense of self.

The use of intense breathing patterns can sometimes lead to wonderful feelings of well-being, access to a greater level of intuition, and a sense of spiritual connection. This same intervention with another client or with the same client at a different period in therapy can result in a collapse of resources. Developing a pathway in the psyche that habituates around the transpersonal realms is an escape from dealing with the daily concerns of grounded reality.

Not Enough Too Late

The other polarity is not making appropriate interventions or providing stimulus too late. An example would be where a client is directing their attention to body awareness and reporting it in the session. They report feeling that they are sinking, begin to speak of feeling very needy, and appear frightened. If left to their "natural process," they may well be regressing into a very early developmental phase and may not have adequate resources to renegotiate whatever unfinished business resides there. They may also be accessing a period of post-traumatic shock in a manner that will re-traumatize them. In these instances, the therapist needs to know how to be a sufficient resource for the client so that the process can slow down and not simply spiral into some reenactment of the original pain. This may require the therapist to touch or hold the client in a particular way. Certain muscle groups can be held or stimulated to hold the client's experience at a more resourceful level so they can maintain the resources to renegotiate the original patterning.

This brings us to a discussion of timing—a very difficult matter to teach.

It is much easier for people to learn the skills necessary to conduct an assessment or an intervention. Developing a sense of timing for when to do what is considered an art by many teachers and trainers of therapists. If the therapist's timing is off, they can do the wrong thing at the right time or vice versa. Knowing when to intervene in such a way that the client is not overwhelmed, and yet is supported to generate the necessary resources to deal with shifting their experience in a positive way, rests on a well-developed knowledge base, good training, and supervision, which results in a solid treatment map of the therapeutic journey. It is the authors' belief and experience that the field of body psychotherapy is presently far too lax in what constitutes professional practice. Notwithstanding many excellent teachers and professional training programs, the whole field of practice of body psychotherapy is largely wide open. The EABP has made significant moves to address this issue. In any emerging field, that openness of explanation is necessary to explore a wide enough range to begin to develop a more unified body of knowledge of theory and practice. The opinion of the authors is that the field of body psychotherapy is moving into a more mature phase and with this, a need for a more serious look at the ground on which it stands and the ethical considerations in its practice.

Recommendations

This leads us to the dilemma facing both the experienced and the novice body psychotherapist. As in any specialized form of therapy, it is necessary to have certain training and skills.

Most counselors will admit that in their more mature years of practice, they are slightly embarrassed about what they didn't know in their early years, despite what they thought at the time was adequate academic knowledge and training. The field of body psychotherapy is so new that there is not a well-developed body of knowledge and training criteria to ensure that the aspiring psychotherapist can rely on solid ground. This speaks to a need to be even more rigorous and diligent in learning the component element of the field, training in the skills necessary in assessment and treatment, and adequate supervision. The following would seem to be a beginning framework for ethical considerations in body psychotherapy for the responsible therapist.

1. The therapist should engage in a study of the theory and practice of body psychotherapy. This should include at least introductory anatomy, physiology, and advanced counseling and psychotherapy capabilities.

2. Given the nature of body psychotherapy, the therapists should engage in obtaining supervision of their work from an experienced body psychotherapist.

3. The therapist should establish a keen appreciation and knowledge of their own body as a tool of mirroring and intervention, and the depth of contact evoked by this consciousness.

4. The therapist, through training and extensive practice supervision, should establish a great degree of skill in sensing their own and their clients' boundaries. This sensitivity to boundaries should be developed both in terms of physical touch, energetic presence and boundaries, and interpersonal boundaries.

5. The therapist should involve him/herself in a very thorough personal therapy experience in the approach they are studying.

6. As a part of the therapist's training, they should explore their own bias toward or away from touch and the impact that may have on their work and various clients.

7. Specific attention should be placed on the therapist's awareness of his/her own nonverbal messages. The therapist should be aware of these "meta" messages.

8. The therapist should give an adequate explanation and education of the process being used and the possibility of a strong emotional response to the proceedings. In no case should touch be sexualized or clients "pushed into an overwhelmed state of being" to resolve their unfinished developmental or shock issues.

References

Bernhardt, P., M. Bentzen, & J. Isaacs. "Waking The Body Ego." (unpublished manuscript.) (Albany, CA: Bodynamic Institute, 1993). See also page 94.

European Body Psychotherapy Association. *Information Brochure* (Lindau, Germany, 1991).

Hall, Edward. *The Hidden Dimension* (New York: Anchor Books, 1990).

Part Three

The Bodynamics Model— Somatic Developmental Psychology

The Bodynamics Model— Addressing Body, Mind, and Spirit

From the broader framework of mind-body approaches in general, and important fundamental principles in training and practice, we move now to an interview with Lisbeth Marcher, who, in collaboration with others, is the founder of the Bodynamic Approach. The article, "Individuation, Mutual Connection, and the Body's Resources," explores her view of the importance to individual development of connection with others and also of the need to balance personal autonomy and togetherness—well-known themes in family system therapy.

In "The Art of Following Structure," she further explains the historical process of the development of Bodynamics theory, emphasizing the contributions other theorists have made to Bodynamics.

Waking the Body Ego, Parts 1 and *2*, then illustrate in some detail the bridge between theory and practice in a number of ways. They offer a model of character structure, approach to assessing developmental and shock trauma, and guidelines in each.

Inherent in the Bodynamic approach is the process of understanding individuality and supporting healthy mutual connection. "The BodyKnot Model" represents a unique contribution in reducing conflict and facilitating individual and interpersonal harmony. Its utilization of body sensation and awareness provides opportunities that will enhance any communication situation.

Centering, grounding, and boundaries are central resources in maintaining relationships, whether in a psychotherapeutic setting or daily life. "Caring for Yourself While Caring for Others" provides a deeper understanding of these essential resources.

"The Therapeutic Power of Peak Experiences" explores the components of peak experience and its contribution to the latest theory and practice trauma model developed by Bodynamic Analysis. Understanding the components of peak experience—that it can be revisited and utilized for personal enhancement as well as its relationship to traumatic events—is presented.

For those interested in an easy-to-utilize body map reading for psychological content, the illustrator of *Psychological Muscle Function* gives a picture that shows clients and therapists alike the areas of the body related to specific developmental tasks. It is a far cry from overly simplistic forms of body language explanations because movements and body sensation (as outlined in the previous article) are included, which can give rise to very profitable psychological discussions.

Individuation, Mutual Connection, and the Body's Resources: An Interview with Lisbeth Marcher

—Peter Bernhardt, M.F.T.

Because of new research into child development, the developmental perspective has captured the attention of the therapeutic community for the last fifteen years, and it is transforming the way therapy is being carried out. Most schools of body psychotherapy have also been deeply impacted by this shift, but most have had to rely on theories that address primarily psychological development to inform their work. In this interview, I discuss the formation of a truly somatically based theory of human development with its founder, Lisbeth Marcher. While this theory complements the ideas of Mahler, Stern, and other modern developmental theorists, it has also arrived at unique conclusions about the nature of being human.

Marcher is a Danish body psychotherapist who has conducted her own extensive research into psychomotor development over the last twenty years. By testing the psychological content of each muscle independently of others, and by studying when each of these muscles first becomes activated in the sequence of psychomotor development, she has acquired enormous range and accuracy in interpreting body structure and process. She is comfortable on the one hand exploring intrauterine, birth, and early infant states, and on the other, having done original research on somatic aspects of peer and group relations, she is at ease exploring the territory of later childhood and adolescence, areas often ignored by other developmental theories. David Boadella, the noted Reichian scholar, has called her "the Scandinavian legacy of Wilhelm Reich" and goes on to say that her system, called Bodynamics, offers one of the most advanced character structure models to come out of the new generation of body therapies emerging in Europe.

In this interview, we focused on what might be called the "metasomatics" of her theory, the over-arching ideas from which she works. One of these is her belief that the driving force in humans is the desire to be connected to others and to the larger oneness that surrounds us. She calls this the drive toward mutual connection and holds that the essential field for this connection resides in the body. Another central idea is that of somatic resource which relates to the potential integrating function of the psychomotor patterns, which she evokes in her clients. It is not enough, she says, to reexperience traumatic situations to heal them. We need then to go on and create a new psychomotor imprint and activate resources hidden in the body. I spoke with her as she was preparing a presentation of her work on rebirthing infants and children at the 1991 pre- and perinatal-psychology conference in Atlanta, Georgia:

PB: *As I see it, body psychotherapy has been in something of an identity crisis for the last ten years. Many therapists I know have distanced themselves from the emotional release work so prevalent in the sixties and seventies, and are moving away from working with the body to a more purely psychotherapeutic stance. On the other hand, I see a number of systems emerging that reeducate or retrain the body, which don't really make the therapeutic—in the sense of resolving "psychological conflicts"—a clearly stated goal. From what I know of your work, it seems that you have managed both to keep therapy at the heart of what you do, and to have kept the body at the center of the therapy process. How is this possible for you?*

LM: It comes from my belief that our basic drive is toward being connected to other people, what I have called the drive toward mutual connection. This means that people who come to me are ultimately struggling to be in relationship. Opening relationships is the essence of therapy, and of life, so I can't abandon that goal. And I can't separate my understanding of relationship from the body and body awareness. It is through body awareness that we sense ourselves *in relation* to the other. The more body awareness we can attain—which includes an awareness of sensation, energy, and emotion—the more we are able to establish deep connections to others. So these two things, mutual connection and body awareness, are inextricably linked for me. Therapy that doesn't deal with body awareness will always lack something. Body awareness work that leaves out relationship will always lack something.

PB: *Your idea of mutual connection seems to have something in common with Reich's idea of two energy streams merging—which he called cosmic superimposition—during the orgastic pulsation. Is it similar?*

LM: I always felt that Reich was wrong to make the sexual experience the core of his idea of relationship. He, like Freud, took sexual energy to be the primary drive inside us. I don't agree. To me, the human experience is much broader than that. I feel it took him down a certain path that he got stuck in—everyone running around trying to have the most intense orgasm, missing all the mutual connection around them. But it would be a mistake to make a caricature out of Reich, to simplify his idea too much. He was really the first to come up with a truly integrated therapy including the body, and his ideas are very important, very strong. And of course, sexuality and the orgasm are profound forms of connectedness and are key aspects to any therapy.

Let me say too, that I don't see myself as a Reichian so much as I see myself in a field that has been defined by Reich. So much of what has followed has been in response to his ideas. My own route to body psychotherapy was actually initially quite independent of Reich's influence. It was only later that I took on and integrated his work, and understood where it could help my thinking.

PB: *How is your work different from Reich's and neo-Reichians'?*

LM: Well, the core of Reich's ideas is pulsation and establishing a free flow of energy in the body through releasing what he calls the "armor," and also through activating the breathing system in a conscious way to build a charge of energy to evoke an energetic/emotional discharge. I don't disagree with Reich's concept of pulsation, but I don't think the best way to get to it is through turning the tap on full-blast and seeing what happens. To me, that is not an integrated therapy. Essential parts of the self get split off in that kind of work. I see the same problem with Stan Grof's Holotropic Breathwork. I admire what he has done in uncovering birth issues, but I don't believe you need to hyperventilate to work through birth trauma. In fact, what happens in that work—having experienced it myself and seen a number of others who have gone through it—is that so many issues from so many age levels come up that they can't be fully integrated. In that sense, I am concerned about what therapy is—what actually helps a person change their life—not just have an intense, unintegrated experience. Therapy is a long term, slow process. We may get better at it, we may deepen it, we may extend its range, but we can't shorten it by much.

PB: *You said so many age levels come up in the holotropic breathing. Can you explain that?*

LM: Well, the way I work is to activate specifically those muscles related to an issue or psychomotor pattern, and not others, because I want to work with just the one issue at a time. This allows it to be experienced more fully and worked through. High activation breathing techniques activate all the muscles from all ages at once, which means that all these issues will pop up at random, like a roman candle, and you don't really know what's going on, where it's coming from. Often the content is split off from the emotion, or something will emerge that is too far away from the person's ability to handle it so that we dissociate from what has emerged. We come away thinking, "that was the deepest thing I've ever experienced," and then we forget about it, or treat it as an icon; we worship emotionality per se, or *Aliveness*, or *Orgasm*, or *Birth*—big things larger than life, larger than our own self. We all want something to follow.

PB: *Isn't your focus on mutual connection just another form of that?*

LM: Well, I'd like to think that the idea of mutual connection is a broad enough, flexible enough way of thinking about human experience that it avoids that. I suppose any theory risks being used to avoid coming to terms with ourselves. And of course, it too is a limited way of thinking where we need to look at life in many different ways.

But I see mutual connection as a way of organizing what so many of us are looking at into a larger picture. I see different people mapping out different aspects of mutual connection. Freud looked at the oedipal situation, and the child's wish to connect to his or her parents; Reich looked at the nature of orgastic connection; Mahler and others looked at the separation/individuation process in early childhood; Klaus and Kennel looked at infant bonding; now we speak of intrauterine bonding; and so on. Each of these stages is important, but it is the whole picture that I want to emphasize. There is no time in our lives when the experience of connectedness is not a crucial aspect, and finally it is a spiritual aspect we are talking about. At the same time, I am fascinated with the different aspects that gain ascendancy at different developmental stages, and as a therapist it is very important and enjoyable to illuminate these particular qualities of mutual connection.

Another place I got confirmation was from the work on Niels Bohr, the Danish physicist, who discovered that when nuclear particles were split, they would move away in opposite directions from each other at the speed of light. But the amazing thing was that these particles would mirror each other exactly, turning right or left in unison instantaneously, without any perceivable force connecting them. This says to me that we are always connected in some way to all life, and we are never alone in an absolute sense. You are always part of a wholeness. For example, at certain ages children appear to want nothing but to be away from their parents, to be independent. But in fact, while they truly seek this independence, they are still desiring a kind of connectedness. One of the tasks of life is to learn to recognize, tolerate, and enjoy a multiplicity of styles of connectedness in ourselves and in others.

PB: *How does this relate to body psychotherapy?*

LM: Well, how is it that we experience this mutual connection? We can know it in our minds, of course, and that is important, but it is through the body, through body awareness that we know it most profoundly. Though maybe I just fell into a dualism that I don't believe in; it is a whole experience. But certainly the body is a huge field of our experience, without which we would live narrow lives. It is also that mutual connection is an energetic process for me, not just an idea—and our body is the conductor for this energy.

PB: *How do you work therapeutically with mutual connection?*

LM: Well, there are many parts to that answer, but the most important part is that I always work with body awareness as the beginning place. By building a careful field of body awareness, you have a base to work from, and it is what ultimately I want people to take away with them, the capacity to sense themselves in different life situations. That *is* mutual connection—the capacity to experience ourselves in relation to others. You might say that what I do is look for the holes in body awareness and from that, I infer a break in mutual connection. I then track that break to the person's present life—in their character structure, in their body, and finally in their own life history. Then I help them work through the emotions that are unresolved there. And finally, what is very important is that I help them find new resources so that they can build the impulse that was missing or blocked. For me, it is not enough to work with the unfinished emotions. We need to find and activate the resources that were given up. In my system, this is done by knowing precisely the developmental movements from different stages, and the specific muscles used at that stage, and activating them.

PB: *You said earlier that a break in this connection in the child leads to a break in their developmental process. What exactly is a break in mutual connection?*

LM: I come to this question from a number of viewpoints, but the most important is the developmental perspective. I've come to believe that the child goes through seven major stages from the womb to adolescence. Each of these stages offers crucial resources to the formation of a whole self, and thus to the maturing of the capacity for mutual connection. I think of each stage as organized around a particular need or right. They are, beginning with the earliest: *the right to exist; the right to have needs; the right to be autonomous; to be intentional, directed and willful; the right to feel loving and sexual feelings; the right to have your own opinions; and finally the right to be a full member of a group without having to be special on the one hand and being able to perform, shine and compete on the other*. Each of these needs or rights is social in nature, that is to say they happen in the context of a relationship. If these needs are thwarted, it is because the parents or the social group can't tolerate something in the child, so there is a break in the sense of connectedness between them: connected in the sense that "I can be me and you can be you and we can be together." We then form a character defense, which, as Reich pointed out, is a compromise we make. I will do this, or give up that, in order to stay connected to you. I will give up my boundaries, or my sexuality or whatever, as long as I can remain a member of this family or this group. But even though we compromise, there is still a break, because we are no longer ourselves, and the only way to have the deep connection with others is when we are ourselves.

PB: *Can you give some examples of breaks in mutual connection?*

LM: The first stage of development takes place in utero, during the birth process and in the first month of life. During this stage, the most central task for the child is coming to sense his/her own existence, physically, psychologically, and spiritually. If there is a trauma in the womb, such as the mother becoming ill, or if the parents are struggling to make psychological space for the child, or if there are any number of difficulties in the birth or the first month or so of life, the child's sense of a secure existence is threatened, and thus there is a disruption in the foundation of mutual connection. After this time, the child may have many good experiences, some which may even begin to heal this basic break. But until these experiences are worked through, the child will always feel a basic struggle to exist. This would certainly create difficulties later in life, feeling connected to other people.

Let me offer an example from later in development. At around eight months, the child's motor skills, and thus his/her ability to explore the world take off—almost explode. Crawling moves to standing and walking, and fine motor skills lead to grasping, picking things up, and to games of give and take. At the same time, the child is learning to move away from mother and develop a sense of personal boundaries. I call this the age of the development of the capacity for autonomy. Here mutual connection means something quite different from what was needed at the existence stage. Here, the child needs a relationship where there is help when needed, but also where he/she is allowed

to explore the world. The child wants someone to share the joy and excitement of this exploration without feeling taken over, and without being expected
to be able to do more than he/she really can do. A break in mutual connection here would lead to either a feeling that the child can never really be on
its own and play in the world, or to a flight into activity to get away from feelings of engulfment or helplessness.

And so a child goes through each stage. A particular aspect of relationship
becomes a focus of development. During the next stage, what I call the *will
stage,* from two to four, the child is learning to *do* things, to plan and complete
tasks, and this leads to a sense of the power to do things—and this leads to the
power to say *no*—but also to choose to do things for another, the beginning of
the feelings of altruism. Parents often confuse this capacity to say *no* with a
power struggle—the child wanting to control them. I certainly don't see it that
way. Of course there are often power struggles, but it is the parents who are
struggling! I don't mean to imply that this is an easy time for parents, but I do
believe there is a way through it that allows the child's sense of will to be
affirmed. Next comes what I call the *love/sexuality stage,* from three to six,
where the child develops a deep sense of romance on the one hand, and sexuality—
more a sensuality at this age—on the other. Often parents promote one aspect
over the other—either affirming the child's love and denying the child's emerging sexuality, or somehow activating the child's sexuality but de-emphasizing
the child's feelings of love. I am not speaking here of incest or sexual abuse,
which I see more as a shock issue rather than a characterological one.

After the *love/sexuality stage* comes the *opinions stage,* between six and eight.
Here cognitive development has brought the child to the place where he or
she develops a view of the world, and starts to have strong beliefs and ideas
of things in a new way. The next stage, from seven to twelve, I call the *soli-
darity/performance stage.* Here the major task, in terms of mutual connection,
is how to be in groups. The child wonders, "Am I good enough to be a member of a group?" and "Can I shine in a group, compete and win and still be
included?" In Denmark, solidarity is very strong, and we are able to support
each other deeply, but beware the person who wants to rise up and have dif-

ferent ideas or really compete. In America, it is somewhat the opposite. There is a lot of support for doing your own thing, but little sense of creating community and deep support.

So this is my map—though there is one thing I would add about breaks in mutual connection, and that is *shock*. If people receive deep shocks, which can come from physical and sexual abuse, severe illnesses, accidents, surgeries, and so on, then this too can create a break in mutual connection. Shock needs to be worked with differently than do "character" issues, issues that evolved gradually in the family and cultural atmosphere.

Again, at each of these stages the child gains resources—cognitive, social, emotional, and psychomotoric. It is a whole integrated process. In my system, Bodynamics, we make particular use of the psychomotor patterns that become active at each stage. There is research that shows that at least in some cases, psychomotor development actually precedes cognitive development, that psychomotor patterns act as a foundation from which other capacities emerge. If there are problems in psychomotor development, there will be problems in cognitive, emotional, and social development. Our theory is that whatever good or bad environmental influences are happening at a given stage, they will be embedded in the psychomotor processes of the grown adult. This connection to the psychomotor process is especially true at the earliest developmental stages, where motor development is so rapid and where language is less a resource.

PB: *Can you say more about how you use the idea of resource in therapy?*

LM: I see the biggest problem in body psychotherapy to be integration. We know through Reich, Lowen, Grof, and others that deep emotion and memory in us are actually relatively accessible. The problem is what actually helps people to change. For me, the answer has come through understanding what "resource" is. Reich was the first to conceive of the muscular "armor" and he saw it as something to be free of, something that restricted the free flow of energy. This is true as far as it goes, but it misses the fact that the armor is in effect one kind of resource in that it helped us to survive. Take it away, and people have no defenses—no resource. Lillemore Johnsen, a Norwegian physiotherapist, was the first to use the term "resource" in the sense that I have come to use it. It came out of her work with poorly functioning clients who seemed to have no resource—no ability to function in the world. She discovered when she did physical therapy with these people, that instead of a predominantly tense muscle pattern, their muscles were in fact undertense, or hyporesponsive. When she used a very gentle kind of touch with these muscles, she found she could reawaken the resigned impulse in the muscle and it could find its lost function; the client then had more resources. She worked a lot with schizophrenics and other hospitalized patients using this approach, and found they got better. This was somewhat the opposite of Reich's rigorous, aggressive touch, which can actually break down what resources a person has.

But even a soft touch brings with it the problem of integration. In my own original training in the Relaxation Method,[1] we used a very fine deep touch that brought up a great deal of emotion in my clients, but the work remained in many ways incomplete. In fact, there too some people nearly had psychotic episodes with the amount of material that was activated.

Seeing Johnsen's work, however, I began to formulate my own ideas. She also worked to understand child development, especially very early development, and this sent me on a journey to map out very clearly the psychological content of different muscles and link them to the time of their first activation.

PB: *How is this actually useful in therapy?*

LM: Well, it is the key to integration. Each time we form a character attitude, it is in relation to our own impulses. At the body level, this means that we either give it up to some degree, and thus form a hypo-responsive muscle, or we fight for it in a rigid way, forming a hyper-responsive muscle. Integration comes when the muscle can come back into its normal "healthy" range of response, neither giving up nor rigidly fighting. We have our own impulses, our own movement toward life, toward mutual connection, but we also come to have choice. The impulse can come to consciousness, we can assess what reality has to offer and make our choice based on knowing what's happening inside us and outside us. You see, character defenses create illusions. I may have the fantasy that it is hopeless to reach out. This comes from a memory I have about bad experiences reaching out in the past, but also I get a feeling in my arm when I reach out that it is hopeless because the hypo-responsive muscle has no life; it wants to give up; it gets no good feeling from reaching. So the muscle confirms the fantasy: "It is too hard, too much to ask for help." But if I can help the person sense that his muscles can actually do it, that this muscle can come to life and allow the impulse to reach to come alive again, then I can work also with the fantasy. Now there are the resources in the body to change the fantasy, and there is the basis for deep lasting change.

I call this *developmental holding*, holding someone in a developmental activity, and working it through until the impulse is reawakened and practiced. In this way, my therapy is very different from therapies that focus just on what happened or didn't happen. For me, integration happens when a new decision is made based on new motor and cognitive abilities or resources. In some ways, it is a lot more boring to watch and it is hard work. The tendency is often to regress to an earlier place to get out of the hard work. In that way, my work is not "process" oriented, because process work usually means regression, which in itself can become a defense.

PB: *Can you give me an example of what some specific resources are?*

LM: Well, the movement of development is toward greater and greater individuation and independence—greater sense of oneself as whole. This takes place in many arenas, in cognitive, emotional, and motoric and perceptual realms. But at a body level, one crucial example is that of learning to create boundaries. I think of boundaries ultimately as an energy field around the body that if we learn to sense, can become a profound resource in our daily life. It is also crucial for a healthy mature capacity for mutual connection. Mutual connection does not have to take place in a merged state. This is one of our greatest confusions. It is possible to have deep profound connections to others while maintaining boundaries. In fact, for adults, boundaried contact is a prerequisite to more merged forms of contact. Especially people with problems from very early in life have never learned to form secure boundaries, and thus always feel invaded, or that they have to give all of themselves in order to be loved or cared for.

Developmentally, we know that certain muscles are activated at certain times that relate to boundary formation—the iliotibial tract is one example in the legs. The triceps in the arms help push people away, and the medial deltoids help create a sense of personal space, and so on. Once we had established that boundaries were an issue with a client, at the appropriate time, we would activate these muscles through touch or movement, and also work with the psychological issues at the same time. Once this is sensed in the body, it then needs to be practiced, and we might give homework on it, try using boundaries in specific ways, and so on. So it is not enough to know you were invaded and have poor boundaries. For full integration, that training is necessary so that new resources become rooted in the body. I also make use of the therapeutic relationship to facilitate this. I am active about supporting these new resources, both with me and in the world. I teach them how to sense their boundaries with me, and I support them to do it in the world. In that way, creating resources has a parenting component, helping to give the messages that were missed when they were children.

PB: *How do you integrate spirituality into your work?*

LM: Again, let me come at that question from a developmental perspective. Children, as I know them, up to the age of about three or four, are directly in contact with spirituality. They see auras, spirits, and are in touch with other manifestations of energy. Then there is a closing that happens at around that time. This is partly from denial in the family and in the culture, but it seems actually to be more a natural developmental process. Why is this so? What is the need to have these things go underground? I don't know the answer to this, but it seems important to respect it. One idea is that spirituality closes as other aspects such as emotion, sexuality, and cognition take a more forward position. Later on, in the teenage years, the child opens again to spiritual explorations. We might say that there is a "spiritual latency period," similar to the natural closing of sexual feelings around age six, which then open again during adolescence.

It is important to respect this natural closing of awareness of spirituality because I think there is a lot of confusion about how we come to spirituality. What I see happening is a lot of people jumping out to their spirituality rather than expanding out to it. Their spirituality is particularly not integrated with their emotions. People try to move to a mental level of mutual connection before they know how to live fully in an emotional kind of mutual connection.

This is what I would call a defensive form of spirituality. Let me explain: If a young child is traumatized during this natural time of opening to spirituality, then his/her experience of spirituality will be affected in some way. It may be that there is a decision to shut it down completely—to close, to stop knowing, because it is too painful or frightening. But there also may be a decision to flee into the spiritual as a way to escape the pain of this world. The decision to go toward spirituality seems more common where there has been early massive trauma or shock—something that brings up strongly the issues of existence. Later in life this person will have remained in touch with their spirituality, but it has become a defense. The problem comes in living fully in a here and now way. They don't have a choice. They are stuck in the spiritual.

For me, in therapy, the integration of spirituality would tend to take place toward the end of therapy, and this is because I work in a specific way developmentally. I work with later issues moving to earlier and earlier developmental stages. This is so that the person can make use of the resources of later ages to go through the intense regressions of the very early stuff—intrauterine or birth trauma and the first year or so of life. So I would first work with someone's issues in getting group support; their ability to have strong opinions; their sexual and heart issues; their right to have strong emotions and so on; before I would work with earlier issues, including spirituality. With some people, the task is to help them open up to energy and spirituality. For others, the task would be to help them learn to have boundaries around their spirituality, so they can have emotions and arguments, and go to the movies without being flooded with past lives or without alienating their friends. I see some people make the same mistake Reich made when he focused so strongly on sexuality. They forget what it is to be a person.

For me the goal of therapy is not the orgasm, not nirvana, but the experience of having choice. I believe that we have the greatest choices, the deepest choices when we are in touch with our bodies and our emotions and our thoughts and our spirituality, and when we don't confuse them. If I were to be a junkie about anything, it would be for body awareness and body experience, because for me, that is how I know myself the best.

PB: *So we might call it your quest for "body reality."*

LM: Yes, body reality. Reality is very deep for me. I really want people to be in their reality because it is the only place from which you can make a clear choice. It is our defense system that creates illusions. Then these illusions create new illusions and so on.

Reference

[1] The Relaxation Method is a very developed system of body awareness and massage originating in Denmark—we know it in the U.S. through Charlotte Selver who pioneered sensory awareness in this country.

The Art of Following Structure— Exploring the Roots of the Bodynamic System: An Interview with Lisbeth Marcher

—Peter Bernhardt, M.F.T.

In a previous interview, Lisbeth Marcher discussed her basic principle of mutual connection and how her commitment to relationship has influenced her thinking. In this interview, undertaken on the occasion of the tenth anniversary of the formation of the Bodynamic Institute, I wanted to get more at the process of discovery she embarked on twenty-five years ago. I also wanted to highlight Marcher's love of structure—her ability to see the underlying architecture of people's behavior. A passionate builder of models, she took on the task of investigating each muscle in the body in order to understand its psychological "content." Out of this process came a number of discoveries that laid the foundation for a new theory of body psychotherapy, which Marcher calls Bodynamic Analysis, or to use a more generic subtitle, "Somatic Developmental Psychology."

There are three key aspects of Marcher's model: The first is the hypothesis that muscles respond to stress in one of two ways, either resignation, resulting in a hypo-response, or over-control, resulting in turn in a hyper-response, i.e., a dual response theory. The second is a theory of a link between motor development and psychological development and an accompanying seven-stage map of this developmental process. The third is a character structure model, comprised of seven types that correspond to the seven developmental stages. Each of these seven character types incorporate two positions, one dominated by the hypo-response and one dominated by the hyper-response.

The most concrete example of Marcher's research can be seen in the Bodymap, which is an outline of the body in which all the muscles in the body are charted. During a Bodymap test, each muscle is tested for degrees of hyper- or hypo-response. The degree of response is charted on a map of the body. Properly interpreted, the Bodymap shows patterns of resignation, resistance, and healthy functioning, and it indicates the impact of environmental stress or trauma at varying stages in the client's growth. This map can be subjected to intensive analysis. It can pinpoint specific character structure issues and specific "functional" strengths and weaknesses: the client's ability to maintain his/her boundaries, how grounded he/she is, his/her ability to tolerate intimate interactions, and even how well he/she is able to think and plan.

The Bodymap shows just how many levels of information Marcher has been able to integrate into her thinking, and emphasizes what is meant by her ability to follow structure—see the superscription of this interview. Students of Bodynamics are often daunted by the sheer mass of information presented in the Bodynamic Model, and some are even tempted to see it as overly rule-bound. In this they have missed the liveliness of Marcher's mind, her willingness to stay with a problem until she has figured out how it all fits together, to discover the underlying structure of experience. For her, it has been fun—a kind of play. Also, she has the kind of personality that has allowed others to be deeply involved in her journey. The Bodynamic Model is still constantly undergoing expansion, refinement, and stimulating new research, much of which has been and continues to be carried out by her colleagues at the main institute in Denmark, and now increasingly in other parts of the world. It is the particular admixture of Marcher's inclusiveness, intellectual playfulness, and profound insight into human problems that has made her my most important teacher.

In this interview, Marcher speaks about the process of linking psychological content to specific motor patterns and specific muscles. She describes some of the mechanisms by which the brain operates, i.e., the mechanisms that tie movement to thought and language. She describes how she moves between levels of observation—from listening to language and thinking styles to observing movement patterns and body posture. Next, she describes how language and movement reflect different character structure issues and different age levels. She also discusses how she uses the principles of muscle activation and a knowledge of hyper- and hypo-responsive muscles in her work. We also review various influences on her thought, not only from her previous training, but also from her early childhood.

PB: *I'd like you to talk some about your personal history. The more I know you, the more I sense that there are events in your life that have been especially important, not only in shaping your direction, but also in giving you some of the tools you would come to need. For example, I know you were a sort of gymnastic child prodigy from a very early age, so that your deep training in the body began very early. I also know you were born in a time of tremendous upheaval in your country and in the world, namely during World War II. I can imagine that these two vastly different events must have had a complicated impact on you.*

LM: As to the war, yes, it had a tremendous impact on me. It was a terrible time in my country and I have very early memories of some of the things that happened. I saw the jackboots marching through our town. When I was three years old, I saw people chased by German soldiers and shot dead in the street, and my family and I were in danger of being shot ourselves, if we had been discovered. My parents were involved in the resistance, and this meant that we had meetings and such at our house that put our family in great danger. I could not know about these meetings, so my parents had to lie to me. But I knew something was going on, and was terribly afraid for my family. The level of terror I felt at that time has left a deep imprint on me. It also led to certain kinds of extrasensory experiences in those years. I had the experience of leaving my body and following family members and their friends on their journeys, tracking them, trying to keep them safe. I wasn't able to talk to anyone about these experiences, because I didn't think anyone could understand such things. In one out-of-body experience, I saw a school bombed and children dying. These events were confirmed later by others. I could recognize people who had been in my house that I had never actually seen. Now, through the understanding of shock that we have developed, I can see just how terrible it was for a child to have to go through these things. In fact, my ability to work with shock comes in part from my having to deal personally with levels of fear that hadn't healed.

As to the gymnast part of it, this was indeed going on simultaneously with the war, and the two are intertwined in some way. When I was two-and-a-half, my older sister, who was twelve at the time, invited me to hang around the gym class she was assisting in. As it turned out, I was quite good at gymnastics. I caught onto things very quickly—more quickly than the others, and was soon taking part myself. It was always fun for me, so I stayed with it. One thing that became clear at that time was that I had the ability to contain myself—to focus and to learn. I could stand back and learn moves by watching closely the movements of the others. This allowed me to excel. It was a pretty healthy situation, because the teacher and my family didn't make too big a deal out of it—it was just fun. I did formal gymnastic training until I was seven, but after that I kept it up on my own.

PB: *What do you think you may have learned as a gymnast that you were able to use later?*

LM: Well, in a way I felt the benefit of it right away, as well as later. This is where the war came into it. In order to do gymnastics well, you have to be extraordinarily centered. I took this part of the training to heart, and practiced it frequently—every day, in fact. Being the kind of child I was, this was not just a mechanical centering, but something I took into my being. In fact, now I think that this ability to center and make use of it under stress helped me to endure the terror of the war. It kept me grounded when I wanted to leave my body. So I guess you could say I have a very early imprint of the power of the body's resources, and the value of conscious exercise of these resources.

Later on, when I was undergoing my training in relaxation therapy, these defenses began to disintegrate, because of the nature of that method. This relaxation work focused on breaking down muscle tension, without realizing that tension is often what holds you together. I'm sure that my centering, however vital a resource it was, was also a kind of defense against shock. What we now know is that shock structure breaks down pretty easily at a certain point because it is so brittle. I was getting a two-hour massage each week, in which the people treating me would go into the hyper-tense muscles and very skillfully and subtly penetrate and stay with the tension until it began to let go. This is fine work for many people, but not for those with a weak defense system for containing shock trauma or early developmental trauma. It was from this traumatic therapy experience that I resolved to modify the relaxation method. I did in fact go through a very rough time. There were times when it was hard for me to hold on to reality. I look pretty solid from the outside, so no one saw how much trouble I was in.

PB: *What other impact did the war have on you, if any?*

LM: Very early I made the decision to do something about all the fear in the world—no less! Especially the unspoken fear. I saw so many things in the war that I began to get another perspective on life. I saw a kind of coherence of things. If you have a spiritual experience, you are not only seeing the separateness of events, but also the wholeness of them. I was seeing how all things are connected, all life is part of the same spiritual energy, the same source, the same ground-spring.

PB: *You had another particular hurdle to overcome—your dyslexia.*

LM: I found out I was dyslexic in the second grade. I started to have stomachaches, but when the doctor examined me, there was nothing physically wrong. I was taken to one of the leading experts in dyslexia in Denmark at that time. He tested me extensively and found that I was dyslexic to such an extent that it constituted a handicap. He said that I would never be able to read and write like other kids. I was very intelligent, but it would be a problem, he said. I was told about all the accomplished people who had been dyslexic, like Niels Bohr and Hans Christian Andersen. My dyslexia never hit me at the psychological level because those around me made it clear that I was okay. The school I went to had a program to deal with dyslexia. Spelling was always my biggest problem, but I was good at expressing my thoughts. I was good at math, and often got top marks, and I did well in physics. But I couldn't read until I was eleven. Then I read my first real book. Things take longer when you're dyslexic; you have to learn new ways of remembering. It's a lot harder to learn languages. Where a normal person goes through one process, I am faced with three or four. My special teacher was very good at helping me overcome these difficulties, and I still use many of the things she taught me. She was always very down-to-earth. She made it very clear that dyslexia was a handicap, and explained what consequences it would have for me. Some professions were closed to me: for example, I could never be a pharmacist, an office manager, a language teacher. When you're dyslexic, you think differently; your brain works differently. If I had had negative experiences with my teachers and my schoolmates, then it would have been much worse for me.

PB: *Your father had been an actor when he was young and made his living as a printer, and your mother had been a high-level amateur athlete and a masseuse. Your father's character especially was a strong influence on you.*

LM: Both of my parents, to my way of thinking, had special qualities. They looked into people's hearts, not at what they were doing. They had the ability to see people as they really were. Both of them were there for people when they really needed help, even if that meant personal danger.

My dad had the most direct influence on my thinking. He had strong socialist ideas. He printed a communist paper and a journal that covered the new thinking about teaching that was emerging at that time. These and many other papers were always in our home. And there was always a lot of intense discussion about current events. If I asked my dad why people acted the way they did, he would describe how people came to different ways of doing things, the impact that class norms had on people. For example, he described why the working class didn't read in the way that we did in our middle class family. He never put people down, and he taught me to see the positive aspects of working class norms—like the emphasis on fellowship and on family life. Having heart was the most important thing to him.

I'll tell you one story about my dad that left a deep impression on me. I remember when I was eight and we were swimming in the sea. I got scared, because the current pulled my feet out from under me. I called for my dad to help me. I think I expected him just to come and get me out of there. But instead, he came up beside me and asked, in a very matter-of-fact, non-judgmental way, "What are you afraid of?" "I can't stand," I said. "So don't stand. Now you are floating, so feel where the current will take you," he said. And I found I could really do what he said, sense myself floating, and then I looked and saw the current would take me to a safe place. So he said, "Just trust your body sense—that you can float and that you will be safe." He taught me that I could use my inner senses to orient myself, that I could know from inside me what was safe or not safe. He taught me to trust myself from deep inside.

PB: *We've had many discussions about Danish culture and how it is different from American culture. What were the key intellectual movements in Denmark that have had an impact on you?*

LM: Well, I think one of the strongest must have been Grundtvig, a Lutheran minister who had a huge impact on Danish culture. By the way, Martin Luther King, Jr., actually went to a school in the U.S. that was based on Grundtvig's principles. Grundtvig started a free church movement in Denmark. He is also the founder of a special kind of non-academic school still flourishing in Denmark—schools where adults go to learn about ways of living, philosophy, literature, religion, and so on, typically after high school graduation. He taught how to have a spiritual life, how to value yourself and to be present in life. This man was very alive, and open to emotions in himself. The most important thing to him was that you had an opinion, even if it created conflict. He emphasized having God *inside* you: being able to sense the physical aspects of God as well as the spiritual aspects. My dad's parents brought him up in this way, so these ideas also came down to me through him. In fact, my dad met Grundtvig when he was a child.

PB: *It's easy to see how these themes are alive in your own work: How to see people's essences, into their hearts on the one hand, and then also to see the influence of culture.*

LM: I think I took that deep inside me: that people need their defense system, and that we have to understand why they do what they do—why one culture develops one way of doing things and others do it in another way; why the nomads need a different character structure than an agrarian culture, for instance; how they have to plan differently and follow their own impulses differently and see the world differently.

Speaking of the impact of culture, I had, in common with all other leftist young people in Europe, and especially in Scandinavia, read Marx. Marx affected the way all Europeans understand power dynamics and social problems—a view quite different from the attitude predominant in America. I also got from Marx the power of the dialectic process, the power of making use of duality rather than getting caught in it.

PB: *How did you come to choose to train in relaxation therapy?*

LM: I had wanted to become a midwife since I was seven. But when I had a closer look at the training, I found it was too strenuous for a single parent, as I was at the time. So I looked around and considered other careers. I looked into physiotherapy and occupational therapy, even considered becoming an accountant because I loved math. Then I found relaxation training, and saw that it was the right thing for me: working with people, and teaching them how to sense the body in a healthy way. I started training as soon as my kids were old enough to go to preschool, when I was twenty-five.

PB: *What influence has the relaxation method had on your way of thinking?*

LM: The training in relaxation method was quite extensive: four years of training in anatomy, kinesiology, massage, and a kind of physical education system. There was also a psychological emphasis in our training. The goal for people coming to us to become trainers in the method was to learn to use their bodies in better ways in their lives. The massage technique we learned went deep, both in the sense of extensive training, and also in the results: our clients experienced profound changes as we probed into personal issues that had been hidden deep in their bodies. It was, however, a system that concentrated only on the hyper-responsive musculature, and thus the outcome for at least some people was the breaking down of their defense system, so they actually functioned less well.

It was my encounter with the ideas of the Norwegian Lillemor Johnsen, her concept of the muscular hypo-response to trauma that filled a big gap in my thinking. Her idea was that it was in the hypo-responsive muscles that a person's underdeveloped resources reside; if we can waken these hypo-responsive muscles, then missing parts of the person come to life. The person begins to build structure, build ego capacity, instead of structure and ego defense being broken down, as happened in the relaxation method. Lillemor's thinking also included another important element for me, which was that she thought developmentally. She thought about which areas of the body were becoming active and which age level, though she did not really pinpoint specific muscles. These ideas, resourcing and thinking developmentally, were very stimulating for me. Johnsen was in fact the one who originated the idea of mapping areas of hyper- and hypo-response in the body. She also mapped areas that were healthy. Her map used a similar system of grading to the one I now use, in that there was a range of four levels of hyper-response, and four levels of hypo-response, and one area of healthy tissue. I even use the same color-coding system as Lillemor: red for hyper, green for neutral or healthy, and blue for hypo. However, for me there were many missing bits in her system, both in terms of therapy and of theory.

Here is where circumstance has played a big role in the discoveries that followed: without my training in the relaxation method, which was extremely detailed when it came to the study of anatomy and the analysis of movement, I never would have been able later to detail the theory in the way that I have. The relaxation method also taught me something of clinical importance, which is a core part of the Bodynamic approach now, and that is the progression from talking about an issue, to seeing very specifically how it is active in a person's life, and finally to creating specific action plans—homework—for people to work with to bring about concrete change in their lives.

PB: *Could you talk about how you came to study each muscle's psychological function or content?*

LM: Well, it began simply by asking some of my friends if they would be willing to have me touch specific muscles, and asking them to talk about what associations came up for them: what images, thoughts, sensations, emotions, and memories. In this way, I began to get data back from them. I had become a teacher in the relaxation school and began to use this situation to do research with clients there. After some initial explorations, I started a project in which I asked trainees to record their work with clients in specific ways. I asked them to chart which muscles they had activated in each session and also to describe what particular psychological issues their clients came up with. I also asked that clients report their experience of each session in writing. Each week, I got about thirty-six letters both from trainees and clients. These letters became the basis for supervision, but they also began to form a kind of database, categorizing what specific psychological function or content related to which specific muscles. I did this for five years. I estimate that I received 10,000 letters in all.

PB: *How did the process of assigning psychological issues to particular muscles actually work?*

LM: Well, it was a long process to find a specific muscle's content. I would get this mass of associations that were by no means clear in the sense of giving me a larger organizing theme. I would sit with the material, thinking and talking about it, and then I would wait for more information to confirm my intuitions. Some muscles were clearer than others when it came to revealing their meaning, in the link between motor function and psychological function. Eventually I began to get a sense of solidity regarding some muscles' psychological function. Part of the challenge was in trusting what people's associations were. Once you get the big picture, of course, it is easy to go back and see what all the fragments and pieces meant. But at the time, people would come up with so many levels of associations. I began to discuss the data with some of my colleagues, many of whom later became my co-founders in the Bodynamic Institute. We began to put together the associations with function in a way that made sense.

Let me describe an example of the process. The *tensor fascia latae* is a muscle in the upper leg. When we touched this muscle, people began to speak about various issues and experiences connected to what we now call containment. Containment is the ability to incorporate feelings, thoughts and sensations in yourself, to keep yourself together, especially under stress. Why did this small muscle in the leg bring up the issues of containment? Finally it became clear that this little muscle serves the function of tensing the fascia sheet that surrounds and contains the leg. So its content was rooted in its function in a very simple and concrete way: *it contains the leg*, so when it is activated, people have the inner experience of holding themselves together, of being more contained. The memories activated when we touch this muscle are there because when we need containment of a specific kind, we activate that muscle particularly. It all fits together. But there is this slow process of going from the very concrete physical function to increasingly abstract, psychological functions.

PB: *Of course, I am particularly fascinated by this progression from the concrete to the very abstract, complicated psychological functions you have connected to each muscle, and how it is possible to do that. It seems so far-fetched, in a way.*

LM: I've recently read some neurological research that may describe the mechanism by which this progression from concrete to abstract takes place (*New York Times,* November 8, 1994, page B5). The neuro-scientists are now saying that higher thought, located in the neo-cortex, may well have evolved directly out of the cerebellum, which is the structure in the brain that has to do with planning and orchestrating movement. This link has been intuitively obvious to people who have studied the body. It is also reflected in the fact that many of our key linguistic metaphors are linked to body experience: *Stand your ground; I can't stand it; backed into a corner; I've got to hand it to you; you're a pain in the neck; to have both feet on the ground; to be stiff-necked, hard-headed or tight-fisted; to get cold feet; etc.* Where do these weird expressions come from, if not that we have some direct link between who we are psychologically and who we are in our bodies? This research helps us think about the specific mechanism by which the link was established in the course of evolution; the complex thinking required to plan and execute movement began to expand the brain's ability to think. But is also means that thinking is set originally in a body language. So when it comes to the progression from concrete muscle function to higher abstract thinking, it reflects the brain's structure. It's as though the brain takes a movement and sees how far it can go with it, how it can make use of it, how it can play with it: "If I move my arm in this way, what happens? What happens when I'm with other people? Oh! If I push them away, I feel better. What happens if I tell them to go away, if I use language to do what I did with my body? Hey, it works!" Thus language begins to extend what begins in the body, and yet it is still rooted there.

PB: *Can we look at some more specific examples of psychological content?*

LM: Well, with some muscles we have an idea of the content, but we don't have as clear a link as we would like. For example, the *galea apponeurotica* is the cap of fascia that covers the head. We can see that it is related to planning, to being able to organize thinking so that the person can retain a plan of action in his mind. When it is palpated, these are the associations that come up, and when people are planning, this tissue activates. But we don't know why—there is no obvious function it serves. One day the link will come, or we will modify our understanding of it.

Another example of the kind of discovery we made, after a long time of being puzzled, is about the *quadratus lumborum*. This is a muscle in the back that runs from the lower ribs to the crest of *iliacus*, the pelvic bone. When this muscle is palpated, people's associations have to do with showing who they are and meeting the world, of exploring and interacting with the world. Sometimes people would describe letting their emotions come out, being able to express their feelings. But there were qualities in the associations that had to do with more than just emotion: they related to a quality of *exploration*, of a sense of *being myself in the world*, of *being able to sense my inner impulses and express them in the world*. We know that this muscle is a secondary breathing muscle, which is to say that it supports the breathing under certain circumstances. But there was more to it than that. The link to exploration came to us when we were practicing certain developmental movements. It turns out that the *quadratus lumborum* is a primary muscle relating to *crawling*. Now crawling begins at about seven to nine months, and this is the first time that the child can really *go out and explore the world*. Up until then, the world comes to the child, more or less. So this is a key muscle involved in the child's process of actively moving out into the world. Aha! Suddenly it all came together. Here was the missing piece that organized all the associations that we were getting. That was very exciting. We also recognized another level of complexity of this muscle and its function. It served as one of the fundamental bridges between the upper and lower body, between the function of standing in the world, which comes from the lower body, and reaching out into the world, which comes from the upper body.

Now we also say that this muscle is one of the muscles that can tell us how well a person is integrating his personal, inner life with his more external life. This last bit came when we began to look at all these factors in terms of organizing character structure. Before we had created the character structure model, I had tried to organize a vast amount of material simply according to the age level of a particular function. It turned out that this was a poor way to organize it. For one thing, there was so much information that the trainees could not manage it. For another, it left out the central organizing impact that came when we finally got the right themes in the right places.

A major insight came to me in response to another mystery that turned up in the course of our research. This is somewhat complicated to explain, so bear with me. When working with a client on a particular issue, we would palpate muscles that we thought were connected to the age level relating to the issue that he was speaking about. Sometimes this palpation was indeed helpful: the person would become more able to access resources within that issue. But there were other times when touching the muscles appeared to be unhelpful. The person would become more confused and vague, and we couldn't really get at the issue. This puzzled me for a long time before I figured out what was going on.

My realization is now a key to our character structure system: What is of relevance is not simply the age at which a muscle *comes into play*, it is the specific theme that a particular muscle activates in relation to that age. Now we simply say that our character structures overlap in time somewhat with the developmental stage that precedes it and the one that comes after it. For example, the autonomy structure phase is eight months to two-and-a-half years. The need structure phase that precedes it runs from one month to one-and-a-half years, an overlap of ten months. What this means in practice is that for ten months or so the need structure muscles and the autonomy muscles are being activated at the same time.

PB: *How does it come about that a muscle becomes hypo- or hyper-responsive?*

LM: Let me use the autonomy phase as an illustration. At this age, there are many ways in which the child begins to test himself in the world, and he is learning a vast amount of new motor behavior. How the world receives and supports this exploration is tremendously important. How much help or intrusion the child gets at various points is vital for his later ability to have his own sense of autonomy: Will he have to fight the world to keep his impulse? Has he been so unsupported that he has had to give up the process of exploration? While there are many muscles that *come into play* at this age, and which also carry some of the same overall issues concerning autonomy, the *quadratus lumborum* is one of the most important, because the ability to crawl, then stand and walk, is so crucial to being able to explore the world.

As to how a muscle becomes hyper or hypo, our basic hypothesis is that if a trauma occurs relatively early in a muscle's critical period, or is relatively intense, the muscle will more likely tend to become hypo-responsive. The impulse in the muscle has been overcome, it cannot hold up under the stress, so it gives up to varying degrees. If the trauma is relatively late within the critical period, when the muscle has established the impulse more securely, or if the trauma is relatively light, we believe that the muscle will more likely become hyper-responsive: it will hold onto the impulse, to control it. A person who has, say, a hypo-responsive *quadratus* might have been severely discouraged in exploration of the world.

I recall one client who had a very difficult time finding what she wanted to do in the world, and she struggled with serious depression. In working with her on this issue, we found that her mother's father had died when she was about one year old. My speculation is that at the critical time when she began to move out into the world, her mother became quite depressed, because she deeply mourned her father. In all likelihood, this client's mother, under normal circumstances, would have been enthusiastic about her daughter's budding explorations. But because she was depressed, she was unable to respond with the kind of joy that the child yearns for. As it turned out, my client had never even crawled. Instead, as some kids do, she moved around by scooting on her butt and went directly to walking without ever really using her *quadratus* muscle. In a way, she never got to have the inner experience of a certain kind of exploration, of joyously and energetically moving out and playing, and thus when she was an adult, could not find her way, could not locate, let alone trust, her impulses to explore the world. So this is an example of the hypo-responsive dynamic. In characterological terms we would say that this person was stuck in the "early autonomy structure;" it is an autonomy-age issue, and the muscles are more hypo, so the trauma more likely occurred early in the phase.

At the hyper-responsive end of the spectrum, I think of a man I know who has a hyper-responsive *quadratus*, as well as other "late autonomy structure" muscle patterns and issues. He has lots of energy to explore the world, and in fact has a very strong impulse to move out into the world, but he has to do it alone. He is very afraid of someone coming in and taking over his enthusiasm or messing with his impulses. He finds it very hard to accept any help, and pushes people away when they offer any. This man had an intrusive mother who would try to take over his impulses, and include herself in his enthusiasm.

PB: *How might you work with a person who had a problem related to this muscle?*

LM: This for me is a question of levels. The simplest thing to say is that eventually you have to go to where the trauma took place and create a new imprint, to heal the injury. But to get there, you have to look at the big picture. First, you need to look at the character structure as a whole, at all the ages and issues a person has, to see when it is best and in what way it is best to approach an issue. The other critical evaluation you have to make is: "How many *resources* does this person have?" By resources I mean how much energy, flexibility, how much observing ego, how much body awareness, and so on. If the person doesn't have a lot of resources, then before you do any really deep character work, you have to develop some in his structure, teach the person how to use his body, how to sense it and so on. I have come to believe that if you do this resource-development part well, you have made it much easier to work with the characterological part. In the two examples I gave, the first person, the hypo-responsive woman, had very little resource. Much of the work would be about helping her to build herself up and to be able to sense herself more; teaching her about grounding, about how to develop aspects of herself that are missing.

As part of the general process of accessing resources, I would in all probability teach her something about motor skills development. I might give her crawling lessons, so that she learned it from the ground up; I might show her how to activate her *quadratus lumborum*. If this proved difficult for her (as in fact it did) I would lead her further back, letting her roll over from her stomach to her back, and back again. I might even start her off with lifting her head, one of an infant's first movements, and thus gradually work our way forward during a series of sessions, leading her through perceptual stages of development in such a way that she always kept in contact with her self, and yet was closely in touch with the content of the movements. This would mean that she could begin to coordinate her movements better, and let more life and sensual awareness into them. This would also activate the psychological themes connected with these movements, thus giving her more energy. Sometimes you can see very big changes in a person's life just from doing this kind of resource work. But you have to be careful not to activate too much at the emotional level while doing it. I am very careful not to regress people psychologically when I am doing this. It can easily become an overwhelming and not very useful experience. Too many issues surface all at once, and if the person has been through many traumas, the process simply grinds to a halt. But to get back to our example: Eventually this person would get to the crawling stage, and we would encourage the crawling impulse, to see if it could emerge as an impulse, not just a task to be done. If we could get this, then we would really have something useful and we would carefully build on it. Eventually the impulse could become stronger. She might begin to get not just the *impulse to crawl*, but also the *impulse to explore*. That is crucial in the sense that here is the link from pure movement to psychological content. Here again she would likely need a lot of support in waking this exploring impulse. She would need me to play with her and provide a rich environment that would make it fun and emotionally and relationally rewarding to be out there in the world. Once we had established this capacity within her, we might then begin to approach her problem of finding her capacity to explore the world more from the psychological, characterological side: what was actually going on at that age, what was her mother like, etc. And from there we could work with creating a new imprint at a deeper relational, emotional level.

PB: *How can you speak about working with the early movements and not work regressively? What do you mean by that?*

LM: Well, here again it is a question of level, and here I suspect we are talking ultimately about levels of organization in the brain. In my work, I have come to distinguish between four levels of body *awareness*: body *sensation,* body *experience,* body *expression,* and body *regression.* When I work to bring out a person's resources, I keep them on the first levels primarily: body sensing and body experience, and help them to encapsulate and set aside the emotions and the strong regressive forces. This may sound somewhat controlling, but people often experience a kind of relief or safety in not having to engage with these powerful forces before they are ready. For many, this is part of what caused the trauma in the first place, being overwhelmed by a storm of pain, fear and helplessness, so not to contain it can be retraumatizing.

If we consider again the man who had the more hyper-responsive *quadratus lumborum* and generally had to keep people away from him, the issue connected to the *quadratus* would be more about a split between his energy as he expresses it with other people, with the world, and how he relates to himself, his private self. He believes he has to protect his most private self from being invaded and thus creates a split between his center, located more in the lower half of the body, and his more relational part, located in the upper body, in his arms and face. He already has plenty of resources. But he has lost the experience of being able to be in himself and to be with other people at the same time. He is always performing when he is with other people, he is controlling his impulses very carefully. Here more pure character structure work needs to be done. You have to help him to believe that you will not invade him, that it is safe to experience himself without performing. At the body level, once you could get there, the task would be to help the *quadratus* soften its tension to allow a flow of sensation to move down into his center. Here you don't go in and break the tension, you go in and meet the resistance in the muscle and talk to it and help it relax a little bit at a time. The confrontation, if there is one, occurs when you point out his defenses to him: resisting any support from others, his patterns of self-isolation. If we stay with the metaphor of crawling, we want to teach him that he doesn't have to push so much with his exploration. People with a lot of late-autonomy issues are often quite overactive and lack other ways of making contact with the world. They become trapped, overheated, and locked into the impulse of exploration. They don't know how not to explore!

So these are two very different ways of working, but they are in a sense both going in the same direction: toward being able to explore the world in a way that is both vital and safe. But to get there, these two people have different paths to take. One needs to be woken up and supported very carefully, the other needs help to get into deeper contact with himself.

PB: *How does your concept of hyper- and hypo-responsiveness fit in with the concept of muscles coming into play or being activated?*

LM: Well, when the child is born, only a very few muscles are active in the sense that a voluntary impulse is active in it. Most muscles are at that time activated through involuntary reflexes. But as the child develops, specific muscles become innervated or awakened by the voluntary branch of the nervous system. These awakened muscles feel very different from those that are not yet awake. We call sleeping muscles "baby muscles," because they have a strange quality to the touch. A baby muscle has energy; it's not dead, but it has little sense of structure. You can't test them for hyper- and hypo-response. When the muscle becomes active, it develops an aliveness, or what we call *responsiveness*. The critical period for imprinting this muscle motorically and psychologically is at the time it first comes awake.

So one meaning of "active" is that the muscle has woken up developmentally and begins being used in accordance with its psychological/functional content. Another meaning of "active" is that later in life a specific issue is surfacing strongly in a person's life and the muscles are being used intensely. This is the case, for example, under stress situations of various kinds, and it is also the case during therapy. At such times, muscles might actually change their responsiveness; i.e., either become more healthy or develop deeper dysfunctions. In some adult individuals who have not really grown up, we find muscles that feel like baby muscles: these people have certain functions within themselves which never really awake.

Thus our whole developmental theory is based on the concept of muscles becoming active. We worked a long time with this concept of becoming active, and further elaborated our data by testing children. Here we started getting a clearer picture of when the specific muscles would become active in the course of the child's motoric development.

The aforementioned problematics concerning the overlapping character structure gave us a lot of trouble until we found this simple solution. It was the same discovery that led to the solution of the question of why some clients became so confused when I activated apparently age-appropriate muscles. These were in fact muscles related to that age, but not to the same theme. It is not enough to say that muscles are relevant to a certain age; one also has to see the theme they are connected with. Once we found the larger themes from which to organize our character structure system, the whole developmental map has become much more comprehensible. And it worked both ways. It was by sifting through all the associations from clients that we could see the larger pattern of themes.

Coming full circle now, back to the *quadratus lumborum*, the issues that it is connected with, and the way people spoke about their inner experience, became part of the heart of what we call the autonomy phase or autonomy structure, for which the key developmental task is to be able to explore the world through following your impulse. We now track that theme, and other sub-themes, through that structure. Here finally all the forces come together: The developmental movements, the palpation, the psychological function.

PB: *I want to return to the nature of character structure and how you work with it. Having heard you go through all these levels of organization, it seems to me that character is where it all comes together. It is the largest box—it contains the most. I personally went through a resistance to thinking in terms of character. I found it rigidifying and kind of boring. Now I understand more why it is so important—for two reasons, I think. One is the organizing aspect, the other is getting something about human endeavor deep into one's core: The need for defenses and also the cost of defenses. I've heard you say that "If you don't go into the point of most pain you can't change." This is fundamentally a statement about the nature of character, isn't it?*

LM: Yes. And character is the greatest puzzle. We can understand existentially why people need to avoid that pain, but on the other hand, we can't understand why they aren't willing to go into it. That is the dilemma seen from the outside.

One of the first big insights for me, and one way I think very differently from other theorists, is that I see the later age levels as much harder, really, to work with than the earlier ones. This is because the ego becomes much stronger as it ripens, and thus when trauma assails the more mature self, the character decisions that result are much more potent, much more resistant to change. To my way of thinking, it is relatively easy to work with birth or early-infancy material, once you can see it and are willing to go in at the re-parenting level— the deep tissue level. Of course working with early issues must be done carefully and the timing must be correct and so on. I don't mean to minimize these issues. But the later character issues are so much more tenacious.

I believe the reason that so many people have been so focused only on the early issues is in the nature of the defenses themselves: we avoid the point of most pain, so we go to where it is relatively less difficult to tolerate. And because of the way the nervous system is organized, it is comparatively easier to bear the pain in the earlier phases—which is one of Freud's core insights: regression. So when we do a lot of process work with people, we tend to get involved with earlier and earlier issues! Both the client and the therapist feel compelled to do this. It is not that there is more pain in the later character structures, per se, but that there is more power in the decisions that emerge from them. When we confront our own issues from later stages, it is also difficult to face the fact that we had more of our own personality involved in the choice to take up a defensive position. This is a different kind of pain than in the earlier issues, where it is clear that as an infant or a small child we had little choice in the defense systems we had to construct.

Maybe this is why I like the metaphor of the coach so much, because the coach, while he has sympathy for you in your suffering, has only one goal: *to get you to the next step*. To move you forward developmentally, to support you, to push you to some place you don't know if you want to go to or can get to. A good coach will take you to the point of the most pain in such a way that you can get through it or over it. This is where we have a lot to offer with the understanding of the hyper- and hypo-response and the levels of muscle dysfunction. If you have this knowledge, you know just how hard or soft you need to be: You don't just follow process, but *follow structure*. I like that—following structure. That is what I do!

PB: *Tell me more about that. How do you follow structure?*

LM: At a certain point in my work, I began to make sure I was always touching both a hyper muscle and a hypo muscle at the same time. This way I was not just releasing tension or building resources, *I was addressing the structure as a whole*. I was trying to speak to and understand the whole structure, not just one part. What I found is that, if instead of going into parts that were the most dysfunctional and provoking them, you began to work with the muscles that are only a little bit out of balance, then the other muscles that contain the deeper, more damaged parts of the self will begin to wake up and say, "Hey, here is someone who is really going to be able to help. I'll consider coming out." In terms of following structure here, I am trying to pick the points in the structure that are ready to move. The trouble with following process alone is that process is like water: it wants to avoid any places that it will get stuck. By looking at the whole structure, the riverbed and the water, you can say: "Hey, if that rock were able to move, then the whole river would flow more freely."

Here we want to work with developmental retainment. It's kind of like finding the rocks in the river and gently moving them. Let's say a woman wants to work on an issue. She wants more contact. This issue shows up in the body as various small reaching movements, say, but when she talks about how hard it is not to have the kind of contact she wants, she makes pushing-away movements or her arms go dead. As she goes into the issue, she tries to activate her resources, those developmental movements that, if they could be completed in a healthy way, would get her what she wants. If she could in fact reach out and pull someone toward her, she would be successful. But in talking about it, her defenses come up—memories of failures or violations are consciously or unconsciously activated. At the body level, hyper- and hypo-responses begin to kick in, and it starts to get hard. Here is where the structure says, "Hey, this is too much work, and it won't change anyway. Let's get out of here." So the easiest route is—normally—downward, to earlier issues. So the client remembers an earlier issue, and both client and therapist say, "Aha!! Here's the real source of the problem—this early stuff. Lets go for it!" So off they go, chasing that issue, and the structure of the initial issue is left basically intact. There has been no change in the movement pattern and the hyper- and hypo-structure related to the problem is still basically there.

Using what we have termed developmental retainment, we stay with the structure. We say, "Yeah, this is hard, but what do you need to get through this? Where is it that these movements want to go if you could get some help with it?" We stay with the movements until the movement pattern completes itself. This is where the structure itself begins to change, because the reasons, the justifications for the structure can't hold up while this fundamentally new information is coming through to the body.

But a caution: We are able to do this because we work very specifically with the particular muscles that are involved in those movements that are incomplete. The more specific you can be, the more you reach—as I've said, the point of the most resistance of the fantasy or the most pain—to those specific parts of the brain that are holding the issue in check. The more general the movements, the less specific the issues that are evoked. This is where the study of the Bodymap research has been so invaluable: We see the whole structure at once.

From the Bodymap we have learned so much about the nature of character, something we could never have gotten to in another way. It is hard to overestimate how important a tool I think this has been for the development of my understanding and of Bodynamic analysis as such.

PB: *You speak about character and character defense as something that to some extent lets you escape pain. This makes me remember what you told me at the beginning of this interview about your experience of the war. You had made a decision to do something about the fear in the world. What has happened to that decision? How have you realized this vision in your life?*

LM: I think the core of my commitment has been that I have really tried to teach people how not to be afraid. Not to be afraid of life. Not to be afraid of anger or pain or fear. And to examine our core decisions in life to see if we are moving toward life, moving toward love, or away from it. People are entitled to defend themselves, yet ultimately to grow we have to go where we cannot defend ourselves. Pain is an inevitable part of choosing life. From being in the war, I saw the worst things that can happen to people, so perhaps that has taught me that I can endure anything. I have lost the need to be protected at some basic level. I also got a gift from my parents, who demonstrated an ability to go into life and to do what you have to do, even if it puts you at risk.

You can't push people to go into their fear and pain, but you can help them get stronger so they can face their emotions and so they can see where they have made choices to limit their life. The worst thing about character structure is that it limits our ability to be in mutual connection with ourselves, with others, and with the world; it keeps us from being able to commit to life. Here I am a bit like Reich. I think Reich chose life. He did it at great cost to himself, but still he did everything he could to be alive. He did it in spite of his character. And his vision of character as *armor,* as something between us and life, still contains a core of truth for me. I don't believe in breaking down the armor, as he did. I have created a system quite different from Reich's in that I help people build more ego strength, but I still believe in the radicality of Reich's quest. At its core, therapy should be a radical process for each person who undertakes it. It should disturb our own individual status quo.

In a way, both Reich and I came out of the wars of Europe, though we were two or three generations apart. A major difference in the influences that shaped us is our respective cultures. The Danish culture has been able to seek its resources and to choose love over power. Reich's culture did not. We are both very political, but he had to work against his culture, and I had the luxury of being able to work with mine. Wars are the stupidest expression of character structure, of choosing power over life. Maybe we both learned something from being witnesses to that.

Waking the Body Ego, Part 1: Core Concepts and Principles

—Peter Bernhardt, M.F.T., Marianne Bentzen, M.A., & Joel Isaacs, Ph.D.

Outline

Part I of this article introduces clinicians to Lisbeth Marcher's Bodynamic Analysis, a somatic developmental psychology that emphasizes working with body awareness as a central tool in strengthening ego functioning. Body awareness, and specifically perception of body sensations, when trained, functions as a bridge between thought, action, and emotion. Use of it enables a client to contain and digest many levels of stimulation and activation of the nervous system. When body awareness is combined with an experience of specific development movements that are related to particular therapeutic issues, clients gain access to significant new levels of resource (previously unavailable skills).

What is the role of a specifically somatic approach in facilitating ego-relatedness? The body constitutes an enormous field of consciousness that is only beginning to be recognized as such by traditional schools of psychology. Along with the brain, the body provides a fundamental resource, or set of tools, for exploring the environment and for integrating experience. Muscle activity has the unique property of being mediated by the voluntary nervous system and therefore reflects the growth of ego/voluntary processes. Body sensation provides a foundation for the body ego, and in turn for *all consciousness*. Developmental deficits and traumatic experiences directly impact consciousness by reducing, distorting, or dissociating the capacity for body sensing. When body awareness is mobilized in working with a developmental trauma, clients gain access to *body memories* that can be integrated into *ego understanding*, which activates spontaneous healing resources.

The focus on activating developmental resources constitutes one of Marcher's fundamental contributions to the theory of somatic therapies. This focus is especially helpful when working with difficult therapeutic concerns, such as deficient ego organization encountered in clients "stuck" in early developmental states. Eight basic principles of working with psychomotor development in the context of the therapeutic relationship are described, starting with deep body awareness as the cornerstone for building the body ego, and ending with the need to distinguish clearly between working with characterological and shock trauma.

Part II of this article will outline the Seven Developmental Stages, the characterological profiles that emerge from developmental problems encountered in utero through the teenage years. It includes brief clinical examples of working with these character structures.

Introduction

Are there those who think that the most intense experiences belong to instinctual and orgiastic events? I do wish to make it quite clear that I believe this to be wrong, and dangerously wrong. The statement leaves out the account of the function of ego-organization. Only if someone is there adding up personal experience into a total that can become a self does instinctual satisfaction avoid being a disrupting factor, or have a meaning beyond its localized meaning as a sample of physiology. ... Psychoanalysts who have rightly emphasized the significance of instinctual experience and reaction to frustration have failed to state with comparable clearness or conviction the tremendous intensity of the non-climactic experience of relating to objects.
—D.W. Winnicott, *Playing and Reality* (1971)

A similar situation exists today in somatic psychotherapies as existed in psychoanalysis when Winnicott wrote the above statement. Somatic approaches to psychotherapy are often most potent in effecting deep emotional release or in activating regression to early infant or child states. Referrals to somatic therapists frequently want to release their anger, or they have a sense that something happened to them when they were very young. They wish to explore this area through somatic work because they haven't been able to reach it through verbal therapies. While these may be appropriate referrals, they also point to a perception about the nature of somatic psychotherapies. For many professionals, somatic practices are not seen as a complete form of psychotherapy, but only as an adjunctive tool. In this article, we present a somatic approach to therapy that emphasizes a broader field of therapeutic action than emotional release or regression, and particularly is concerned with ego-formative experiences reactivated through specific qualities of body awareness.

Marcher's work utilizes her highly precise understanding of infant and child development, especially psychomotor development, which allows her to apprehend adult developmental issues through movement, posture, and language. By working somatically, she is able to energize and resolve these issues fully and rapidly. She has evolved a long-term somatic developmental therapy that builds psychomotor resources, a process we have termed "waking the body ego." Marcher views the drive for connection with others as the cornerstone of her metapsychology. In her view, the function of development is to bring more and more resources to relatedness. While relatedness begins before the child's ego has fully formed, Marcher believes that our connection to others ultimately must involve the ego. It is the function of therapy to strengthen the capacity for ego-relatedness.

Historical Perspective

Wilhelm Reich was one of the first modern Western thinkers to develop a theory of the interaction between psychological/emotional issues and the body. Although his work has had enormous impact on the many somatic therapies, Marcher's work did not initially develop out of Reich's system. Instead, her work has its roots in the interrelated fields of education and health emerging from the Scandinavian countries (some of which, however, were influenced by Reich's presence in Norway in the 1930s, and vice versa). This includes especially the work of the Norwegian psychiatrist Braatoy, who described the interaction between motor movements and psychological issues. His methods of treatment were based in neurological explanations of these interactions (De Nervose Sinn). In addition to her extensive training in a physical education system influential in Denmark, Marcher was influenced by the work of Lille-mor Johnsen, a Norwegian physiotherapist with whom she studied. While Reich conceptualized muscular armor primarily as *muscular tension* that bound energy, Johnsen realized that muscles also gave up and became flaccid in response to overwhelming stress—that they could develop *hypotension*. Reich's therapeutic techniques entailed an aggressive assault on the muscular armor to release blocked energy. Johnsen emphasized working with hypotensive muscles using an extremely subtle touch. This allowed her to awaken and energize muscles containing undeveloped psychological functions. She thereby gained access to very early stages of development, including intrauterine, birth, and infant states, and she began correlating which muscle groups were active at which specific ages.

Marcher worked along similar lines, and through extensive empirical research, determined exactly which psychomotor patterns become active in which developmental stages. Becoming active means that the pattern comes under *conscious control,* since the muscles themselves are active before the patterns are established. Furthermore, Marcher has correlated each individual muscle with its specific "psychological content." For example, in observing the stages an infant and young child goes through in developing a mature grip, she has noted that each stage requires the mastery of new muscles. This somatic mastery is paralleled by new levels of cognitive and psychological organization. Thus, while the ability to grip gives rise to the psychological experience of mastery and reality testing, *its specific content shifts* throughout development, as new capacities for discrimination emerge. For example, an early experience could be of being able to "hold onto something," and a later experience of being able to "grasp something" cognitively.

Marcher has integrated both Reich's and Johnsen's differing discoveries by synthesizing a new understanding of muscular response capabilities: muscles have a dual response to stress—they can become either hyper- or hypo-responsive. If a stressor is relatively minor or occurs when somatic organization is already well established, the defensive response in the muscle is likely to be hyper-responsive. If the stressor is relatively massive, or occurs early in the organizational process, the response is more likely to be hypo-responsive. By systematically testing the elasticity of the muscles, a process called Bodymapping, a trained therapist produces a highly specific map of the course of a person's development, revealing the degree and amount of hypo-responsive, hyper-responsive, or healthy muscle activity at a given age of development. Analysis of the Bodymap also reveals the basic nature of environmental impingements and an assessment of resources and strengths.

Marcher's therapeutic system, Bodynamic Analysis, is a somatic developmental psychology that synthesizes knowledge from many different domains: physical therapy, research with developmentally delayed children, advanced body awareness systems, developmental psychology, sports psychology, and depth psychotherapy systems. Anatomy, physiology, and psychomotor development, along with psychological and emotional development, are integrated with relational psychologies and issues of transference and counter-transference. The map of child development extends from intrauterine life to latency and adolescence, and its use requires practitioners to master a large breadth of knowledge.

The Body Ego

Psychodynamic Perspectives

Conceptualizations of the body ego extend along a continuum of psychodynamic perspectives. Freud stated that the ego was originally a body ego (ego and id). Others have spoken about the role of the body in the development of the concept of reality (Fenichel). Still others have emphasized relational aspects of the body, including experience of inside and outside and body boundaries, me and not me, and the function of the body in primary bonding (Winnicott). Others think of the body ego in terms of formation of the self, including body image and developing a sense of having an interior. Some, drawing from self psychology, prefer the term "body self" to body ego (Krueger).

Somatic Therapy Approaches

Wilhelm Reich's work evolved to the point where he was primarily interested in helping his patients release their blocks to vegetative discharge (emotion and spontaneous movement), and to the life energy (orgone) underlying vegetative discharge. These blocks or character defenses were structures to be gotten rid of—configurations that only distorted the life energy. He did not view the ego as a positive organizing force, but more as an obstruction or hindrance to the healthy energetic core. He believed that more contact with the core allows the spontaneous emergence of self-regulation (of the life force). His model of health is based on the principle that pulsation, the alternation of ebb and flow, is the primary regulating mechanism of energetic systems, and that this principle functioned across species, even across living and non-living matter.

As a scientist, Reich finally was no longer only concerned with the specifically human problems of self-formation and ego development. His early work on character structure is, however, crucial to the concept of ego structure, and is the basis of much subsequent work by other researchers. Alexander Lowen, one of Reich's main followers and the co-founder of Bioenergetics, was influenced by ego psychology's emphasis on the ego's need to protect itself. Lowen introduced the concept of grounding as a central developmental task, one related to the emergence of a healthy self. However, he too saw the major goal of therapy as the breaking down of character (ego) defenses. Stanley Keleman was among the first to emphasize the organizing principles of somatic structure, especially the drive toward greater organization in motivating human behavior. His work focuses on learning to sense oneself deeply and participate in the formative process, rather than attempting to break down structure.

Although several schools of somatic psychotherapies have incorporated varying levels of focus on ego structuring and the client's active participation in learning boundary formation, containment, grounding, etc, the term "body ego" remains rarely used. Somatic therapies have had difficulty finding a language that conveys to traditional psychologists the power and importance of somatic work. This is an area that Bodynamic Analysis, and this article in particular, addresses by articulating a useful metapsychology of what makes somatic therapy successful.

The Link Between Cognitive Development and Sensory-Motor Integration

Sensory-motor development plays a crucial role in the evolution of the ego's synthesizing functions. Cognitive development is actually contingent on certain aspects of motor development. For example, movement patterning plays a key function in lateralization of brain functions. Delays in creeping, crawling, or fine motor skills often signal delays in cognitive development. Piaget (1952) designated the first two years as the sensory-motor period of cognitive development. Ayers (1979), a physical therapist, identified an array of learning disorders that have their basis in poor sensory-motor integration. These include the inability to metabolize auditory, visual, and kinesthetic stimuli, as well as an inability to sense vestibular sensations related to gravity. She identifies these problems as originating in early developmental difficulties including intrauterine and birth traumas, and works with them, in part, by activating developmental motor patterns.

The Link Between Affective/Relational Experience and Body Awareness

If sensory-motor problems lead to cognitive delays and deficits, do they also affect the development of object relations? Here we find that *the relational and affective realms impact sensory-motor behavior.* Mahler (1975) noted succinctly that, "The first step is a first step away from mother." If this is so, it is easy to imagine how a child's emerging autonomy would be affected differently by different styles of mothering. An overprotective mother, who cannot easily tolerate a child's explorations, may inhibit a child's freedom of movement in subtle or obvious ways. Conversely, a mother who dislikes the total dependency of the infant's early months may demand independent movement at the expense of nurturing contact. In both cases, the child's whole self receives an imprint. Specifically in the sensory-motor realm, the child of the overprotective mother may give up the activity of moving away, while the child of the under-nurturing mother may experience walking as a conflicted activity. In both cases, the muscles related to these behaviors receive an imprint that remains in the body. This is a basic component of Marcher's somatic developmental theory. At the muscular level, the body has two basic responses to a large or repeated stressor: it either becomes resigned (what we call hypo-responsive), or it holds back in an over-controlled or rigid manner (hyper-responsive). A muscle that is not compromised in either direction has a neutral elasticity and the associated movement and psychological resource remain available to the child. The closer a muscle is to neutral elasticity, the more aware a person will be about the particular psychological issues connected to that muscle.

Bodynamic somatic developmental psychology places an emphasis on strengthening ego structure through building body awareness. Body awareness, and specifically perception of body sensations, when trained, functions as a bridge between thought, action, and emotion. Use of it enables a client to contain and integrate many levels of stimulation and activation of the nervous system. The healthy body ego is characterized, in part, by a large percentage of muscles that are either neutral or relatively light in their hyper- or hypo-responsive tendencies. When the various tissues of the body have been greatly disturbed by developmental or shock trauma, body consciousness (i.e., sensation, emotion) becomes distorted, diminished, or repressed. In working with the body ego, the somatic therapist helps the client differentiate various levels of body awareness. This increasing sensory differentiation improves the client's ability to test reality, develop a healthy and cohesive body image, distinguish inside and outside, enjoy a felt sense of being, and sense a source from which the self originates.

As an example, we will use the experience of Mary F., a client who talked about feeling ill and also feeling that she just had to take care of a relative who was in town. While she talked, her posture became more slumped, with her shoulders falling forward. When asked to bring her attention to her body, she became aware of being burdened by a responsibility she clearly did not want. Support to her mid-back helped her to feel stronger in herself, and practicing the movement of rotating her shoulders up and back diminished the feeling of having no choice about her relative staying with her. As she learned to sense what clearly felt good in her own body, she changed her posture. We supported her verbal expression of the decision she wanted to make, helped her sense the muscles that supported this decision, and began developing her body as a resource that supported her staying connected to herself while with her relative. Her usual pattern would have been to take care of the relative and be resentful and withdrawn. Instead, they found an alternative place for the relative to stay, and made plans to be together in a way that worked for both of them.

Principles of Somatic Developmental Psychology

Psychomotor Resource

Piaget (1952) described the mechanism of equilibrium-disequilibrium as a central principle of the nature of all development. In this concept, an organism attains a particular stable level of organization to which new input creates disequilibrium. Ideally, the organism assimilates and accommodates to the new input and a new, higher level of organization is acquired. Ayers' model of sensory-motor integration describes a very similar mechanism relating specifically to psychomotor development: "The greatest sensory motor organization occurs during adaptive responses... in addition each adaptive response leads to further integration of the sensations that arise from making that response. A well-organized adaptive response leaves the brain in a more organized state." The capacity to adapt to new stimuli is a key component of a healthy body ego. Marcher's concept of "psychomotor resource" describes the capacities both to integrate new experience and to respond to disequilibrium. At each stage of development, new motor capacities provide new possibilities for interacting with the world, and change the child's emerging consciousness. New motor development implies new sensory experiences—"reality" becomes a bigger place.

The concept of psychomotor resource is crucial to the practice of Marcher's somatic developmental psychology. Activating resources in clients is a main function of therapy. What is a motor resource? For example, again with Mary F., by helping her consciously to move her *levator scapulae* we were developing a motor resource. This muscle, when collapsed, rolled her shoulders forward and she took on burdens, but when the muscle was activated she was able to find new options for helping her relative without sacrificing herself.

As a muscle comes under conscious, voluntary control, enabling a new, voluntary motor activity, it brings new tools for exploring the world and thus it is a resource. Activating resources in therapy means bringing a particular motor activity into play by "talking" with those specific muscles in the client, in the context of working on the psychological issues to which the muscles are related. In motoric terms, psychopathology is viewed as a loss or a rigidification of resource to the point of diminished functionality, and this perspective has important implications for therapy. With Mary F., her habitual pattern was to give in to the demands of others and give up her own needs, without being conscious of doing so. By building motor and ego resources in her present-day life, we help her to develop aspects of her ego that were not developed as a child, when she lived with a particularly violent father and a passive mother.

Particularly within the Reichian tradition, there has been the tendency to view character as pejorative—as "armoring" that must be confronted and broken down. This perspective fails to recognize that character is often determined by *deficiencies* in defense structure, not just by rigidities. It also treats protective developmental processes as dysfunctional. With Mary F., it was adaptive behavior and made sense to protect herself by taking care of her father's needs, as crazy as they were and as difficult as doing this was. Taking care of him kept her from being physically attacked. But as an adult, she didn't know how *not to* take care of others, even when she herself needed care.

In order for the ego to develop, the child must learn to contain increasing amounts of energy to be used for protecting the self against overwhelming external stimuli, and for distancing the self from internal stimuli that cannot be integrated. The child naturally learns to suppress various impulses (e.g., feelings of love or hate) and knowledge (e.g., of sexuality or spirituality) in order to proceed with pressing developmental concerns. Each of these issues re-emerge later in life when the ego has matured, and the experiences can be tolerated within the structure of the developed self. Working from a resource perspective permits the therapist and client to join together in addressing the specific conflicts that keep a given resource from becoming fully functional.

Mutual Connection

In Marcher's view, the driving force in human beings is the desire to experience increasing levels of open-hearted connection to others and to the world around us, a concept she calls "mutual connection." Healthy relationships are characterized by a clearer awareness of reality. As human development evolves collectively and in the life of the individual, the healthy individuated self moves naturally toward greater grounding in reality and greater connectedness with the world. This connection occurs through the ego and through the body ego based on body sensation. Psychomotor activity cannot be separated from relations to the world, because sensory-motor development always takes place in relation to the world. As we mature from child to adult, the early developmental patterning in the body and in the psyche often determines our behavior and responses in new relationships.

Trauma and Disconnection

Developmental trauma and shock (high impact) trauma directly impact body processes and the forming body ego. A healthy organism is able to metabolize some degree of trauma and attain a new, even higher level of organization. If the child cannot metabolize insults, the body ego begins to lose important areas of functioning, and further growth is impeded. Typically, the sensory field becomes inhibited, reduced, or split off, and reality testing, body image, emotional diversity, and perception of motor capacity are concomitantly diminished or distorted. Disruptions occur in learning, motor coordination, and pleasure in body functioning, and in the ability to establish clear body boundaries and trust in physical contact. Similarly, disturbances are registered in the areas of need satisfaction, impulse formation and control, intentionality, and in the organism's sense of secure existence. Some of these were seen in the case of Mary F., who, in addition to the psychological problems already mentioned, often had back and neck problems, didn't like her posture, and never moved her shoulders when she danced.

The Sensory Field and the Process of Change

Sensory information is often neglected as a tool for deep structural changes in clients when compared to working with emotion or cognitive insight. We have found that attention to sensory input pays high therapeutic dividends, however. Major structural change can occur by focusing primarily on sensory activity and by *facilitating the integration of sensation with emotion and cognitive insight*. For example, by supporting Mary F.'s muscles and also teaching her how to use them, she learned to tense the *latisimus dorsi* to give herself a feeling of support, and the *levator scapulae* so as not to unconsciously take on burdens. She became more aware of when she collapsed and when she took on burdens, and she found it easier to make different somatic and behavioral decisions.

Some of the most powerful experiences encountered in this work occur when a client is strongly aware of body sensation while simultaneously enacting a relevant developmental movement. As the movement becomes more fluid, a feedback loop is created with sensation providing information to the motor pattern, which in turn allows for subtler adjustments in movement. This cycle continues to generate more sensory information, again informing movement, culminating in a peak experience that becomes a new imprint at the neuromuscular level and creates new psychomotor resources. Muscle activity devoid of sensory awareness does not lead to lasting change, physically or psychologically.

Developmental Lines of Psychomotor Resource

The notion of lines of ego development was first introduced by Anna Freud. Marcher describes ten developmental lines or somatic ego functions: *Making Connection; Positioning; Balancing; Centering; Grounding and Reality Testing; Forming Boundaries; Thinking; Managing Energy; Self-Expression;* and *Patterns of Interpersonal Contact.* These ego functions emerge in the earliest intrauterine and perinatal infant and evolve simultaneously through different stages of development, at differing rates. Motor development, for example, is largely complete by age seven or eight, but continues to undergo refinements through adolescence.

Marcher has divided the period between intrauterine life and twelve years of age into seven developmental stages: *existence* (2nd trimester to 3 months), *need* (zero to 18 months), *autonomy* (8 months to 2.5 years), *will* (2 to 4 years), *love/sexuality* (3 to 6 years), *opinion forming* (5 to 9 years), and *solidarity/performance* (6 to 12 years), described in detail in Part II. Specific motor functions have been linked to specific psychological functions in each of the seven developmental stages, by observing, where possible, how the ten aspects of body ego mature. These seven stages have areas of overlap, and various muscle groups also have overlapping functions. Additionally, other systems are also involved in these processes: nervous system, organ tissues, language, etc.— all are integrated in the course of development. *But muscle activity has the unique property of being mediated by the voluntary nervous system and therefore reflects the growth of ego/voluntary processes.* What follows are very brief descriptions of several of the somatic ego functions.

Grounding and Reality Testing

The fetus is grounded initially through contact with the mother's body in the womb. During birth, the baby uses a powerful pushing reflex in the legs to assist in moving through the birth canal. Once outside the womb, the baby cannot yet use its legs and grounding is experienced on the belly, a position she often finds for herself. Typically, at six months, the baby has learned to sit and can then begin to experience grounding from the floor of the pelvis. As the child learns to creep and crawl around eight to nine months, and learns to stand at about ten months, specific muscle groups are activated, developing additional resources for grounding. Still later, more muscles are used to assist in stabilizing and gaining endurance in standing. Between three and six years, the changes are more subtle as the child begins to shift its weight, using newly activated muscles in the pelvis. The body continues to play a role even as the locus of grounding shifts to the cognitive area (opinion forming) and to relationships with peers and in groups (solidarity/performance).

Balancing

Acquiring balance begins with the falling (Moro) reflex in the newborn and continues with the project of learning to balance the head on the body with the suboccipital muscles. Later, the baby learns to roll as she experiments with gravity and balance. During creeping, crawling, and standing, the child is learning to balance left/right and top/bottom parts of the body. At this time, the psychological task is to balance the child's own needs with the expectations he experiences in his relationships. During the oedipal phase, the child is balancing heart feelings with sensual and sexual feelings, and internalizing the norms of his family and culture. Between ages five and eight, the child is learning how to hold itself in the upper back, and this is related to balancing her own opinions with those of others. During late latency, the child is taking balance to its physical zenith through intensive practice and mastery of physical prowess, and it is also a time when the child is learning to balance his needs for mastery with the needs of his groups.

Making Connections

Connectedness in utero is encoded through the umbilicus and through the fascial attachments in the fetus's upper back (which typically rests against the uterine wall). Through the experience of this bonding, an infant will feel more or less secure in relationships and in the world. A muscle that registers the baby's basic imprint of bonding is the *serratus anterior* (uppermost portion), which is used in breathing and in reaching, and is an area frequently touched by caregivers. Throughout life, experiences of bonding are connected to breathing and to close physical contact. Later, a deep muscle in the torso, the psoas, which initiates leg movements and integrates whole body movements, is involved in the child's physical bonding as well as in the child's sense of his or her own center. Between three and six years, a breathing muscle connected to the heart area, the *serratus posterior superior,* allows the child more conscious awareness of feelings of love. Later still, the *serratus posterior inferior,* also connected to the heart and thorax through fascial attachments, comes into play by expanding the breathing system. This allows more sensation in the heart area, and is related to bonding with peers and groups outside the home.

Forming Boundaries

The child in utero and in earliest infancy has little or no boundary, and therefore no sense of itself as distinct from the mother. First to develop are energetic boundaries, as an infant learns to distinguish their own energy field from that of others. A baby can begin to differentiate by pushing away with his arms (triceps), a movement that says "no." Later on, muscles in the shoulders come into play, helping the child to make space for herself and to throw off unwanted expectations. These help her to sense herself while still remaining in contact. Without an adequate sense of boundary, she might always feel invaded or that she has to give up herself to be in close relationship. The sense of physical boundaries continues to develop and strengthen throughout latency. Boundaries are an area for which the problematic developmental stage(s) can often be pinpointed simply from the verbal description of the adult problem. Many adults with weak boundaries must learn that boundaries are not barriers to intimacy.

Thinking

The body is not usually associated with cognitive development, though research has shown that motor development is linked to cognitive processes. Conversely, if certain motor milestones are not successfully resolved, cognitive deficits become evident. At a more subtle level, we can often observe significant body activity during thinking processes. The muscles of the face are engaged as the child begins to explore sound and speech. Words, a cornerstone of cognitive functioning, are actually *felt in* and *organized by* the body. Cognitive development is mediated through touching, reaching, pointing, and grasping. These activities allow the child to form an internalized, three-dimensional model of the outer world. Developing muscles in the back of the neck mediate a new capacity for focusing attention. Portions of a fascial sheath on top of the head (the galia aponeurosis) come into play, first facilitating short-term planning, and later long-term planning, which is a leap in cognitive ability. During this same time period, the child can learn to form and hold an opinion. This has been correlated with fine muscles in the hand, used for opposition of both thumb and little finger, which are active when expressing opinions. Hypo-responsiveness in these muscles corresponds to difficulty holding an opinion, while hyper-responsiveness corresponds to rigidly holding onto opinions, even in the face of contradictory facts.

Principles of Working with Psychomotor Development in Therapy

A psychotherapeutic model requires a method of tracking the flow of unconscious material, and so working with transference is of central importance. Following our core notion of mutual connection, the therapist's task is to recognize breaks in object relatedness and engage the client in an investigation of the missing elements. As an overall stance, we are active and involved in interactions with the client. For example, we are likely to enact the role of parent to embody the other half of the developmental sequence that is unfolding, or to function as a coach by encouraging movement patterns.

Marcher's model offers a broad, yet highly specific map of child development from intrauterine states through adolescence. Each developmental task is associated with specific body experiences and motor patterns. By understanding and activating specific psychomotor patterns, we can access equally specific developmental situations through body awareness, touch, and movement: intrauterine and birth states, creeping, crawling, grasping, give-and-take games, early visual/kinesthetic integration, etc. With regard to the later developmental stages, we can recognize specific motor behaviors and body positions that correspond to the cognitive and socialization patterns of children forming peer groups.

There are *eight basic principles* of working with psychomotor development:

1. Distinguishing levels of body awareness.

2. Engaging already established resources within the client.

3. Observing the developmental motor patterns that accompany psychological issues.

4. Working from later developmental stages to earlier ones in the overall course of therapy, and drawing resources from later stages to support earlier deficits.

5. Engaging a developmental motor sequence by first establishing precursor movements and bringing those movements forward.

6. Holding a client to one developmental stage and specific motor pattern until the resources in that pattern are activated and a new imprint is established.

7. Working with character regressively.

8. Differentiating shock trauma from developmental trauma.

1. Distinguishing Levels of Body Awareness

In exploring the phenomenology of body awareness, we have found it useful to delineate four discrete categories: (a) *body sensation,* (b) *body experience,* (c) *emotional expression,* and (d) *regression.* These categories allow clinicians to choose the entry category they feel will be most productive for the client, and to channel the flow of a session. This control allows the therapist to build resources, where needed, before the client enters emotional or regressive states. By virtue of the powerful nature of memories stored in the body, somatic therapies can quickly uncover very early or traumatic material releasing vivid emotions. However, this cathartic regression is not always desirable. Experience has shown us that activating memories and emotions, without preparatory and follow-up work, does not promote the kind of ego integration that leads to lasting structural changes.

a. **Body sensation:** Awareness of temperature, level of tension/flaccidity, proprioception and kinesthetic sense of location, position, movement, vestibular sense; gravity (weight, balance), touch, perception of energy (tingling, flow, etc.), physical pain, intention, preparatory movements; senses of sight, hearing, smell, taste.

b. **Body experience:** Emotions of anger, grief, shame, joy, fear, sexuality. Associative processes connected to body sensations; body memory, image, and fantasy (distortions in body image, size, shape, strength, etc.). All other forms of activity from unconscious, e.g., imagery, thoughts.

c. **Expression:** Emotional release, vegetative discharge, pulsation. Completed intention movements. Charged verbalization, making sounds.

    d. **Regression:** Body movements, cognitive and emotional expression consistent with specific age level (or levels). Regression can be to recent past or even back to intrauterine levels.

Initially, Marcher helps the client differentiate body sensation from body experience. Body sensation is related to here-and-now reality, and once awareness of it is established, the client has a baseline for evaluating new sensations. These new sensations, such as increased pressure, tingling, pain, etc., often indicate that important issues are being activated. Also, some clients are living in what amounts to a body fantasy. They have no direct access to their sensations, which are continually filtered through unconscious fantasies, e.g., of being happy, powerless, totally loved, etc. Other clients may not be capable of rich body experience. They are stuck in sensation only, not recognizing their emotions, for example.

The following are examples of each type of language:

    a. **Body sensation language:** I sense tension in my shoulders. My feet and hands are cold. I can sense movement in my wrists when I turn my hand. My chest feels warm. I can feel muscles letting go, muscles tightening up. I can sense how thick my leg is. That tension is on the surface; this one is deep. I sense the weight of my arm as I lift it. I'm out of balance, and I want to right myself.

    b. **Body experience language:** I feel relaxed. I'm nervous, anxious. I've got butterflies in my stomach. Something's eating at me inside. I'm freezing. I could melt into the chair. I've got a steel plate in my chest. I've got no skin. My heart is broken. My head could explode. I could cry forever. I'm so angry I could kill. There's a hole inside of me. I feel empty. I feel like a computer. I'm a monster. I feel fat. I'm spinning out of control. I'm so strong, no one could ever hurt me.

2. Engaging Already Established Resources

From the Bodynamic point of view, character structure represents the natural process of a person coming to terms with his or her environment. Character represents an "adapted self," an achievement deserving recognition and, at times, reinforcement. As such, no matter how dysfunctional, it is a resource state to some degree. By recognizing and supporting the notion of healthy defenses, the therapist acknowledges the core integrity of the individual's reality. Identifying and using a client's sources of strength as a foundation for therapeutic work means joining with his or her level of ego development. This joining, in turn, facilitates the client's expansion into other more ego-alien realms. Also, clients typically have areas of genuine health, as measured by the responsiveness and flexibility in the body. Awareness of these resources in both therapist and client aids in negotiating the difficult waters often encountered in the therapeutic process. With certain clients, in fact, the initial goal may be one of expanding their adapted self, because their inner core appears to be too fragile to endure significant stress until an adequate level of ego structuring has been attained. We find this approach to be particularly important with some borderline personalities. The adapted self can be built to the point where a client has enough stability and resources in his life so that he can face his deficiencies without decompensating.

3. Observing the Developmental Motor Patterns That Accompany Psychological Issues

As clients talk about the specific issues that concern them, we watch the body for the emergence of movement, posture, and language patterns that may tell us which age level or levels are predominating. If many age levels are present, we choose the one that feels most accessible or workable. When the client explores these particular movements, he may find that motor impulses and feelings that were unrecognized in the past now become activated and expressed. After these feelings have been expressed and related cognitive issues worked through, the motor pattern in the muscles needs to be retrained. For example, it is not enough for a person who as a child had given up reaching out and drawing in nurturing supplies, simply to reexperience the feelings of deprivation that led to resignation. While this is an essential first step, if it remains the only step, it becomes a reenactment of the trauma, and resources, at best, are incompletely activated. The person's "inner map of the world" is not changed and hyper- and hypo- muscles will tend to return to their chronic patterns.

If this first step is followed by a retraining of the age-relevant psychomotor activities (here it would be reaching out for and pulling someone close), a new imprint of *muscular response* and *interpersonal resource* is made, which can then be integrated into daily life. Thus retraining involves three basic steps: 1) reactivating the original situation; 2) retraining the psychomotor pattern in an environment where the impulse reaches a successful emotional and physical conclusion; 3) practicing the new imprint in life with the support of the client's social network and the therapist.

4. Working from Later to Earlier

Working with later developmental issues before early ones enables us to build resources before delving into more primitive material. Children find their own resources to help them manage the developmental roadblocks they encounter: they use transitional objects to soothe feelings of separation, or enter fantasies to compensate for feelings of inferiority, and find adults and friends to fill gaps in their parents' mirroring of them. However, some children are not able to find such resources; either the environment is impoverished or the parenting too depriving or overbearing.

In Bodynamic therapy, clients can make use of later developmental resources before approaching earlier issues that often entail deep feelings of helplessness and dependency. For example, the task of making friends, while based on many, very early experiences of attachment, begins relatively late along the developmental sequence, usually peaking between the ages of seven to twelve years, during what we call the solidarity/performance stage. When clients have a poor social network, we often begin by exploring their history of making friends and attempting to resolve some of the conflicts that arose during this age period. By resolving these conflicts, clients often begin making new friends, and typically these friendships deepen, allowing more contact needs to be met. This in turn helps to activate contact issues in therapy and acts as a resource for the client in the therapeutic process. By contrast, analytic therapies emphasize healing the transference relationship with the therapist, with the expectation that the new awareness gained from this process will then transfer to the client's other relationships.

Another resource from later development (ages five through eight) is the acquisition of cognitive abilities—the training of the mind to think, ask questions and attempt to solve problems. Clients who have an inadequately developed observing ego need to cultivate these basic cognitive skills before working with early issues. Here we help clients learn how to express strong opinions, verbalize their thinking, be able to think critically, and articulate their observations of inner and outer events. Without these abilities, clients are likely to become submerged in body sensations and emotions, which then remain chaotic and inarticulate.

Paradoxically, it is often difficult to keep a client focused on later age issues of latency and adolescence, because children this age are highly developed, yet still dependent, immature, and more acutely aware of their vulnerability. Issues from the teenage years can be some of the hardest to engage by virtue of the strength of the matured ego in defending itself. In contrast, through the use of developmental movements and body memory, relatively easy access can be gained to earlier developmental stages.

5. Engaging a developmental motor sequence

Noted Danish physical therapist Britte Holle trained developmentally delayed children to attain their delayed motor skills by first working with the movements that preceded the delayed ones. This approach precludes overwhelming children by asking them to perform movements that are beyond their abilities to activate. In her work, for example, a child with poor walking abilities might need first to return to creeping and crawling in order to solidify walking abilities. If creeping and crawling are not well established, the child might have to go back to the even earlier stage of rolling. Taking children back to their area of confidence and capability, and *then* moving forward, allows the resources contained in this earlier stage to be brought forward in a natural way.

Bodynamics has adopted this approach in working with adult psychological issues. We often make a conscious choice *not* to work regressively. This means that we do not push to identify the underlying emotional content or the traumatic event; we do not attempt to process the emotional layer. Rather, we primarily start with body sensing and body experiencing levels. In this way, clients learn to sense and understand their overall emotional experience, even though the emphasis is on training them to sense or to move in an emotionally supportive environment. Clients often experience the process of engaging a new movement as difficult, painful, and awkward. They want to give up; they feel it is stupid when asked, for example, to creep or crawl. Structural changes occur, however, when the client is able to explore a previously unavailable movement while also aware of her body sensations. Once this takes place, the client has a new resource, a new tool with which to manage the world. The body ego has access to new "territory" to integrate into its landscape. Often this is experienced as a paradigm shift: the world becomes a new place—with new possibilities! Both the learning stage of frustration and disequilibrium and the excitement stage mirror normal child development. As children attain new abilities, their world is altered and the experience is one of excitement.

This aspect of our work requires knowledge of child development as well as developmental anatomy. The more specifically we can awaken the appropriate muscle, the more sure we are of engaging the resource in a lasting way. We call this process "resourcing the client." As a result of this process, there is a sense of accomplishment—a body self to draw on, together with the experience of support from the therapist, with which to face deep despair, terror, anger, loneliness, or resignation. It is one of the ways we prepare for character work in which we will more deeply explore the emotional issues that created the deficit in the first place. We avoid having clients confront or engage their early life traumas from a deficient state. Resourcing the client is especially important for those who have inadequate ego development and few life-functioning skills.

6. Developmental holding

"Developmental holding" or "containment" is an approach related to activating resources. In this process clients are *contained* at one specific age level until they have renegotiated an issue psychologically and somatically. Holding or containing addresses a problematic tendency of clients to continue regressing to earlier and earlier issues. While it is often assumed that the earlier issue is related to or the cause of the later one, it is not necessarily the case. The client may simply feel safer or more familiar with the earlier issue. This problem is not limited to body psychotherapies. Often one memory leads to an earlier memory, which then leads to an even earlier one.

As a technique, developmental holding emerged from our experience with hypo-responsive, resigned muscle patterns. Resigned muscles either receive weak impulses or none at all. Psychologically this is experienced as "I can't do it," "It's impossible," "It hurts too much," "I don't have the energy," and so on. In effect, a belief about reality has been imprinted in the muscle. This belief is reinforced each time the muscle tries to function. What the muscle does not know is that the original traumatic situation is no longer imminent and that the constraint is now entirely internal. The constraint is real, however, in the sense that the muscle is not trained to contain the impulse. Under stress, the body can either use other resources or adjacent muscles in trying to compensate for it deficiencies, or it may sense other areas of weakness that confirm the hopelessness of the situation. The task in attempting to activate these muscles is to "convince them" that it is safe, in essence, to come out into the sun and live, to awaken the lost impulse. This may mean regressing to earlier levels of development or moving to later ones.

The therapist's task in these developmental holding situations is a precarious one of encouraging, supporting, and even insisting through persistence that the muscles begin the process of waking up. This containment requires sensitivity to the level of activation that may be overwhelming, and to other elements that may be necessary if the client is to experience the strength to awaken impulses. Some muscles can be so hypo-responsive, so resigned, that they should not be worked with until other resources have been restored. Here, even if you engage the muscle and its contents, it will tend to slip back into hypo-responsiveness. The same potential problems exist for hyper-responsive muscles, though the emotional qualities are reversed: "I will do it," "I have to do it," "You can't stop me," "I must do it this way," etc. Here, the emphasis is on getting the muscle to relax, to let go of the necessity for action or for a particular action. The client needs support to sense that support exists—that other alternatives exist, different from the historical choices that no longer apply.

When the client does have sufficient resources to proceed, developmental holding means staying with her through her frustration and resignation and maintaining the focus on an issue in one specific developmental stage, until that issue is resolved and new resources have been established. For example, consider a client who is having difficulty getting close contact and support. If the muscles for *reaching out and pulling in* nurturing are resigned, he will either not attempt this activity or fail to recognize that it is even a possibility. Assuming that trust is established to work at this level, the therapist can begin to activate the relevant muscles (coracobrachialis and biceps for reaching, biceps for pulling toward, small muscles in hand for bringing in close to the body) by gently provoking the specific muscles or by having the client practice certain movements slowly and asking him to describe his sense impressions and experience. Not uncommonly, the client initially experiences the exercise as mechanical, and does not sense anything happening or states that it is too difficult. The therapist encourages the client to continue, and if she is activating the right muscles for the issue, awareness begins to build and the client begins to sense his psychological issues connected to *reaching out and pulling in.*

This is an important beginning, but more is usually necessary. Emotions and memories may begin to surface. The temptation may be to explore these, and indeed at some point, they should be explored. However, it is important to remember that at the body level, the client has only just begun the work of establishing this motor pattern as a resource. Now the client needs to have a successful experience of *reaching out and pulling in.* It is not enough to practice the movements in an emotionally neutral environment—the situation must feel real. Here the therapist is experienced in the transference both as coach and as libidinal object, for it is the therapist who is on the other end of the client's hand, providing contact.

The therapist is also making sure that the muscles in the arm and hand are activating, and looking for any signs that an opposite impulse is emerging—for example, the impulse to push away. It may be that this client was invaded as well as insufficiently nurtured, and that the two impulses of *reaching* and *pushing* need to emerge at the same time. There may be many small impasses on the way to this simple but crucial developmental activity. All such conflicts or impasses need to be cleared until the client is able to have an unconflicted experience of this simple activity—a successful experience of *reaching out and pulling in*. Only then do we say that the client has established a new imprint.

Here, establishing the new imprint was most important, and leads to more structural change than would have taken place if we had focused only on the experience of deficit, or on the process of releasing emotions associated with past unsuccessful experiences of *reaching out and pulling in*. We can assume that there is unexpressed deep crying, anger, and loneliness within this person, which still needs to be released. Having had a successful *reaching out and pulling in* experience does not automatically dissipate this sadness. Our experience is that there is less likelihood of decompensation or retraumatization if the resource has been established first.

7. Working with Character Regressively

The concept of regression has varied application among the different schools of psychology. In analytic thinking, it typically is used to describe a primitive defensive maneuver aimed at avoiding conflict. Psychodynamically, a "regressed patient" is one who is stuck in early developmental states—he or she can't seem to grow up. Thus, the term regression generally carries a pejorative connotation of very early or infantile behavior that is out of control in an adult. If there is a general weakness in analytic verbal therapies, it is having less access to age levels preceding verbal development. Recent developmental research has been focused on pre-oedipal states, even birth and intrauterine states. We share the excitement in the discoveries of this long ignored territory, but also regard later developmental issues, all the way through adolescence, as crucial areas of therapeutic focus. Thus, in Bodynamics, when we speak of regressing a client, we refer to the reexperiencing in session of emotions, memories, body sensations, etc., from a broad spectrum of age levels, and in particular from the seven developmental stages.

When working regressively with an issue or memory, we attempt to hold the client to that particular issue, and to the age level or levels from which the issue originates. Initially, we may enlist the client's observing ego by making an agreement clarifying the scope of the work on this issue. Then, should the client later feel pulled toward other issues or age levels, we might say: "We can focus on that another time, but I think we should stay with this issue for now." The process of developmental holding is sustained by responding to and reinforcing only those themes and phrasings in the client's description of her experience that relate to the particular issue and age level. Similarly, we observe body posture and intention movements and encourage only those specific patterns that relate to the designated age. We can further secure containment and focus by stimulating muscles related to this specific age and issue.

It is our experience that, while preparatory work is crucial, healing finally takes place when a person is regressed back to the age level at which the original disturbance happened. While the psychodynamic view is that the client uses his or her adult state to parent the injured child state, we tend to work directly with the child ego state. Ultimately, the ego is healed through a direct positive experience of the missing relational and behavioral elements. An adult who received little physical contact as a child may have gotten much support later on, and thereby learned to cope with his deficit. For the deepest layers of trust and inner sense of self to develop, however, that person needs the experience of positive physical contact while regressed to the age of deprivation. For example, an adult whose curiosity was crushed when he was a child may only be able to recapture the fullness of his impulses by experiencing the joy of learning to crawl and explore, with the therapist present as an excited and supportive fellow traveler. Our approach was developed using the Bodymap diagnostic test, which gives us specific information about when a specific developmental problem originated and how the child responded. While the approach is at odds with much of the analytic mainstream, there exist significant exceptions such as the ongoing debate about "corrective emotional experiences," an issue that refuses to go away.

8. Distinguishing Shock and Developmental Trauma (Character)

Developmental trauma includes harmful relational demands or deficits in early social environment, and usually emerges from chronic relationship interactions within the family. Examples include inadequate mirroring, inability to tolerate emotions, humiliation, lack of physical touching, authoritarian demands, etc. In order to master or better tolerate these interactions, the child slowly generates *character defenses*. Since the child has the opportunity to practice and refine these defenses, they represent an active solution to the problem and include an element of (partly unconscious) choice.

While character trauma involves low or moderate levels of nervous system activation, shock trauma is characterized by brief, sudden, massive impacts upon the individual. While character defenses employ a relatively high level of cognitive choice, shock trauma is registered quite differently in the body and psyche. By contrast, shock activates more reflexive levels of the nervous system, including the extreme survival mechanisms of tonic immobility and dissociation, or the flight-or-fight reflex. Shock trauma requires a significantly different treatment approach. Techniques that are useful in working with character issues (cathartic techniques or analysis of resistance) can be retraumatizing here if they overstimulate the already compromised nervous system/psyche.

Earlier, we identified the capacity to adapt to new stimuli as a key function of a healthy body ego. Regarding the effects of trauma within the nervous system, we quote Peter Levine: "A healthy nervous system, when confronted with a stimulus, goes into a state of disequilibrium and will then reorder at a higher level of integration. A nervous system that has been highly disorganized by trauma has lost its ability to adapt to a normal level of stimulus, and is not capable of reorganizing." To moderate stimulation and not overload the nervous system, the therapist cautiously introduces small levels of activation and helps the client develop a new level of homeostatic control. These techniques are called "titration" and "renegotiation." Other techniques involve the client visualizing actual supportive people and a secure environment that existed for him around the time of the traumatic event. One method of titration is having the client run physically on a mat while imagining moving in space and time from the traumatic situation to the supportive people in the secure environment. He or she only "stays" in the experience of the traumatic situation until autonomic nervous system signs indicate the onset of dissociation or tonic immobility.

While it has long been acknowledged that physical and sexual abuse constitute shock traumas, it is less well known that "purely physical" events, such

DEVELOPMENTAL TRAUMA

- Typically formed through repeated social interactions with caregivers.

- Mild or moderate nervous system activation.

- Generates moderate psychological defensive responses (character structure patterns) mediated through voluntary nervous system.

- Ego mediated.

- Character structure resilient to moderate amounts of stress.

- Therapy may include more stress.

SHOCK TRAUMA

- Typically formed through brief, intense experiences outside the range of normal social interactions.

- High nervous system activation.

- Generates extreme psychological defensive reactions of either fight/flight reflexes and/or dissociation/tonic immobility.

- Mediated through involuntary nervous system.

- Lacks ego organization.

- Shock structure may fragment under even small amounts of stress.

- Therapy requires careful modulation of level of stimulation. No cathartic techniques until underlying structure is understood.

as bicycle falls, tonsillectomies, high fevers, hospitalizations, moving to a new area, etc., also can deeply compromise development. Shock issues related to these types of injurious events are not spontaneously talked about in therapy, partly because they are not remembered or recognized as important. When characterological therapy becomes blocked or resists completion, unresolved shock may be the cause. Long-term symptoms of unresolved shock can appear in the form of phobias, depression, emotional constriction, "borderline" or "psychotic" behavior, etc. Clients with shock issues may decompensate in the course of therapy, seemingly for no apparent reason. An understanding of the dynamic effects of shock trauma is extremely useful in untangling a wide range of complex client profiles.

Summary

The healthy body ego has the ability to utilize sensation as a form of reality testing and as a medium for integrating stimulation from the environment. Marcher emphasizes the sensation level because it forms a bridge between cognitive and expressive forms of psychotherapy, as sensory integration is a key component in the formation of a direct experience (a felt sense) of the self. The Bodynamic approach is to build the body ego by developing body awareness, which then serves as the foundation for work with developmental movement, activation of resource states, emotional expression, and activation of full regressive states.

Waking the body ego requires a highly specific knowledge of motor development as it interfaces with psychological development. The body ego becomes distorted by patterns of muscular tension and resignation, representing unresolved developmental movements. By engaging these movement patterns in the context of therapy, the psychological issues connected to them emerge and may be resolved.

Marcher and her colleagues have developed a comprehensive diagnostic tool, the Bodymap, that enables the Bodynamic therapist to test therapeutic strategies for their effectiveness. The Bodymap is an excellent research tool in somatic theory, as well as in comparing somatic psychologies to more traditional psychological approaches.

References

Ayers, A Jean. *Sensory Integration and the Child* (Los Angeles: Western Psychological Services, 1979).

Bentzen, Marianne, & Peter Bernhardt. *Working with Psychomotor Development* (Albany, CA: Bodynamic Institute, 1992).

Bernhardt, P., & L. Marcher. (1992). "Individuation, Mutual Connection and the Body's Resources: An Interview with Lisbeth Marcher." *Pre and Peri-natal Psychology Journal* 6(4). See also page XX of this book.

Bernhardt, P. (1992). "Somatic Approaches to Shock: A Review of the Work of the Bodynamic Institute and Peter Levine." Monograph from the Bodynamic Institute. See also page XXX of this book.

Boadella, David. (1990). "Somatic Psychotherapy: Its Roots and Traditions, A Personal Perspective." *Energy & Character.*

Britte, Holle. *Motor Development in Children: Normal and Retarded* (Oxford: Blackwell Scientific Publication, 1976).

Johnsen, Lillimor. *Integrated Respiration Therapy* (No publisher listed, 1981).

Jørgensen, Steen. (1991). "Bodynamic Analytic Work With Post-Traumatic Stress." *Energy & Character.*

Krueger, David W. *Body Self and Psychological Self: A Developmental and Clinical Integration of Disorders of the Self* (New York: Brunner/Mazel, 1989).

Levine, Peter. "Transforming Trauma, Giving the Body Its Due." In Maxine Sheets-Johnstone, (Ed.) *Giving the Body Its Due (Suny Series)* (New York: State University of New York Press, 1992).

Mahler, M.S., F. Pine, & A. Bergman. *The Psychological Birth of the Human Infant* (London: Huthchinson, 1975).

Marcher, L., & L. Ollars. (1990). "The Bodynamic Analytic Imprint Method of Rebirth." *Energy & Character.*

Morris, G., & A. Teicher. (1990). "To Touch or Not to Touch." *Psychotherapy* 25:492–500.

Ollars, Lenart. "Reliability of Bodymap test" (Danish version). Bodynamic Institute, Denmark.

Piaget, J. *The Origins of Intelligence in the Child* (New York: International Universities Press, 1952).

Sarnoff, Charles. *Latency* (New York: Jason Aronson, 1976).

Winnicott, D.W. *Playing and Reality* (London: Tavestock Publications, 1971).

Waking the Body Ego, Part 2: Psychomotor Development and Character Structure

—*Peter Bernhardt, M.F.T., Marianne Bentzen, M.A., & Joel Isaacs, Ph.D.*

Abstract

In Part I of this article, the basic concepts of Lisbeth Marcher's Bodynamic Analysis were presented, along with some of the principles and methods of therapeutic treatment developed by Marcher and her colleagues at the Bodynamic Institute in Denmark.

In Part II, we focus on the seven distinguishable stages of human development that Marcher considers essential to the understanding of character structure formation. We will describe developmental motor activity along with our understanding of the child's psychological experience of these activities. We will outline the ten lines of body ego development, and give brief case situations and examples from child development.

Overview

Bodynamic Analysis has developed a theory of character structure that distinguishes seven basic stages in child development. The stages span the age range from in utero through twelve years of age. In this article we also discuss adolescence. The stages are named for the central issue or theme dealt with during the respective age period. There is some overlap between stages, and of course there are individual differences between children. (See page 162 for Table of Character Structures). The stages are:

Table of Character Structures

2nd trimester	Existence	3 months
1 month	Need	1½ years
8 months	Autonomy	2½ years
2 years	Will	4 years
3 years	Love/Sexuality	6 years
5 years	Opinions	8 years
7 years	Solidarity/Performance	12 years

While the formulation of these stages is unique in important ways, they are also based on or incorporate some of the work of a number of other theorists. (Principally, they include Wilhelm Reich, Alexander Lowen, Frank Lake, Britta Holle, Lillemor Johnson, Margaret Mahler, Jean Piaget, and David Boadella.) Reich pioneered the understanding of character structure in terms of body structure. He formulated several character types based on the concept of character armor or rigidity. Lowen expanded on Reich's work, particularly with the earlier developmental types of Oral and Schizoid. Lake took character structure still earlier, into birth and intrauterine life. He hypothesized a basic duality to character structure formation in his notion of the schizo-hysteric split that can occur in utero or during birth if stress becomes too great. In this event, there are two options or strategies for the self to survive: one is the schizoid withdrawal away from the body, stress, and contact; the other is the hysteric's flight into contact, intensity, and emotionality. In a very different context, Lillemor Johnsen was becoming aware of a dual response of muscles to stress: they could become hypotonic or hypertonic. Working in Norway, often with severely disturbed patients, she observed that many of these people were characterized mainly by a hypotonicity of the muscles, rather than the hypertonicity associated with Reich's concept of muscular armor.

The Bodynamic Analytic model of character brought great clarity to the study of character by applying the concept of a dual response to stress to all developmental stages. Drawing from Reich, Piaget, Holle, Lake, and the observation and theory of motor development in children, each character structure was seen to actually have three basic positions: *healthy, early,* or *late.* Our theory is that, for a given individual, whether the relevant muscles respond to the stress with neutral, hypo-, or hyper-responsiveness depends on two factors: the intensity of the stress, and the timing of the stress within the emerging developmental process. If the stress is within the limits that the particular individual can tolerate, the elasticity of the muscles will remain neutral. This neutral responsiveness corresponds to a vitality and flexibility toward the psychomotor task involved. If a developmental stage has a preponderance of neutral responsive muscles, we say that the individual is in the *healthy* position for that stage. As an example, the healthy position for the Existence character level is characterized by a security in existing. In our therapeutic work with this person, we will remember that she has the resources appropriate to this stage, and that these can be counted on to help resolve the more troubled stages.

If the stress in a given developmental stage is early and/or relatively massive, resources are likely to be overwhelmed, and the related muscles will be *hypo-*responsive. This corresponds to psychological resignation in relation to that specific psychomotor task. When a given developmental stage has a preponderance of hypo-responsive muscles, we say that the individual is in the *early* position for that character structure. The early position for the Need character structure, for example, is characterized by a despairing attitude toward need fulfillment. In general, the early position is characterized by a relative lack of the appropriate resources, and by a lower energy for the related tasks than either the healthy or late positions. In therapy on this character level, this person will have to learn how to do things, and will have to practice these in their life.

If the stress in a given developmental stage is later and/or lighter, resources are challenged but not necessarily overwhelmed, and the related muscles will be *hyper-*responsive. This corresponds to psychological rigidity, resistance, control, holding back, or fighting, in relation to that psychomotor task. When an individual has a preponderance of hyper-responsive muscles in a particular stage, we say that the individual is in the *late* position for that character level. The late position for the Love/Sexuality stage, for example, is characterized by seductiveness. Therapy on a character level where the person is in the late position often involves confronting their behavior in specific ways.

As an example of an early psychomotor task, let us examine the impulse to creep and crawl that develops between seven and ten months of age. If a child is supported in this activity and only experiences stress within her limits, she will have a vitality and excitement about crawling. Additionally, she will have resources in the related psychological areas of self-motivation, curiosity, and directedness. If the child is traumatized relatively early in this motor sequence, her muscles will have had little time to establish a strong pattern of creeping or crawling. The pattern is more easily interrupted, leading to hypo-responsive muscles. If the thwarting comes later in the sequence, when the child has already established a capacity for crawling, her pattern will be more difficult to disrupt, making it more likely that she would sustain the impulse to crawl. Now, however, from having had to fight to maintain the impulse, or from holding back the already established impulse, the muscles involved in crawling will be relatively hyper-responsive.

Stern (1985) makes a central point regarding the value of attributing later pathology to specific stages or critical periods of development. He believes that it is more useful and more congruent with his research to recognize that the themes with which individuals struggle are active across the spectrum of development, and are not located in one specific age level. Our somatic developmental psychology at once agrees and disagrees with this viewpoint. On the one hand, our theory is based on the detailed observation that certain muscles are activated (come under *voluntary* control) at specific ages or critical periods. We do believe that the first imprint typically occurs within a specific period, and in therapy we put weight on understanding these crucial periods. On the other hand, we recognize that certain themes are present throughout development, and that it is the history of the theme in totality that must be taken into account. For example, many character issues initially evolve in utero or during birth. These early experiences will affect how similar issues are dealt with later on. Also, we know from the study of Bodymaps (a Bodynamic diagnostic tool) that events later in life can impact the responsiveness of muscle associated with psychomotor movements from specific early periods. Adolescence, for example, is generally a time when character structure issues resurface. At this time, they will either be pushed deeper into dysfunction (move away from neutral responsiveness and resourceful activity) in response to negative experience, or be moved more toward health (a lighter, more neutral resourceful activity) in response to a positive experience. Shocks and traumatic experiences later in adult life will also change muscle response, as will positive experiences.

Thus, while we believe that there are critical periods for core issues, we also observe a recognizable thematic thread active and mutable throughout life. To widen the scope of the developmental issue even further, we (as both parents and researchers), have observed that a developmental stage is rarely initiated without a precursor period. In this period, the child enters into typical activities and interactions of the next stage, for a few days or weeks, some months before that developmental stage opens. Further, developmental stages begin at different times from one child to the next, and adjacent stages overlap somewhat. We find that the Bodymap can be a useful tool for assessing a child's actual maturity, since the activity in the muscles will give an accurate picture of the developmental resources available to the child.

Mutual Connection

The overarching concept, or organizing principle, of Bodynamic Analysis is that humans, in their development, inherently move toward greater and greater connectedness with others and the world. Marcher calls this drive *mutual connection,* and sees it as our most basic motivation. This concept is expressed from a different point of view by Maturana and Varela in their scientific treatise, *The Tree of Knowledge:* "This is the biological foundation of social phenomena: without love, without acceptance of others living beside us, there is no social process and, therefore, no humanness."

In a healthy development, mutual connection grows in breadth as the child acquires an increasing variety and depth of resources and tools for the realization of this connection. During each developmental stage, the focus of connection in the parent-child relationship occurs around a particular theme. In the first stage, the *focus* is on developing a secure sense of existence; in the second, on a sense that our needs can be met; in the third, on exploring the world, and being autonomous; in the fourth, on having our own power, our own intentionality or will, and still being loved; in the fifth, on being able to have deep romantic and sexual/sensual feelings; in the sixth, on forming deep beliefs and opinions about the world and reality, and expressing them; in the seventh, on being a member of a group without needing to be special, but also with our uniqueness valued.

If we take the Opinion structure as an example, it is a time when the child is helped to form beliefs and to express them verbally. In a healthy development, the child learns that she can have her opinion and others can have theirs, and there can still be a connection; that differing opinions do not imply separation. She can stand up for her opinions and still be separate enough from them to take in new information and change. Health in this stage might be expressed as: "I may not be right, but I know what I think."

Implicitly, the character structures come about through *breaks* in mutual connection. Every time there is a break in mutual connection, there is a break in development. A break in mutual connection occurs whenever a child is placed in a dilemma of having to give up an impulse or resource in order to maintain contact, or having to give up contact in order to keep the impulse. The early and late character position for each stage are the ways the child attempts to maintain a connection to self and other. A child in the early position of a character structure will tend to withdraw from connection to maintain a sense of self. An adult in the early Need structure, for example, waits for you to come to them if their needs are to be filled. It may look as if they are indifferent about the contact, but they are really waiting for you to come to them. The later positions in each structure fight for contact, but will often give up maintaining a sense of self. While they fight for contact, they don't trust the contact and thus don't let it in. For example, the late Need structure will distrust or denigrate the things that are offered to them. Additionally, the fighting often breaks the contact, since from the outside it may be perceived as pushing away. So we can see that both early and late positions have compromised their abilities to simultaneously be in contact and have a clear sense of themselves.

The Seven Developmental Stages

The Existence Structure: Second Trimester to Three Months Old

Theme: Building a secure sense of being.

Early position: Called the mental existence structure, characterized by a withdrawal from life.

Late position: Called the emotional existence structure, characterized by a flight toward life.

Healthy position: Characterized by a secure sense of being, of belonging in the world. This person feels loved and accepted for simply being alive.

> **Starts** with the beginning of the second trimester when the prenate has established all basic reflexes: breathing, heartbeat, sucking, swallowing, and others. This corresponds to a beginning sense of core, which might be expressed as, "I have a core and I'm different from that which surrounds me."
>
> **Ends** with the inhibition of the gripping and rooting reflexes, and the ability to support one's own head, allowing the activities of nursing, grasping, and orientation to come under voluntary control.
>
> **Focus** of the existence process: The child is experiencing her basic sense of being and how she is received, particularly by the mother and family, and also by the world. At the physical level (including gender), at the level of personhood or self, and at the level of spirit or soul, this sense of being welcomed or not welcomed for existing is deeply imprinted. This imprint forms the basic self-concept from which the personality develops.

Psychodynamically speaking, the basic task in this period is to achieve a secure sense of existence. Physically, emotionally, and psychologically, the child experiences and evaluates the security of her existence, how well she is loved and is welcomed, and whether the field of human energy and attention around her is stable and reliable. At the purely physical level, if severe stress is present during the first months of pregnancy, the child's life may be threatened or she may be physically deformed. However, whether the traumatic state is early or late, or an ongoing stress throughout pregnancy, it is experienced by the child as life threatening, resulting in insecurity about existence and a mistrust of reality as stable.

Intrauterine Development

The *first trimester* is characterized by pulsatory movements at the cellular level, as the blastula moves down the fallopian tube toward implantation, and an incredible formation process unfolds at a furious rate during cellular division. All basic organs are formed during these brief months. The first movements in the organism are global—opening movements toward pleasant stimuli, and twisting movements away from unpleasant, noxious stimuli. These movements are reflexive in nature.

In the *second and third trimesters,* the fetus develops and grows at a rapid rate, and the spaciousness of the womb gradually diminishes. The prenate child can now move her head and arms independently, and the startle reflex (a movement with head and arms extending in response to sudden unpleasant stimuli) begins. After birth, this reflex is commonly activated by unexpected noises and loss of support to the head. Strong insecurity of a physical or emotional nature will result in a constant state of alert or a giving up of the startle reflex, and may later be observed in the child or adult as *cephalic blocking*, a dysfunctional response of the suboccipital muscle group activated by the startle reflex. Both the hyper and the hypo response in the suboccipital muscle group attachments indicate a problem in establishing a secure sense of existence. This dysfunction in responsiveness is palpable in the tendon attachments of the muscles involved rather than in the muscles themselves. This seems to be the case whenever the developmental activity affected is reflexive rather than voluntary.

During the *third trimester,* the child is more responsive to events occurring around the mother. The mother herself is more physically changed and impacted by the pregnancy now, and more aware that there is a separate being inside of her. This may change her attitude toward the fetus. The mother may also be more sensitive to how people view her. Since from implantation, mother and prenate are chemically and hormonally connected, the mother's emotional state and reactions to her own life and her pregnancy, as well as her responses to other people's feelings about her pregnancy, are imparted to the prenate through her energy field, through the umbilical cord, as well as through the subtle alterations of her body rhythms and movement patterns.

Overall in uterine development, it is the excitatory nervous system that is active, while the inhibitory has not yet become active. Here the connective tissues (fascia, tendons, ligaments) are the main physical structures that can function in an inhibitory role (apart from the spatial restriction of the womb itself). While in later developmental stages the voluntary muscle is mainly responsible for the inhibition of impulses, during intrauterine development, neither the nervous system nor muscle tissue have developed sufficiently for this inhibitory function to occur. Thus, in working with issues from this time, we look primarily to the fascia rather than muscle for hyper and hypo patterns to indicate character patterns.

Theories of Early Character Formation

Lake (1966) was the first to propose a polarity in early character formation. Previously, the primary understanding of character formation from earliest life has been described by Reich and Lowen as the schizoid character type. The schizoid character is defined by massive withdrawal of energy from the body into the mind and away from contact with others and the world. Lake began to analyze the idea of "flight *into* the body" at the age of early infancy (which he calls the hysterical character structure, as distinct from the Bioenergetic description of a later, more rigid structure of the same name), where the child desperately flings herself toward intense contact and high emotional charge in an attempt to ensure her own continuing existence, and that of the world. Reich and Lowen categorize this as an oedipal "hysterical" structure found in women, having developed from the female child being rejected by the mother. In this theory, she then turns to the father as the primary source of contact and gratification, offering herself sexually to ensure the stability of this source. Bioenergetics theory does not describe this character formation in men. Boadella compares these two views in depth in his article *Stress and Character* (1974).

Lake's concept was that under severe stress, what he called "transmarginal stress," the fetus could split its unity into either the schizoid or the hysteric position, in order to maintain a sense of its own integrity. This concept was instrumental in Marcher's development of a system having three positions: *early, late, and healthy*. For this stage of development, the early position corresponds to the schizoid, the late to the hysteric, and the healthy to the unsplit structure.

The Mental Existence Position (Lake's Schizoid)

The mental existence position (early existence) is thought to develop in the second trimester in utero. At this time, the fetus has few mechanisms with which to protect itself, primarily contracting or relaxing the fascia. If the stress experienced by the fetus becomes transmarginal, the protective response is to pull the energy out of the muscles and periphery and into the head and the spine. This splitting of the energy reduces the felt anxiety, pain, and despair at the cost of giving up a great part of connection to the mother (and the world). As reported by adults, the experience of the environment in the womb is one of not being wanted or loved, and that the world is not a welcoming, hospitable place. The person has a resigned approach to living, not wanting to participate fully in the world as it is. This view, that *resignation* is the central dynamic in the mental existence position, is congruent with Lake, but opposed to Lowen's and Lewis's view that tension is the predominant somatic response to severe and long-term existential threat at this age level. There is, however, general agreement that the mental existence position, or schizoid personality, experiences "I" as a feeling predominantly in the head and in a thin line of inner life along the spine. The schizoid personality feels unsafe with high emotional charge, interpersonal contact, and liveliness. This is understood as a "flight *from* the body" in terror of the overwhelming threat of annihilation from the parents or the world, and a withdrawal into the relative safety and stillness of the world of the mind.

The Emotional Existence Position (Lake's Hysteric)

If the fetus has had a good enough experience for the first two trimesters, the environment of the womb will have been sensed as good (or good enough). As the fetus continues to grow in the third trimester, it has a growing impact on the life and experience of the mother, and this can be disruptive for the mother. However, if the emotional climate changes, or a traumatic event occurs and transmarginal stress is experienced, the imprint of the world being good will tend to remain. Should the fetus undergo a splitting of energy to protect itself, the fetus will most likely not withdraw from contact and the world, but will pull its energy out of the head and into the body, the muscles, and the periphery.

In the emotional structure, there is the sense of having lost paradise, and of desperately wanting to regain it. There is an emphasis on emotion and action, and a clinging to relationships and involvement in the world. The "I" feeling is predominantly in the body, in emotional flow and the desire for contact. In this case, the flow of energy into the head is experienced as strange and unsafe, and later, clear thinking in relation to stressful relationships is impaired.

Birth

The outstanding single event during the existence stage of development is the birth process. Birth is the transition from umbilical connection to visual, oral, and tactile bonding; from physical, energetic, and chemical unity to physical separateness, and hopefully, energetic unity. The birth itself is also an outstanding example of a psychomotor process. Birth is triggered by a chemical from the prenate, and during the process the fetus actively pushes its way through the birth canal. Birth complications often show up later in life as a general difficulty with initiating or completing projects, or with having sense of direction in life. The inner rhythm of readiness to initiate a great task and proceeding to do so, and then triumphantly completing it, was not securely established. Conversely, a child who has successfully come through *part* of the birthing process will retain this as a resource, even if later stages of the birth prove traumatic.

Bonding after Birth

An early bonding reflex is the gripping reflex in the hands. In Bodynamic Analysis, birth and early bonding reflexes are often evoked in the reworking of early trauma. As shown in the following case, seemingly small interventions of this kind may have an extraordinary impact on the client's basic experience of reality. In an introductory workshop, the participants in a paired exercise were guided to imitate the gripping reflex of an infant. The instruction was for the first person to use the little finger of the hand to grasp the outstretched finger of his helper. When the therapist came to one particular group, the man doing the gripping reflex said he didn't get much from the exercise. The therapist asked him to repeat the movement, and observed that he was not using the little finger, which is the finger that initiates the infant's reflexive movement. When this was corrected and the participant's hand supported through touch, he faded into a light trance and his hand started moving involuntarily. Later he described having had an unusual and wonderful experience—he felt the movement to have been initiated by therapist, who moved his arm and hand in a way that felt absolutely natural and right, and made him feel very peaceful. His thinking processes afterwards were quieter and less chaotic than he could ever remember. In fact, the therapist had not initiated any movement, but only followed the small movements initiated by the participant.

This is an example of an adult having the experience appropriate to a very young infant who is met with correct mirroring—the infant experiences the other person as doing things that make it feel good or bad. The infant's own activities are often without ego-identification or any sense of causality (except when in distress, where protective reflexes are activated, and an 'I' awareness is forced to develop prematurely). This case also emphasizes the power of activating the specific muscles involved in a given movement. Activating the precise motor pattern renders early experiences easily available, without requiring deep emotional regression. This is a common clinical experience in Bodynamic Analysis.

Finally, the above example shows the lack of a sense of personal boundary typical of regression to intrauterine and neonate times. Reports from adult and child clients indicate that the pre- and neonate child has the sense of being surrounded by energy, rather than by a physical container. Energetically, the child still experiences herself as unified with the mother.

Need Structure: Birth to Eighteen Months Old

Theme: Sensing needs and acquiring basic satisfaction.

Early position: Despairing. Child cannot recognize needs or own the ability to fulfill them.

Late position: Mistrusting. Child confuses needs; is sure that others won't give what they need, or they will give the wrong thing.

Healthy position: Self-satisfying. Child is able to identify her own needs, act to have them met, and delay gratification when necessary.

> **Starts** with the first voluntary suckling movements and intentional gripping. Since the need age is largely characterized by the establishment of voluntary control over reflexive action, the onset of the Need age is defined by the inhibition of these primary reflexes. This denotes early boundary formation.
>
> **Ends** when the neural connections to the fingers and hands have developed enough to make them more sensitive to shape than the mouth. Until that happens, the mouth will remain the primary organ of exploration.
>
> **Focus** of the need processes: Through interaction with the primary caretakers, the child is learning to recognize and differentiate its own needs, to act to get them met, to take in and absorb, to feel satiated, and to handle delay of need fulfillment. This process is interactional, and the child depends on deep connection and precise mirroring to put meaning to its inner sensations.

A basic principle of somatic developmental psychology is that the attainment of voluntary activity is central to ego formation. One of the key dynamics of the Need stage is the movement from reflex systems to voluntary systems. This is most evident in the seeking of nourishment. Sucking begins as a reflex in utero during the Existence stage. Soon after birth, the infant learns to suck voluntarily. Researchers have identified the beginning of pauses in the sucking patterns of month-old infants as indications of voluntary activity. By five to six months, the sucking reflex disappears and sucking should be voluntary. This is a major milestone in the process of need gratification. By gradually attaining control over her sucking behavior, the child becomes an active participant in her need gratification.

The basic skills of need gratification, in the order of development, are: the ability to express need and to take in nourishment and assimilate it; the ability to differentiate needs and recognize satiation; and the ability to satisfy one's needs by one's own actions. The establishment of these skills makes possible the postponement of needs.

During the later phase of the Need stage, the child learns to delay gratification. While delayed gratification is often spoken about as something convenient for adults, seen from the point of view of the child's natural movement toward increased self-control, delaying gratification gives the child an increased sense of self in its interaction with mother. The child also has an investment in delayed gratification because other things are becoming more interesting! Who can be bothered to eat in such an exciting world? The breast becomes more of a fast food restaurant for the infant on the go. Creeping, crawling, looking, and reaching are all rapid in coming.

In the later part of the Need stage, there is a tension between being able to establish a secure, nurturing base with mother, and moving out into the world. This is the overlap between the Need stage and the next stage of establishment of autonomy. A child at ten months may be so involved in crawling that she won't stop even when exhausted and whiny—she is struggling to balance the impulse to learn with the need for rest and food. The actions of the surrounding adults strongly affect her ability to establish this balance. An overprotected or depressed child at this age may get stuck in unsatisfactory attempts at need satisfaction if the drive to move out into the world is restrained, and a child forced into premature self-reliance may give up attending to basic needs for rest and nourishment.

When the child is hungry, changes in her movement patterns or crying should bring a caring adult with food. The subsequent excited feeding activity slowly gives way to fullness. The experience of her needs and her perception of the primary adult's willingness to discover and fulfill those needs are crucial elements of bonding at this age. Through that willingness, the child becomes able to differentiate her needs and to feel satiated. This is experienced by the child through visceral proprioceptive sensations and autonomic states. As this pattern is internalized over time, the child learns to accept her needs, and also forms deep bonds. The autonomy that comes with her growing motor abilities allows her to satisfy more of her own needs, and this lessens the dependency on her mother.

In this state of great dependence, the quality of the parents' mirroring determines the clarity with which the child understands herself and the world. The following interaction between mother and three-month-old child is an example of this: Observing the infant crying, the mother checks all the basics—hunger, diaper state, last sleep, bowel movement, temperature, and out-of-reach objects of interest. She walks the child, holds her, bounces her, sees if she wants to play with something—all to no avail. Finally, she lifts the screaming child at arms length in front of her and says: "I can't understand what you're trying to say to me." The child stops in mid-scream and gazes directly at her mother, apparently satisfied with this direct contact. We can't know what the original need was, but we do know that whether or not it was met, the contact made was satisfactory, and the child felt recognized and secure.

In the Existence example talked about earlier, the workshop participant was working with his gripping reflex and the result was a peaceful, trance-like state. Clinical material from children and adults tends to show that the visual impressions of the first months of life—the early Need stage—have a quality similar to that described by clairvoyants. Children and adults in touch with early perceptions describe seeing clouds of color that they associate to personality qualities and emotions of the person they see. Work in the Need stage with voluntary movement often brings clearer, more directed movements and consciousness. In the following example, voluntary gripping has begun to prevail over reflexive gripping. A client was trying to resolve a feeling of overwhelm and loneliness related to a difficult situation at work. The therapist asked him to make a conscious gripping movement (from Need age: three to five months), starting with the little finger using a specific muscle (*flexor dig-iti minimi*), and adding ring and third finger. At first, he failed to use the specific muscles involved and gripped only loosely, leading to a nebulous, unclear feeling. When he began using the correct muscles, he got a clear sense of what he wanted and needed in the work situation. This sudden clarity gave him an immediate sense of empowerment, a feeling of being able to guide his actions according to his needs, instead of only according to outer requirements. This is a basic ego skill: the ability to recognize one's own needs and act toward their fulfillment.

In comparison to the Existence example, the client here stayed quite aware, and experienced no reflexive activity in his hand or arm. Indeed, the sense of empowerment came directly from the experience of precise, voluntary gripping, from the experience of precise requirements and the possibility of meeting them. This brief re-patterning exemplifies a healthy experience of the infant's development during the first six months. It was activated as a resource relating to a present day issue. It is clear that this resource was preconscious, and also close to consciousness; the client could not initially access the clarity brought forth by the gripping movement, but was able to access this resource almost at once when he "got" the right movement. This demonstrates what we believe to be an essential part of therapy—the ability of the therapist to stimulate access to resource states close to consciousness, rather than bringing up material that is deeply unconscious and more difficult to integrate. For the infant, this corresponds to the difference between good and bad mirroring from a parent or caretaker. Good mirroring, necessary for the establishment of a good sense of self, recognizes when a baby needs nurturing, and when to let her explore and practice her growing capabilities. It is in the latter that she finds excitement and a sense of personal accomplishment.

The Need stage child continues to refine and develop her ability for voluntary movement. The capacity to orient and move toward things brings an enormous feeling of empowerment: "I can see something I want to handle, but I can't reach it from here. How do I get there?" This initiates the activities of rolling, creeping, and crawling. The previously mastered skills of voluntary gripping, rooting, and sucking has given her a sense of solidity or clarity in her own needs. These felt needs determine direction and intent. The new skills of locomotion are the foundation of her ability to maintain a sense of direction. This foundation builds on the cornerstone of the birth experience, of what happened the first time she used her power to go in the direction she wanted. Her approach to crawling will be colored by this previous experience. If birth was a thwarting experience for her, she will hesitate to mobilize the sheer strength and determination required to move out toward what she wants and needs. If birth was exhilarating and empowering, she will move with confidence. Locomotion will give her an opportunity to reevaluate the satisfactions of going into the world under her own steam. A good experience here will modify a poor imprint from birth, and a bad experience will confirm and strengthen it, and vice versa, for the good birth imprint.

Boundaries

A child first develops a sense of his or her own boundaries from the way they are handled. Boundary development thus depends on the boundaries of the parents or caretaking adults. A crucial element in acquiring self-containment is the child's experience of the parent containing his or her own needs in the service of the child. If the child's parents are able to respond in a caring and containing way to her needs and upsets, and do not attempt to fulfill their own needs through the parenting bond, the child will acquire an inner map in which its own needs and feelings are securely contained by an adult energy.

The decline of the Need stage of development occurs at about one-and-a-half to two years of age, when the fingertips develop a sensitivity that surpasses that of the mouth and lips. The child uses the mouth less and less as a primary tool for getting information about the world, and is increasingly interested in exploring the world through touch.

The Autonomy Structure: Eight Months to Two-and-a-Half Years Old

Theme: Organizing the impulse toward activity.

Early position: Non-verbal activity changing. The child's own impulses and feelings are easily lost or go unrecognized. She changes focus non-verbally and without noticing.

Late autonomy position: Verbal activity changing. The child actively and verbally changes the focus of attention to avoid noticing unpleasant feelings, particularly helplessness.

Healthy autonomy position: Emotionally autonomous. The child notices her impulses and feelings, owns them, and can act upon them.

> **Starts** at eight months with the onset of creeping, which is one of the first skills (along with rolling) the child acquires to move herself out into the world. Previously, objects had been pulled toward her. Another sign is a new level of eye-hand coordination, allowing her to choose which objects to reach for, rather than just reaching. Binocular vision is being established at seven months, allowing a greater expansion in the visual field. Her hand is now able to grasp tiny objects between the thumb and first two fingers, developing a pincer grip that is practiced with specific focus of vision and attention.
>
> **Ends** with the onset of abstract reasoning, such as the ability to sort things by shape ("put all the ones like this one here, and all the ones like that one there"), and the ability to distinguish unseen objects (e.g., touching a previously seen plaything under the table). The child understands language well enough to follow requests made without gestures. She also has the ability to control her anal sphincter without using her hamstring muscles, making it possible to sit on the potty without support. Her walking is characterized by basic foot articulation.
>
> **Focus** of the autonomy processes: The key words here are differentiation and reality sense. The child is developing her ability to differentiate options of activity, recognize and follow her imagination and impulses, and distinguish and express feelings and emotions. She is also establishing independence and autonomy through her ability to move out into the world under her own steam; reality-testing her sense of herself and the world by exploring and practicing; and balancing security (baseline needs) and adventure, through rapprochement activities. She is also

learning to balance her own needs and impulses against the expectations of others.

While the Need stage is characterized by learning to become self-directed in the process of need satisfaction, the stage of Autonomy witnesses an explosion of activity directed to exploring the world. The child follows her impulses and acts for the pleasure of activity. Several threads of development come together to make this possible. Intrapsychically, the development of an internal image of the external world gives the child's impulse a focus. This coincides with an increasing capacity for object constancy. Psychomotorically, she acquires a huge array of new skills that must be integrated and reality tested. Interpersonally, in the process of this reality testing, she needs, but often does not want, appropriate help from her parents. Overprotective parenting leaves the child unable to find or struggle with her emerging skills, or leaves her feeling engulfed. Parenting can also be characterized by an expectation that the child can do too much by herself, such as dressing without help at the age of one-and-a-half, or insistent encouragement to stand or do things too soon. This pushes her to accelerate her own pacing in order to be accepted, and can leave her feeling that she cannot get help when she feels it is needed.

An important contribution of Bodynamic Analysis to character theory is the clarity that it has brought to the Autonomy stage. Again, this comes from the observation and correlation of how movement patterns and activities normal to this age become set in personality patterns that appear later in life. This is the stage in which a basic imprint toward impulses and activity is set. The basic motoric and cognitive style of this age is called *activity changing,* since the child acquires an enormous range of new motor skills, and practices them one after the other. If the child is frustrated early or strongly in this stage, there is a tendency to lose the impulse toward activity. This is the early position. When consciousness of impulse formation is lost, the child will grow up with an inner passivity to starting activities, and with little or no pleasure in them. As an adult, they will often passively resist direction and change.

In the late Autonomy position, where the frustration was milder or later, the child will use the impulse to do things as a defense against feelings of helplessness or engulfment. This child will actively change activity, or change topics in conversation, in order to fend off unwanted feelings. The use of impulse as a defense is often seen in highly overactive people who hold several jobs, are members of many clubs, and have many friends, but who lack centered, contactful relationships.

In the Bioenergetic characterology, Lowen has chosen the name "psychopathic" to describe the character type that emerges at this age. He describes a charming, manipulative character whose goals are primarily selfish, who is unable to be empathetic, and so on. While there is an element of this in the Autonomy character, the whole aspect of the need for protection is lost. While many people may *feel* manipulated by an individual who does not truly know what she wants (early), or by one who changes the subject frequently (late), these habits have been learned as a method of self-protection. In addition, the description of the Lowen's psychopath confounds the passive and active positions, and this is a source of great confusion. Finally, we believe that the "true" psychopath, a person who is unable to feel any empathy or remorse, is not related to this stage. That personality disorder actually has its origins in severe, early intrauterine trauma.

Independent—and Needing Help

During this age period, the child begins to establish bounded contact with mother, rather than the merging flow that characterized previous contact. The mother should respond to this with both adequate attention to the child, and with sufficient joy in the child's new independence and accomplishments. The separation is prefigured in the child's nascent motor ability to let go, starting at eight months, and in her absorption in exploring the world. The child is so deeply involved in this experience that she will continue practicing standing or playing with new objects even when she is extremely tired or hungry. With this activity, she redefines her relationship to her mother, since she is dis-identifying herself with her needs, learning to delay basic need-gratification, and identifying herself more with her passionate activity. Mahler calls this the "love affair with the world."

If the child perceives her parents accepting and supporting these changes, she will feel accepted in her emotions and activities. "My activity and my fascina-tion *is* me" is the inner sense, and parents must understand this to respond with adequate mirroring. Later in this stage, the child gradually separates her sense of self from the things and activities that fascinate her, as well as from her parents' guidance. She should finish this stage with a sense of "being myself, with my own feelings, that no one can take away from me; and my own activ-ities, which I sometimes need help to accomplish."

Reality Testing

With the onset of locomotion, an explosive period of development occurs. Starting at about eight months, when the child begins to creep, she becomes able to move herself *to* objects, since developments in her visual perception have already rendered the surroundings more visible. As the child's intentions and impulses solidify, these forays become more powerful and directed. By ten or eleven months, she is able to imagine something she would like to do, and immediately try to do it. A sense of reality is established by actually handling things and being able to deal with the experiences. The infant needs help so that she isn't overwhelmed by painful experiences. Through handling and experimentation, the child is constantly matching her perceptual impression and her inner images against what she does and can do.

Since the child is just learning what she actually is capable of doing, these images will often be quite out of touch with her capabilities. An example of this is an eleven-month-old boy watching mother vacuum. He was delighted with the thought of imitating her, and tried to take over the machine. His mother let him play with it, but even so, he was devastated. He was barely able to move it, and completely unable to manipulate it as his mother had done. His image was being reality-tested, and it proved unrealistic. Since the boy is still merged with his image formation, he experiences the destruction of his image as a strong disruption in his being. To be able to detach his sense of self from his image formation is one of the natural tasks of this age level.

This problem of a gap between an image of what we can do and what we can actually do is often described as a problem of Narcissism. For Mahler, the "practicing stage," peaking at eighteen months, is the cornerstone of a healthy formation of a narcissistic self-image, coming from the child's intense excitement ("Look what I can do!"). Marcher, who is in fundamental agreement with Mahler in some of her observations, has emphasized the development of "emotional autonomy." Marcher emphasizes that in this stage the child is learning to recognize emotions as separate from the core self, and as separate from the events that trigger the emotions. To the child, this means that other people cannot "take away" his or her feelings or impulses. It also means that these feelings or impulses can change, even dramatically, without threatening the sense of core self. Bodynamic Analysis sees the Autonomy structure as a cornerstone for understanding narcissistic and borderline personalities (Bentzen, M., 1996 manuscript).

One of the main tasks of the Autonomy stage is to balance all of the abilities being rapidly developed. The multiplicity of developments gives the child her first experiences of balancing a large degree of self-dependence, surrender to her own protective reflexes (the falling reflex, for example), and the need for help in her endeavors, as well as the desire for pleasurable contact with people and things. This kind of balance can be seen in adults in the familiar trust exercise of falling and being caught by a partner. The balance between trust, physical balance, and falling is one that troubles many people.

The following is an example of the impact of fear of falling on the basic sense of reality. In working with the falling reflex, an adult woman was terrified of allowing herself to fall backward from a sitting position, even when she knew she could catch herself with her arms behind her. In renegotiating this, by having the therapist sit behind her and catch her a few times, she experienced a marked drop in her baseline fear level. She also felt that the floor had suddenly become real—she could trust it to not vanish without notice. She also sensed being able to be more "real" with people present, and that she did not have to hide inner feelings of helplessness. This corresponds to a primary issue of the Autonomy stage, balancing social self and inner self.

In the above example, changes in the client's perception of the floor come about through working with her balance, her trust in the therapist, and her falling reflex. This illustrates how closely linked grounding and balance are in many stages of life, and especially at this age. As the child learns to sit and stand, she establishes a completely new relationship to the ground, which allows her to use the same form of locomotion as the older people around her. Her delight in being able to do this stems partly from the sheer joy of accomplishment, and partly from her feeling of being more like others. In this shift, new reflexes are activated. Sensory impulses from the soles of her feet help keep her body in an upright position. Her relationship to gravity and to the floor parallels her emerging sense of reality. On the one hand, the floor is the support upon which she can sit down and rest for a while, and on the other hand, the floor is also hurtful if descent from the vertical occurs too suddenly. The act of standing up and walking reflects this dual nature of the child's relation to the floor. She gets support from it and needs to be safe with it, and at the same time, she lifts herself away from it in order to explore her environment. Interestingly, this physical process reflects a similar development in the cognitive realm. At the cognitive level, the child is deeply engaged in relating to actual things and people. She is exploring the factualness of them. On the other hand, she is also forming images of events that are not real and not factual, e.g., "me vacuum-cleaning." Here, too, a sudden descent from the passionate unreal idea may be painful. The realization that "I can't manage the vacuum cleaner" shatters her self-image for the present.

Center of Self

The *see-reach* reflex from the Need stage becomes inhibited during Autonomy and the child is able to pause and consider when examining objects. She begins to discriminate between different activities. At the same time, she begins to form internal images and to develop object constancy. When the child first sees someone performing an activity, she begins to mirror the person, and to form an internal image of the activity. The formation of an internal image is a key to organizing internal impulses, many of which are developing at the same time. The child develops the ability to respond to inner desire, kinesthetic sensations, images that have become short- or long-term goals, and input of any kind from the outside world. The child's passionate fascination is the driving force directing her activity. Organizing the child's activities is the impulse to move toward excitement and away from discomfort.

While centering in the Existence and Need phases of development is connected to the core sensations of being and being satisfied, in the Autonomy age, the child is establishing a center of movement, impulse, and desire. Learning to negotiate the upright position, she begins to acquire an inner sense of her physical center of balance (usually located approximately one inch in front of the upper part of the sacrum). Good connectedness with this inner zone gives the child a sense of stability, both in terms of emotional upheavals and in the face of changing outer situations. This is crucial because the child is still merged with what she perceives and is interested in. If an object that she is intently involved in exploring, say a china vase, is suddenly removed from her grasp, she experiences a tearing or vanishing of a part of herself. She does not yet experience any boundaries between herself and the object. As she learns to sense the sacral center of balance, emotional balance becomes easier to reestablish. In adults, this center is utilized in all forms of martial arts, self-defense practices, and meditative practices, as well as in most sports. This reflects an age-old knowledge of the importance of sensing the center of balance in order to maintain physical and emotional equilibrium under stress.

The Will Structure: Two to Four Years Old

Theme: To make choices and choose directions; to be powerful in feeling and in action.

Early position: Self-sacrificing. The child gives up her own sense of power and choice in order to please or serve others.

Late position: Judgmental. The child feels self-directed when she is exercising power over others. She is critical of others.

Healthy position: Assertive. The child acts comfortably with her own power and feels comfortable with other people's power.

> **Starts** with the beginnings of abstract reasoning, such as the ability to sort objects by shape. In walking, the child has basic foot articulation and she begins to master conscious changes of direction while walking. She becomes able to make grinding movements while chewing food.
>
> **Ends** with a fully developed walk and run. The child is able to run with

an instant of floating in the air, and able to change direction fluidly while moving rapidly. She has the motor skills to dress alone, and can begin to choose which clothes to wear. She is self-regulating in her toilet activities, needing occasional help.

Focus: Before the onset of this age, the child is certainly involved in voluntary action, but she does not make conscious, willed choices. This stage, from two to four years of age, is the primary time for learning choice and control. The child is now focused on her ability to choose and effect short term planning, and on exploring her physical and interpersonal power, her will and persistence, along with value judgments about good and bad.

Overview

Between the ages of two to four years, the child is constantly involved in gross motor activity: running, jumping, kicking, throwing things, and learning to negotiate changes in direction. She first becomes able to negotiate a change of direction without stopping to do it. The child is also exploring the contact she can get with parents and other adults when using her power and will to assert herself.

Bonding

A new level of bonding can occur as the child explores using her full power. She learns whether she can feel loved and respected, and whether she can still love and respect those with whom she clashes. This includes clashes about "wrong behavior," such as the struggles about whether it is okay or not to bite or hit, the typical expressions of anger at this age. The child is learning that it is possible, and even okay, to have wildly divergent feelings about the same person or thing at the same time. Take for example, a boy of three, who, after a furious argument with his mother, retired to his room crying. When his mother followed and asked why, he said, "Because you don't love me anymore." She said, "Of course I love you. I was very angry with you. That was why I yelled. But I still love you even when I'm very angry". During their next fight, the boy paused for an instant in middle of a furious retort and said, "I still love you, even though I'm angry with you right now." This example describes the complexity of experiencing emotions and bonding, while growing into full self-assertion and power.

Balance

The child between ages two and four is becoming able to maintain balance while engaging in complex gross motor activity such as running, jumping, getting onto high objects, and getting off again. She is also able to do two quite complex things at the same time, such as steer a tricycle and pedal it.

These skills parallel the child's ability to maintain emotional balance in situations of sudden change. For example, when the child has demanded her favorite breakfast food and something else is forthcoming, she protests vehemently. This is her attempt to regain emotional balance in her chosen actions, namely eating the *right* breakfast. The job of the parent is not to avoid these outbursts, nor to squelch them, but to continue holding the normal boundary when reasonable and necessary. Most adults will recognize in themselves the child's problem here: "I wanted it *this* way, damn it!" And all parents will recognize the difficulties of dealing with children in this stage! In the physical realm, an act of balance with interpersonal aspects is the child's ability to remain standing even when physically pushed or pulled—something she will experience from both peers and adults. This develops concurrently with her ability to keep her balance both physically and psychologically in verbal battles. It is not uncommon for a child of this age, when emotionally upset, to consciously fall and hurt herself.

Boundaries of the Body Ego

This age sees the final stages of the basic formation of ego boundaries. Boundaries have both the function of separating and protecting the child (and *her* things) from the outside world and other people, and that of containing energy in her organism and personality. The child is avidly experimenting with her powers of expression—of outlet, as well as the power of containment—of holding in. Traditionally, this stage is discussed as an anal phase, and certainly the child practices the mastery of anal and urological motor skills. Until approximately age two, unattended potty-sitting is a very insecure activity. The child cannot yet relax the pelvic floor and also simultaneously guard against falling by maintaining tension in the hip extensors.

At approximately two-and-a-half years, the swallowing reflex dissipates. This has been active from birth, making the child automatically swallow anything that is placed sufficiently far back in her mouth. The onset of abdominal breathing occurs at the same time, bringing the contraction of the diaphragm under her voluntary control. These developmental milestones give the child new options about body boundaries in areas that up to now have been largely reflexive. She can now choose to hold back swallowing, defecating, vomiting, and even breathing.

The emphasis on power and containment shows in the emotional and interactional world as well. The child will stubbornly maintain a feeling state—for example, anger—that would previously have faded or changed. In similar ways, she establishes ownership over toys and control over forbidden as well as allowed activities. The two-year-old may touch all the "no" things in the kitchen in a mad dash round the room, only pausing for the required parental "No!"—reestablishing the forbiddenness of touching by actually touching. This is not exactly naughtiness, but rather an exercise of understanding, personal willpower, self-directedness, and independence, as well as a challenge of the boundaries and containment provided by the mother. That outer boundary, the "No!" is essential for the child's own boundary development. Later in the learning process, the child will tell *herself* "No!"—taking over the role of self-correction while still doing the forbidden thing. Still later, having mastered the rule of, say, not eating food that has been dropped on the floor, she will practice correcting others—children as well as adult transgressors of "proper" behavior. In adults who had difficulties at this stage of development—habitual self-correction, other-correction, or both, is often an ingrained character trait.

Direction

The main tasks to be mastered during these years involve choice and power. Having explored, as it were, the options and possibilities open to her at the previous age level, the child now makes powerful and definite choices about what to do and where to go. Motorically, this manifests as mastering the ability to turn. Early in this stage, the child must stop forward movement before turning, and then start moving again. This rapidly becomes practice in turning while walking and running. As her ability to remain focused on one thing expands, she will spend longer times in that activity. At around two years, this attention span is usually no more than two minutes, though the activity is still chosen with passionate intensity, and already something to fight about. For example, when getting into a car at her own pace and in her own way, it is a great disruption to suddenly be required to stop playing and get into the her seat "NOW." At the beginning of this stage, it is extremely difficult for the child to manage an interruption of this type. The child is passionately involved in doing it "MY WAY!" And indeed these years are widely known for the ongoing struggle between parents and children about whether the child gets to do things her own way. The experiences she has had with choices at this age will shape her adult choices of existential direction, as well as the paths of everyday life.

Love/Sexuality Structure: Three to Six Years Old

Theme: To balance feelings of love with sensual/sexual feelings.

Early position: Romantic. The child denies her own sensual and sexual feelings and identifies with her romantic or heart feelings.

Late position: Seductive. The child denies romantic or heart feelings and identifies with her sensual and sexual feelings and actions.

Healthy position: Balance between love and sexuality. The child can feel either or both of these feelings, and act on them with appropriate care.

> **Starts** with the child's ability to connect her own gender with the shape of her genitals, triggering conscious establishment of gender identity, and also gender-focused games and interactions. The child also imitates gender-specific dress and mannerisms. Related motor skills are the rotation of hips and fine-tuning of hip stabilization in walking and running.
>
> **Ends** with the transfer of primary sexual/sensual intimacy with same

and opposite sex from adults to age peers (often designated "puppy love"). Gender differences in motor skills crystallize (boys better at overhand throws, girls better at skipping).

Focus: Gender role identification, exploring and getting containment and boundaries around feelings of love and sexuality. This is done through role-playing and through body-exploration games. Learning to balance love and sexual/sensual feelings first with (mostly) opposite sex parent, then with other adult, and finally with age peers.

Bonding

At this age, the child begins having sensual feelings and love/heart feelings at same time. A child may sit on a parent or snuggle, and use this physical contact to excite herself sexually/sensually. Another common action is to jump up and hang onto the parent with both arms and legs. The child is not being promiscuous; she is exploring new awarenesses and feeling states. She does this with the people that she most loves in the world—who are also the people she feels sexual excitement about. The child bonds in sensual love to each parent alternately. She is capable of fully perceiving triadic relationships, and she is as an active agent in such situations. This awareness, as well as gender role formation and the awakening of genital feelings in an interpersonal context, gives rise to fantasies about being with one parent when the other parent "has grown old and died." If the parents' boundaries are kept, the child's interest will soon turn to people her own age. These romances with peers should not be seen as "just puppy love" but as a crucial and lasting imprint of how to bond in sensual and intimate relationships. Relationships from this age, if not disrupted by external circumstances, will often last for life.

Gender Role Balance

Beginning around age three, the child's physical and psychological balance becomes strongly influenced by the development of gender role patterns. He or she plays and practices extreme gender roles (cowboy hero, nurse) and swaggers or minces accordingly. At the same time, he/she is learning to walk with lumbar rotation. The child begins to push off with the foot when walking, and is capable of performing spring jumps, skipping, or standing on one leg. These motor developments are all utilized in the gender role games. The games slowly become ritualized, as the child finds one or several roles that suit him or her. The child uses her same-sex parent as a model in this exploratory play, as well as older siblings, other adults, and models from TV and the surrounding world. The full range of gender-related movements and action patterns may be seen in children at play, often to the consternation of parents. Drawing her favorite fantasy figures (princess, Batman) is also popular, since fine motor control is developing. This includes an adult writing grip, making it much easier to create good likenesses.

Previously mostly aware of dyadic relationships, the child now grasps the triadic nature of having two parents, or being one of two or more children. This opens the possibility of hierarchies, and with them the question: *"Who do you love most, me or ___?"* as the child explores the different dyadic relationships it has in the family and attempts to place herself in the hierarchy. The ideal placement is to be clearly lower than mom and dad and unable to set them against each other; having a unique relationship with each, but with a secure feeling of being loved by both, and reasonably equal with siblings. In this process, the child will find her physical and interpersonal balance, and her balance between loving and sexual/sensual feelings and expression. If the family is one in which loving feelings are allowed but sexual ones are not, or vice-versa, the child may suppress one pole accordingly. This is very problematic as an adult, since the suppressed side is usually expressed unconsciously.

As mentioned above, the child is learning to stand on one leg during this stage, and severe emotional disruption may manifest as a literal loss of balance. Witness the case of six-year-old boy who started falling significantly more often, sometimes even allowing himself to drop and be hurt, after his parents divorced and began a vengeful incestuous relationship with him. By falling, he was demonstrating both his loss of balance in his interpersonal world and his giving up even trying to "keep his footing" under the circumstances.

Intimate Boundaries

In this stage, the practice of boundary formation and containment is in service of both the emerging gender role and the balance of sexual and loving feelings for others. In her early delight with pleasurable genital feelings and sex-role discovery, the child wants to share this wonder with her parents, as well as with others. She needs to be met with her parents' love, appreciation, and clear boundaries. The appropriate response from each parent is to assure the child that she will, in fact, never be able to take over the other parent's place, and that her sexuality and gender are appreciated, but not open to exploration with the parent. This will initially make her feel angry and hurt. She will also soon feel cared about, and can then safely direct these feelings toward adult friends of the family. When she meets the same response there, she will finally turn to her own age group. There she will typically find an intimate same-sex friend and opposite-sex "love."

An example comes to mind of the four-year-old girl who loudly announced that she was going to stand on her head on her father's shoulders "with *no pants on at all*, all the way down the street!" Through the parents' recognition and acceptance of the excitement she felt about this fantasy, and through their refusal to let her do it, she learns that sexual excitement and imagery are fine, but they are not necessarily to be acted upon. This is a step in learning to contain such feelings and to choose who to share them with. Likewise, through responses to her loving actions and desire for sensual and genital contact, the child learns which of her feelings are acceptable, and also which she should or should not identify with. It is worth noting that the child may be identified with the unacceptable to the exclusion of the acceptable, as well as the other way around. This was the case for the three-year-old whose mother refused to hold her hand when walking in the street "because people might think we are lesbians." Although the term "lesbian" was incomprehensible to her, the underlying message was clear and impactful—wanting to be intimate with mother is bad and sexual. The choice of being intimate and not sexual (right now) was not available. As a grown woman, she was completely identified with being sexual, laboriously re-labeling it good instead of bad. Only then did she realize that vulnerable, non-sexual intimacy was not even in her repertoire of possibilities. This demonstrates how an unhealthy personal gender role may be formed. Some feelings and actions are labelled "me" along with "good" or "bad," while others, equally valid, are labelled "not-me."

Gender Play and Vocational Fantasies

A child's sense of inner direction often relates to his or her early gender role formation. Through games and play, the child practices what kind of woman she is going to be. She role plays certain attributes and imagines different possibilities: having six kids like Mrs. Johnson, wearing a fur coat like Mrs. Peterson, or living by herself like Ms. Brown. Since the child is trying all these different options on for size, she usually changes her declared future identity often, even several times a day. She does not connect her desire today to be a veterinarian with the fantasy yesterday of becoming a lawyer, and may be quite non-plussed by an adult saying, "But I thought you said you wanted to be . . . ." Later in this stage, she is capable of remembering and comparing her own different impulses. This often ends with one choice becoming stable, showing that she has formed a stable inner vision. Adults tend to regard this fantasy activity as amusing and of little real importance. However, like the choice of the first boy- or girlfriend, it may be passionate and deeply felt, and strongly formative in the developing personality of the child. To our knowledge, no research has ever been done on how many people actually choose a job related to this early choice.

Opinion Structure: Five to Nine Years Old

Theme: To form opinions and express them verbally.

Early Position: Sullen. The child can't form or can't articulate opinions, and passively opposes opinions of others.

Late position: Opinionated. The child is identified with being "right," and will fight to maintain the correctness of her own opinion.

Healthy position: Opinion embodying. The child can express opinions and reality-test them. She can argue for her opinions and also can concede or change her mind when new evidence is presented.

Starts with the ability to think simply and rationally. The child asks the meaning of unknown words, and the reasons for things, e.g., "What holds the sun up?" At a psychomotor level, this is related to being able to use the thumb in opposition.

Ends with the ability to negotiate and compare different "truths" and rules in school, at home, with peer groups, in friends' homes, with other families, and with strangers. This corresponds to having grasped complex game rules at play.

Focus: Forming a cognitive, rational map of the world. Bitter fights may ensue about Santa Claus and the Tooth Fairy, and where babies come from. The child is learning different sets of behavior for different social contexts. She forms her own opinions about reality and rules of behavior; and learns to argue for them, to take in new information, and to change her opinions accordingly.

Balancing Love and Disagreement

During this age, the child begins to discover that people she is connected to can have differing opinions and views of the world. At first, she will compare and choose those opinions that tend to give her the boundaries and contact she wants. In certain games, for example, she will keep rearranging the rules so she wins. Later, she starts recognizing and forming opinions that conform to what she holds to be right or true. Both these processes bring her into conflict, first and foremost with her parents, as she tries to deepen the bond with her family, while sometimes violently disagreeing with their opinions or rules.

Peer Groups and Game Rules

As the child becomes aware of the different rules she encounters in different places (preschool, school, visiting grandparents, friends' homes, at work with parents, etc.), she learns to balance herself in relation to these different requirements. Through her posture and movement, she may clash with outer authority, since she will slouch, stand restlessly, walk on the outside of her shoes, and generally make a nuisance of herself in many adults' terms. She stands and moves in these ways to stretch rapidly growing joints and muscles, and often is clumsy since she may be growing as much as one millimeter a day.

The earlier passion of sensual love and emphasis on own gender shifts into passion of interacting with ideas. Emerging from the intimacy of gender-based contact to parents, adults, and peers, she becomes more interested in peer activity. She commonly has one best peer-age friend of each sex, and her play with them is often submerged in larger group play.

Balancing games, gross motor games, and group games are very popular. This is also an age of intense peer group exploration, when group games really come into focus. The group members are not so much choosing each other, however, as they are united in the choice of a game. In the beginning, the children are unable to comprehend that games can be played with slightly different rules, and they will bring their quarrels to the adult caretakers to get judgment passed about "right" rules. Later, as they experience the changing norms of different groups, they can more quickly find their emotional and physical balance with new ways of doing things.

Left to themselves, children's discovery of conflicting rules often goes something like this: Playing hide and seek, one child will insist that another child is "found," while the other passionately disagrees. For both, it's as if the bottom falls out of the world. It is incomprehensible that there can be another set of rules: "That's not how it is!" "That's not fair!" "Is too!" fly through the air. Pretty soon, the others will gather to help decide the issue. The children who "lose" will sometimes leave the group—in disgust—for a shorter or longer period of time. We can also recognize this same passion in panel discussions on TV networks across the world—being identified with your opinions can have far reaching consequences.

Personal Boundaries and Group Boundaries

For a time, the child is assimilating and comparing these seemingly different worlds, as expressed in the statement: "Why can't we do that? John's parents don't mind!" Later, she starts to form her own opinions and views. Typically, this first happens in areas where she disagrees: "That's not fair! Why can't we do it this way?" Here, the child has become its own authority, and refers to its own opinion rather than to "John's parents." Similarly to the disagreement above about the rules of hide and seek, one or more children may refuse to play because the others have "stupid rules." Here, group boundaries are formed about which rules to play by: "The others wanted to play it this silly way, so Anna and me went off and played by ourselves!" Personal boundaries are enforced by the child's willingness to fight for her own opinion. The ability of a group to contain and process is based on the individuals' ability to do so. Many opinion-age ways of dealing with conflict are well known in adult interest groups—from science, to politics, to religion. A group that has resolved the issues from this age level will usually be able to contain, respect, and resolve its differences without splitting apart.

An adult client who was working with this stage of development realized that he had not even thought about really forming and standing for his opinions during twenty years of various therapies. In his group discussions and professional interactions, this often gave him a curiously lifeless quality. During the course of a session, he came to an adult's healthy and integrated version of this age: "I can speak the truth as I see it." This sentence is a good example of a firm but flexible boundary; it displays the integrity and will involved in forming and speaking one's own opinions, as well as a willingness to change if new information is received.

Sense of Direction in Life

Having made a choice of future profession, or at least practiced such choosing, the child goes on to practice stating and living by what she feels to be right and reasonable codes of behavior, articles of faith, and general working rules for the world. At the same time, she is learning an attitude toward opinions; how to form them, their relationship to observable reality, whether they can be changed or negotiated and how to do that, what to do with differences of opinion, etc. The child's sense of direction manifests in her developing physical ability to map and explore the world around her. She starts to move around independently, visiting other children or making trips to, say, the local grocery store for candy. This expanding exploration of her territory parallels the exploring she did when creeping in the family living room. At the same time, she is forming an internal map of her society, of the permissiveness, status, and rules of local families, stores, groups, and organizations. She finds ways to relate to these that establish her as a person in her own right—in her social context, much as she did earlier in her family.

Solidarity/Performance: Seven to Twelve Years Old

Theme: To balance being one's best with being a member of a group.

Early position: Leveling. The child identifies with the group and tries to keep everyone at the same level, so that no one stands out.

Late position: Competitive. The child competes with others for best position or for results, and occasionally competes with herself.

Healthy position: Balancing self and group. The child can perform, can support others in performing, or just relax.

> **Starts** with a shifting of attention from rules of games to performance in games, personal excellence, and competition. Physically, this corresponds to the new abilities to push off from the ground with feet, legs, and buttocks, and also to the development of an adult writing grip.

> **Ends** with the establishment of a balance between personal ego boundary and group identity. This corresponds to the perceptual and motor skills of three-dimensional drawing and fluid writing, as well as the full development of fine motor tuning of gross motor skills.

> **Focus** of the Solidarity /Performance age is on the balance between personal identity and close intimates on the one hand, and large group identification, function, and hierarchy on the other. The child goes through periods of strong group identity and mob behavior, as well as intensely competitive periods and total absorption in acquiring high-status skills and objects.

Bonding and Group Identity

The child has now learned to have intimate contact with both adults and peers. She has learned to negotiate rules of games as well as acceptable behavior with others, and she has established herself with several best friends. She will now start co-creating group identity with the other members, and move in the complex groupings and hierarchies that exist between them. Whereas in the Opinion stage, group membership meant knowing and following the rules, here the emphasis is on conformity and/or excellence. What is important is whether you fit in and are good at playing the game, throwing the ball, jumping the longest, or whatever activity the peer group considers important. Fierce competitiveness evolves around the central activity, and the activity itself becomes a vehicle of that emphasis.

The other main aspect of this group-bonding period is that of allegiance and solidarity. In a healthy group, each member is expected to support the bids of others for excellence, and to be loyal to them through success or failure. A loyal group, for example, will cover for each other and band together against adults trying to discover and punish a group member for some misdemeanor. As the group matures through internal and external interaction and conflict, the individuals slowly find their own place in the group. They learn to utilize the strengths and weaknesses in their particular constellation of individuals and relationships. Successful maturation at this level is the basis for good teamwork in any society, whether in organizational management or hunter-gatherer harvesting.

The group bonding process involves close physical contact—including wrestling, horsing around, pushing and pulling games, laying around in heaps, or talking about the world. There is also the shy, intimate contact of holding hands and falling in love. There is frequent intense physical contact at this age, some of it sexual in nature, and most of it decidedly not. In fact, a child can be ostracized from a group if she is not able to separate sensual from sexual contact. Children of this age are very aware of their nascent sexuality, and are creating group norms about courting and gender-appropriate behavior. Often, these group norms do not match the rules or actual behavior learned at home, and the child will struggle to adapt to and/or shape the group's rules as best she can.

Balancing Identity and Social Boundaries

There is a great deal of age overlap between the Opinion and Solidarity/Performance structures, the more so because children have quite different rates and forms of development. From around age seven, the child has developed the skills and the ability to play complex games, and can seriously begin to develop performance abilities and group solidarity. She can practice specific skills, such as skateboarding or piano lessons for hours a day, week after week, driven by nothing more than her own desire for accomplishment.

A child this age is learning to have fine control of gross motor activity. For example, long jumps in the six-year-old average $2^{1}/_{2}$ to 3 feet, whereas the twelve-year-old can jump twice as far. This drastic improvement is not due only to added strength, but also to improved motor coordination. These motor skills are also important for social interaction; being good at things is "cool." Most popular physical games of this age group have a heavy emphasis on balancing skills: refined versions of jump-roping, tag, follow-the-leader, skateboarding, etc. Interpersonally, the child is negotiating equally complex tasks of balance by learning to relate loyally, and with a clearly defined sense of self—to best friends, to the group as a whole with its changing patterns, and to the larger context of school and community. If the child feels that she is ostracized and punished for excelling, and accepted and praised for underachieving and supporting others, she will establish herself as a leveler in group interaction.

Personal Containment and Fine-Tuning Motor Skills

During these years, the child becomes aware of hierarchies in her peer group, and learns to act on this awareness. Her personal boundary develops from this new awareness, since she is now more consciously shaping her own personality. How to walk and talk, what clothes to wear, who to look up to or down on, and even her own feelings of self-worth are more consciously decided. These are learned and shaped through group interactions with peers, and group responses to her skills and actions.

The child becomes more able to contain and focus her energy, as evidenced by her tenacity in learning certain skills. A typical child of this age will practice extremely difficult motor skills, such as skateboard jumping, for hours, every day of the week, for months. Often, she will cooperate with peers to make a track, and they will then be absorbed in their own individual training, with a bit of discussion about how to do some specific stunt, and the occasional argument about one person "hogging" the track. This demonstrates an extremely high capacity to contain frustration, since many of the skills practiced are so difficult that it literally takes months of intensive practice to do them well. Friends and family will be called in to admire only when she feels she has mastered the skill she wishes to present. Even in this performance situation, the child shows a good grasp of containing excitement: performing lesser skills first and building to a climax with the newest trick.

Adolescence: Thirteen to Nineteen Years Old

Theme: To make the transition from being a dependent child to being an independent adult.

Position: There is not yet a clearly differentiated early, late, and healthy position for this stage. In moving toward forming the adult personality, adolescence involves all of the early character structures. The character formation of this stage is both extremely complex and extremely deep.

Starts with the hormonal changes that trigger the growth of secondary sexual characteristics. This initiates changes in the sexual feelings, involving an intense interest in necking and intercourse, and in the social rules and judgments surrounding such behavior. This period witnesses a growth spurt in the bones, and the hip joints become able to extend fully for the first time. This makes it necessary to change the way the pelvis is carried.

Ends with the solid establishment of the basic adult size and hormonal homeostasis. This corresponds to an inner solidifying of character structure in which the experiences from the various developmental stages knit together in a consistent, if not necessarily coherent, pattern.

Focus is on the attainment of adult personal function at all levels: social, professional, economic, status, interpersonal, sexual, and whatever else seems essential to the individual. This involves an unconscious fusion of earlier character formation and developmental experience into a functioning whole.

Bonding and Sexuality

As the child moves into the teenage years, hormonal changes bring on intense sexual feelings as well as frequent wild swings of mood and self-confidence. During this period, the adolescent is concerned with how desirable she is, and with how to establish an intimate relationship. She will repeat central themes of bonding, which she has previously experienced, blending resourceful and traumatic experiences into a cohesive belief and feeling system. Her emerging understanding of relationships will be influenced by what actually takes place during her forays into erotic intimacy. This brings the possibility of renegotiating past traumatic bonding experiences, in the emerging trust and caring of a new, loving, and respectful relationship. In more unfortunate cases, the adolescent moving toward peers with imbalanced desires or insufficient self-containment—or just pure bad luck—will often suffer further trauma that tend to reinforce previous negative imprints.

Adolescence is a time when character structure issues will either become more entrenched and embedded, or will soften and open. This process can be studied by comparing old and new Bodymaps of children followed into adolescence. Muscle patterns indeed become either more dysfunctional (hypo or hyper), or they become more resourced (less hyper or hypo, more neutral) during adolescence.

Inner Balance and the Melting Pot of Adolescence

Unpredictable growth spurts and neurological reorganization, as well as hormonal changes, play havoc with the youth's physical and emotional balance. And indeed, the hormonal cycle, adjusting to a monthly pattern for women and less researched and understood hormonal rhythms for men, is one of the main changes that needs to be negotiated. The adolescent adjusts to the development of secondary gender characteristics, and starts to hold her body in a way that fits her feelings about herself and her emerging mature sexuality. Balance is further disturbed by the recurrence of all preadolescent stages and the difficulties of development encountered then. The youth may literally be in an argumentative nine-year-old position when making a statement in a discussion, and at the same time, vulnerable to feeling her existence threatened by the time the answer comes. This is hard on the emotional balance, both for her and everyone around her. The problem is usually compounded by the fact that none of the people involved understand what is going on, and everyone keeps hoping for "reasonable" behavior from the others. The adolescent is further developing her observing ego at this time, and tends to recognize the inconsistencies in her parents' responses to her, *before* recognizing her own inconsistencies toward them.

Boundaries and Self-Dependence

Boundary issues during adolescence are concerned largely with separating from the family-of-origin, and the creation of a separate life and separate relationships as a developing adult—with a sometimes alarmingly developing body. This is an age of locked doors, "Adults Prohibited" signs, and violent arguments about all manner of household and personal boundaries and responsibilities. Because of the intra-psychic renegotiation of all previous developmental stages, boundaries become quite difficult to manage. One classic of this age is the struggle for the bathroom; the teenager will violently oppose other family members trying to dislodge her from whatever arcane activities she is engaged in—or their trying to share the space, since she perceives this as a serious violation of her boundaries. She will complain bitterly about these injustices, not realizing that she more or less holds the bathroom under siege, to the practical exclusion of any other family member's use of it. The problem smoothes out as the personal boundaries re-solidify, once again allowing her to balance her need for personal space against the needs of others.

Another important boundary development concerns the becoming of an adult sexual being. The adolescent must learn to negotiate relationships with this new component of her own and others' sexual desires. She must learn how and when to show or not show her developing sexual attributes, and how to relate in sexually acceptable ways. At times, she will have to act quite forcefully to protect her own sexual boundaries.

Summary

In summarizing this article (including Part I), it is useful to view Bodynamic Analysis in terms of the questions it has attempted to answer. The first and obvious question is how to present a very large amount of developmental information and empirical knowledge of psychomotor function in a form that is useable by psychotherapists. The format chosen was the character structure system as developed by Reich and Lowen, and later by Lake and Boadella. The contribution of Bodynamic Analysis is a clarification and extension of this description of human development. Development in each stage has been separated into an early, a late, and a healthy position, and these are correlated with muscle responsiveness. With the delineation of the Opinion, Solidarity/Performance, and Teenage structures, the character description has been extended a number of years.

A deeper and systematic understanding of the origins of hypo-responsive muscles, and their experience by the adult, has allowed for a therapeutic system that can focus on the building of missing or needed resources. This is the dialectic counterpart of the historical emphasis on breaking down defenses, character, and armor.

With the development of the Bodymap, an empirically derived, reproducible diagnostic tool, the therapist now has an assessment of the client's resources as well as the nature and extent of their developmental, shock, and birth trauma. This is a veritable map that continually suggests and informs a therapeutic strategy. The use of the Bodymap has enabled Bodynamic Analysis to formulate a systematic approach to body-oriented psychotherapy. One aspect of this is to use the muscles and knowledge of developmental stages to hold a client to one issue, from one developmental stage, until there is resolution. This helps a client to resolve early issues with the tools appropriate to that developmental stage. In addition, we can help a client who is missing early resources to develop these resources in later stages. This greatly facilitates regressive work, making it shorter and more integrative, while lessening the impact of regressed periods on the client's present life.

In addition to using the expanded character structure model, a client can

BODYNAMIC CHARACTER STRUCTURE

FREUD	ERIKSON	LOWEN	AGE	STRUC-TURAL Issues	HYPO-RESPONSE Predominant EARLY Position	HYPER-RESPONSE Predominant LATE Position	BALANCED RESPONSE Predominant HEALTHY Position	Cross-Structural Issues
Genital	Puberty		Teenage					
Latency	Latency	Four variations of rigidity	7-12 Years	Solidarity/ Performance	Levelling	Competitive	Balancing Self and Group	Cognitive Integration
			5-8 Years	Opinions	Sullen	Opinionated	Opinion-embodying	
Phalliic	Infantil-Genital Locomotor		3-6 Years	Love/ Sexuality	Romantic	Seductive	Balancing Heart and Sexuality	Sex-Role Identification
Anal	Anal-Urethral Muscular	Masochistic	2-4 Years	Will	Self Sacrificing	Judging	Assertive	
		Psychopathic	8 Mo. -2½ Yrs.	Autonomy	Non-verbal Activity Changing	Verbal Activity Changing	Emotionally Autonomous	Boundary Formation
Oral	Oral-Respiratory Sensory-Kinesthetic	Oral	1 Mo. -1½ Yrs.	Need	Despairing	Distrustful	Self Satisfying	
		Schizoid	2nd Trimester - 3 Mo.	Existence	Mental	Emotional	Secure Being	

also be seen in terms of ten somatic ego functions (e.g., centering, grounding, boundary formation, energy management, etc.). The clients' resources, as well as deficits in each of these areas, can be obtained from an analysis of the Bodymap. The individual muscles or groups of muscles related to a problem area can be brought into play in therapy sessions when the specific ego function is involved. As a resource is developed, the clients' appreciation of themselves, and of the presenting problem, changes. We then look anew at the presenting problem from this perspective.

Through knowing the developmental origins of each character structure, as well as the healthy and positive traits of each structure, an empathic attitude is fostered toward the client. An attempt is made to see the complexity of the character structures involved, as well as their interaction. An attribute of Bodynamic Analysis is its breadth coupled with its precision. The precision allows a client to feel accurately perceived, while the broadness helps them to not feel categorized.

References

Boadella, David. (1974). "Stress and Character Structure." *Energy & Character* 5(2).

Holle, B. *Motor Development in Children: Normal and Retarded* (Oxford: Blackwell Scientific Publication, 1976).

Johnsen, L. *Integrated Respiration Therapy* (no publisher listed, 1981).

Lake, Frank. *Clinical Theology* (New York: Crossroad, 1966).

Lowen, Alexander. *Language of the Body* (New York: Collier Books, 1958).

Mahler, Margaret S., F. Pine, & A. Bergman. *The Psychological Birth of the Human Infant* (London: Hutchinson, 1975).

Maturana, Humberto R., & Francisco J. Varela. *The Tree of Knowledge* (Berkeley, CA: Shambala, 1987).

Piaget, J. *The Origins of Intelligence in the Child* (New York: International Universities Press, 1952).

Reich, Wilhelm. *Character Analysis* (New York: Touchstone, 1933, 1972).

Stern, Daniel N. *The Interpersonal World of the Infant* (New York: Basic Books, 1985).

The BodyKnot Model: A Tool for Personal Development, Communication, and Conflict Resolution

—Erik Jarlnaes, M.A., & Lisbeth Marcher

In 2001, Erik Jarlnaes was a member of the planning committee for the European Congress for Body Psychotherapy. One of the themes of the congress was communication. He undertook a survey among members of the many different schools of body psychotherapy about whether they used a special model of communication during their teaching and client work.

To his astonishment, more than half of them said no. The most frequent answer was that they just followed the client's process. This suggested to Jarlnaes that most of the members' communication models were not expressly conscious and thus not part of a planned interaction to teach clients and students how to improve their communication skills.

This article is based on a Somatic Developmental Psychology model known as Bodynamic Analysis. In the Bodynamic system, we assume that personal problems not only derive from malfunctions in character development in childhood but also from the lack of learning social and interpersonal skills. Teaching clients communication skills is thus an important part of therapy. Thus we found it crucial to develop a specific model of communication, which we call the BodyKnot Model.

Our model was originally inspired by the awareness model from Gestalt Therapy that explored the questions of what "I see, I imagine, and I feel." These questions were of great assistance in our work from 1970 onward. We were also influenced by the work of Carl Rogers. He developed a way of connecting with his clients by repeating aloud what he heard the client say. The ability to accurately state what the client had expressed became a special therapeutic tool, which also influenced our model. To indicate that we had created our own model, we coined the term BodyKnot in 1989.

The BodyKnot model functions on various levels:

As a method for personal development, by bringing into consciousness people's habitual ways of thinking of themselves and others.

As a communication model, a method for the improvement and deepening of contact between people.

As a method of conflict solution, e.g., in family relations, workplace disagreements, or in major international crises.

In this article, we will present a model of understanding the level of possible contact or conflict in interaction between people. We will present the Body-Knot Model in three levels of detail, together with examples of its application. This will enable the reader to learn the model in stages. The first step will present the more condensed **basic** model, prepared for daily use. The **complete** model will then be outlined in Step 2. In the third step, we will present a more complete **analysis** of the dynamic relationship between anxiety, trust, and the levels of contact.

Step 1: The Basic BodyKnot Model

In daily educational and therapeutic situations, we often use a more condensed and subtle edition of the BodyKnot Model. This basic edition teaches essential social skills of communication that many clients and students lack— skills that are needed for situations when emotional stress and pressure levels are high. The numbered elements in this basic model also correspond to the elements in the more complete model that follows as Step 2 later in this article. After looking at both models, you may choose to do it your way, since it is not a linear model. It is better explained if the five numbers are put in a circle in order to demonstrate that all elements can come first. There is no correct order, but they all come into play when you are striving for an ideal contact situation.

BodyKnot Element	Statement/Expression
1. Five Senses—Facts	I see/I hear you say (facts) ... give me an example ... I hear a high pitch ... specifically you said ...
2. Interpretation of Facts	I believe you think ... I imagine that it means ... the meaning has to be ... I experience that you ... I perceive you as ... happy/angry ... I "hear" that ...
3/4. Personal Statement with	I feel good ... I am touched ... I like that ... I become
Some Physical, Bodily,	insecure ... it hurts ... I feel strange ... I like it
and/or Emotional Content	a little ... I experience myself as stupid ...
5. Inner impulse—Need—Want	It makes me want to ... I wish to ... I need to ... I would like to ... In order to change that I need to ... my impulse is ...
8. Action (doing and saying)	So I am saying ... I am doing ... will you take part in the talking ... I am requesting ... I am demanding that ...

The following diagram shows the interactive nature of these elements. A person can start from any of the elements and move directly to any another element as they choose.

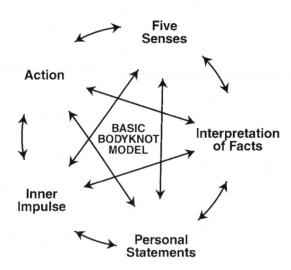

When we choose to teach this edition to clients we emphasize a number of points: Concerning point 1, the **Five Senses—Facts,** please learn to focus on "facts." Every time you frown, get confused, or get a knot in the stomach, it is probably because you are not sure you are talking of the same issue, or you are under attack (by "you" sentences). Therefore, ask for specifics, ask for an example, and ask for the facts. This will not only make you come to a common understanding, but you will also get breathing time while you "force" the other to be more specific. To learn this as a reflex impulse will support a survival impulse.

Concerning point 2, the **Interpretation of Facts,** we teach how to say and respond to what you have heard or seen—check the understanding—or ask for an interpretation, or willingly give it yourself. We also emphasize how it is possible to change the facts through effective interpretation.

Concerning point 3/4, the **Personal Statement,** we tell the client how important it is just to say something—verbalize something—and that little is better than nothing. The tendency in our society is to be very intellectual without sharing the inner world, especially when under pressure (high intensity). It is important to teach that something *is* there, that they may be uncomfortable in giving it words, and that they must verbalize minor personal statements that are not fully revealing.

Finally, we also take time to point out that sentences like "that was beautiful" and "it is great" are *not* personal statements. Two people, A and B, will use "I" and "you" about themselves, and they will use "that" and "it" about something that is "between" them. The unconscious illusion is: *The less personal, the less they can be attacked.*

In point 5, **Inner Impulse—Need—Want**, we point out that we use many different words because they refer to different developmental age levels. The important thing is to try them because this will give you enough experience to make the best choice of words when you are in the situation. Sometimes it is also necessary to talk about what to do when there is no awareness of a need. Often, the problem is that the gap from personal statements to "need" is so big that nothing comes to mind. In this case, we teach them to get away from the feeling state (which often is negative) into a positive one—and suddenly it is much easier to determine what they want or need.

In relation to number 8, the **Action (doing and saying)**, we are teaching that it is not always enough to say what you want or need. This is especially the case when the intensity is high, because a want or need is communicated indirectly to another person, and it is assumed that the other "should" know it. But again, under pressure this insight may disappear. Therefore, it must be stated in a question whether or not the other will take her part in redeeming the situation.

Finally, for training purposes, I ask clients to deliberately listen to how other people are using their language, and *not* using it, and then systematically including more and more words from the different elements.

In a group setting, here is an example of an exercise to teach people the importance of "personal statements": I form a group of four to seven people and they discuss something that is of high relevance. The exercise may last half an hour, or expand into an hour. The only job for the participants is to deliberately include one personal statement every time one speaks about the issue, e.g., if A wants to say "You look like you are perspiring," then this is not enough. A has to find the personal statement (what goes on inside to make him/her say that) and then add something like, "It makes me feel warm also." When one person forgets this, the other members of the group must stop and ask for the personal statement before they can continue.

When this is happening and everyone constantly says something personal, the contact level rises dramatically so that everyone can sense it. For some, this contact becomes so emotional that they burst into tears; they are touched and they want more. On the other hand, some of them reach their limits for personal exposure and interpersonal contact.

We will now move further in the development of this exploration. Some success in practicing the basic model will aid in utilizing the next level of effective communication.

Step 2: The BodyKnot Model

The following nine elements must eventually all be present in the communication process for the level of contact to stay healthy and alive (and succeed). The linear order of the elements describes a/the natural development of a communication process but may vary randomly.

0. Context, Background, and Basic Mood

Context refers to the external framework in which the event took place: Who are you with? What is the purpose? Is there a deadline? Meeting with customers from a different culture is an example of a situation where the context is very significant. A Dane, for instance, is accustomed to maintaining a certain physical distance during negotiations. A Saudi Arabian, on the contrary, wants to be physically close in order to decide whether the dealings should lead to a yes. Being ignorant of this culturally based phenomenon might easily cause the deal to be lost. Being aware of the immediate context creates a readiness for solving possible problems.

The background is the personal history (feeling "baggage" from the past), which we all carry with us. Experiences gained early in life—manifested in recent opinions and values—mean that new perceptions become "filtered" into familiar categories of experience and interpretations as such.

BodyKnot Element	Statement/Expression
0. Context, Background, and Basic Mood	I was angry when I came . . . my background makes me see things this way . . .
1. Five Senses—Facts	I see/you say (facts) . . . give me an example . . . I hear a high pitch . . . specifically you said . . .
2. Interpretation of Facts	I believe you think . . . I imagine that it means . . . the meaning has to be . . . I experience that you . . . I perceive you as happy/angry . . . I "hear" that
3. Body Sensing Statements	I sense relief . . . it hurts in my belly . . . I become heavy . . . I tense up here . . . I experience my strength here . . . I am cold in my shoulder
4. Emotional Statement	I am angry/happy/jealous . . . I feel ashamed/ sad/afraid/ . . . I am proud of myself
5. Inner Impulse Toward Action . . . Need—Want—Desire	It makes me want to . . . I want . . . need to . . . I would like to . . . In order to change that I need to . . . my impulse is . . .
6. Analysis and Calculating Consequences	If A . . . then B will happen but if not, then . . . on the one side . . . we can now choose between . . . the consequences of choosing A will be . . . and B . . .
7. Choice	I am choosing . . . I choose to let go of B . . . The choice is between A and B . . . I take A and let go of B
8. Getting Choice Into Action and Expression	So I am saying . . . I am asking you to do so, will you . . . I am doing . . . will you take part in the meeting . . . I would like a hand from you, will you . . . so, I am requesting . . . I am demanding that . . .

The basic mood encompasses one's mood at the point of entering a contact situation. It is usually a good idea to keep one's basic mood and current mood separated. An example:

A is angry (from a fight at home) coming to work. B is very happy and shares an important event with A, but A talks back in an angry way—not because of B but because of his own basic mood. This may spoil the contact unless B notices A's emotional state, or A understands the reason for his anger, and shares this with B.

One way of using this context is to have morning rounds in groups that need to develop contact in order to work well together—bring the other members up to speed about the ability to be present for the team.

1. Five Senses—Facts

External sense perceptions are the facts from the outside world, which can be perceived by the individual through her five senses: sight, hearing, smell, taste, and touch. The point is to arrive at raw data freed from interpretation. This will make it possible for two people to realize if and when they are talking about the same situation.

Examples: I see that you are stretching upwards. I can hear that your breathing is fast. I notice that your hand is trembling. I can hear (and see) your finger tapping.

In order to improve a communication situation, it is recommended that each person describe specifically what they are sensing and also ask for specific examples from the other person, instead of general descriptions.

2. Interpretation of Facts

How does one make sense of all the perceptions? That's the question. Interpretations can be expressed through many common words, for instance: guess, think, believe, experience, body-experience, imagine, suppose, translate, the meaning is, imply, judge, and indicate. The words feel and hear are often used (and misused) as metaphors for interpretation, but it is important to distinguish "sensing words" from "interpreting words."

Here is an example, based on facts, without muddled or hidden messages:

I can see that you are stretching upwards and I imagine that you are doing that because you are tired of sitting still. I can see that your hand is trembling, and I guess it is because you are scared, is that true?

Sometimes we see second- (and third-) degree interpretations (the interpretation is being interpreted). An example:

B notices that A is changing position in the chair into sitting more straight.

B is stating the (first) interpretation that A is dissatisfied and therefore (second) would like to get up from her chair. A answers: "I am quite satisfied." B: "No, you are not, because in my experience, 'quite' means that you are not satisfied." A: "Well for me it means that it is okay."

Differentiation Between Facts and Interpretations

One of the major threats to the communication process—and the contact—is the tendency to confuse facts with interpretations. Here is one example: A and B are colleagues. The level of contact is low and when A suddenly says, "You are angry," B replies back, "No," but A insists and B, being hurt, keeps saying "No." While this is going on, the level of contact falls toward zero.

One way out of this mix-up is to find out why A thinks B is angry. Interpretation builds on facts, and therefore we need to ask A what he noticed specifically in B that made him believe B was angry. A might reply that B was frowning while they spoke. This gives B a chance to check this out: Can he recognize this in himself? Can he sense if it is true that he was frowning? If yes, he might add that this still does not mean that he is angry. "This is not anger," says B, "but this is what I do look like when I have to choose among different alternatives."

The intensity, already at this point, has fallen; the interpretation has been checked. Most often, it is this easy; sometimes it takes some repetitions before trust has been reestablished between the two. If B *cannot* recognize that he is frowning, he has to say so. Then there might be a dialogue about this, and a request from B to A that he points it out the next time it happens.

3. Body Sensing Statements

Sensation is another word for internal sense perceptions as they manifest in the body. It may be physical pleasure or discomfort in various parts of the body, or autonomic reactions as heat or cold, changes in the pulse, or bowel movement. The body sensations also encompass balance, sensing of the muscles (tensions, vibration), and their location.

As part of the effort to attain the clearest possible communication, it is important to train your ability to verbalize the body sensations specifically and accurately. Body sensations cannot be wrong, but the meaning assigned to them can be. For instance, investigating your internal sense perception can take place in this way: In certain situations, a person can experience that "something is contracting in my gut." Step 1 is to consciously accept the phenomenon. Step 2 is to find out what causes the body sensation. Is it something in the interaction with another person, or is it the fact that the wallpaper in the room reminds you of something that happened in another room at another time?

Naming and locating the body sensations creates a physical container, which makes it easier to contain related emotions, ideas, and interpretations. For instance, the body sensation leading to a statement, "I experience that my head is about to explode," can be that a violent pressure exists in the temples (but nowhere else in the head) and that the muscles at the side of the neck are very tense. In this case, the actual sensations are less scary than the ideas it gives rise to. At the same time, identifying the actual sensation makes it possible to find out what caused the muscles to tighten. Was it a certain movement or did something happen in the situation causing the muscles to contract violently? Was it a reaction caused by an external chemical agent (coffee, tobacco, alcohol, etc)?

If you ask someone what he experiences in a given situation, the answer will very often combine emotion and external/internal sense perceptions – e.g., "I feel great and on top of the world." Sensations vanish into experiences and so it becomes difficult to have a precise communication. If instead you ask the question, "What are you sensing?" you will normally get answers that indicate body sensations far more precisely.

Here are examples of clear and unclear communication:

Clear Communication—Body Sensations:
I can feel myself collapsing in the chair
I feel a restless vibration
My blood is running cold

Unclear Communication—Body Experience:
I feel heavy
I cannot feel myself

4. Emotional Statement

Emotion is the feeling reaction that follows or co-exists with body sensations. We are dealing with eight basic emotions: joy, sorrow, anger, fear, sexuality, shame, disgust, and pride—all of which can be present in several degrees of intensity, separately or combined. It is important for us to note that we consider all emotions positively.

To practice expressing the strength or combination of the emotions can be a very educating experience. It is a good idea to state the percentage with which you experience each of the eight basic emotions in a given situation. It is possible to be just 1% happy, 2% angry or 5% sexually aroused. It is, however, also possible to feel 0% of all emotions. Reporting that "nothing happens" is okay too, because our experience is that this will make you more aware of what you really feel, and then you will start to crawl up on the number scale.

Combined (compound) emotions can be excitement, jealousy, hurt, bitter, pleased, suspicious, embarrassed, etc. When clients need to learn about basic emotions, these blended emotions are taken apart and described as percentage compositions of the eight basic emotions. A given person might, for instance, describe jealousy like this: 30% shame, 30% anger, 30% fear, 6% sorrow, and 4% sexuality.

In order to create clear communication about emotions, it is important that the underlying facts and interpretations are made explicit. If, for instance, you say, "I am scared of you," this is not clear because it does not refer to facts. The other person is "made wrong" and she will have to imagine what it is all about. Often interpretations run wild—confusion and lack of precision in the contact will result.

In the following, the previous examples are expanded further, so that emotion is now given a clear expression:

"I can see that you are stretching upwards. I imagine that you are tired, and I can feel myself collapsing in the chair and that I am a bit depressed."

"I can hear that you are breathing out slowly, and my interpretation is that you are becoming focused inside yourself, and I feel restlessness in my legs and then I get angry."

"I can see that your hand is trembling; my interpretation is that you are getting scared. I can feel my own blood running cold and I get scared, too."

"I can hear you are tapping on the table with your fingers, and I imagine that you are impatient, I experience tension in my thighs and rapid vibrations in my upper arms and I am feeling happy."

3/4. Personal Statements

Both body sensing statements (sensations) and emotional statements (emotions) happen inside the individual. In order to improve communication (and contact) it is important to learn to name both the sensations and the emotions. This will change the whole level of contact, will increase the trust, and thus decrease the level of anxiety.

In practical application, it is often more important to make the clients (or participants in a group) manifest/say/share some personal statement rather than say nothing. People will hesitate because they believe they must find the right words, and differentiate sensations from emotions. This can be achieved at a later time.

This is why we fuse **Sensations** and **Emotions** and call them **Personal Statements**.

Examples of the fusion of sensations and emotions: "I like that," "I am not really content," and "I miss something."

It is emphasized that each participant has to use the word "I" whereas depersonalizing words like "it," "that," and "one" are discouraged. Examples: "It looks good" versus "I like it." The difference in impact is very clearly felt by both the listener and the speaker.

Based on what is happening (or said or understood), a personal reaction always comes: stiffening, holding breath, knot in the solar plexus, a smile, pleasure, apprehension, etc. It is part of our experience that every time a personal statement is said, the contact level goes up (slowly or quickly depending of the starting point, but always up). So it is worth getting to know what to say here.

If the personal statement includes something physical, bodily, and/or emotional, it works—the contact opens up.

For many people this is easy to do when there is *no* conflict in the air, but this easiness disappears when there are conflicts.

When teaching, I tell the participants about possibilities that are physical—like tension, cold and warm, lack of tension, vibrations, movements—and add where in the body they might be located. I try to stay away from energetic statements because I want the conversation to be as physical as possible.

I also teach them to say a small personal statement like, "I like that (a little), I am not really content, I miss something." People have many things going on inside; however, they are not used to putting words to it.

We talk about the rise and fall of an emotion, and how quickly the emotion can change. We talk about how certain emotions have been taboo in the family-of-origin, how one learns to contain emotions, and when it is important to learn to expand the use of one or two emotions.

Many people are afraid of their own anger. Anger is a difficult emotion, but joy can also be difficult. Some people were stopped as children when they were simply happy—stopped so effectively that they became focused on their intellect rather than their emotions. Then, when later in life they find themselves in a happy situation, they could become afraid or sad.

Previously, we talked of percentage. An emotion has the capacity to unfold 100%, but how much have you learned to unfold? It is okay to say "1% joy or anger or ..." This is important for many because often the norm is that you have to fully sense it before you can name it. Small percentages are needed to get started.

5. Inner Impulse Toward Action . . . Need—Want—Desire

An action impulse will arise from body sensations and emotions whether it happens consciously or unconsciously. The action impulse precedes a possible action. However, the action often is not in accordance with the impulse. Indeed, clarifying an original impulse, which is then not acted upon, can often lead to a more precise communication.

Some impulses are not acted on and not even verbalized. Two examples:

A feels like withdrawing from a difficult situation, but chooses to stay in order to get a better, more complete idea of the situation.

B feels the desire to allow a sexual attraction to unfold but chooses not to let this happen because the other person is in an established relationship and wants this existing relationship to continue and deepen.

It can be very important to dwell on action impulses, especially if you abstain from passing judgment on the consequences. In some cases, the nature of the action impulse is better described as avoidance than desire. Therefore, a cautious and defensive lifestyle can be changed so that the person himself makes the decisions and is in control of his direction in life.

It is important to distinguish between impulses and wishes on the one side and the actual actions on the other. Impulses are allowed. You do not have to act out all impulses, so to dare to sense them, and name them without having to act them out, can be very rewarding.

For many people the defense mechanism, when they do not want to act on an impulse, is to immediately erase it from consciousness. This leaves them without contact to their original wishes. Furthermore, the difficulty may be that a person has an opinion—a hidden norm. If they cannot articulate the impulse clearly, they may believe they have no right to it. In this case, the person exploring the impulse may discard it as having no value. We believe that speaking to impulses, even if they are in a formative stage, will lead a person to a better understanding of their own needs. However, in our view, it is acceptable to feel an impulse without having to share it.

In the title of this section, we used several different words to be used in dif-

ferent situations. "Tune in" is our recommendation, and pick the most suit-
able word—impulses, needs, wants, desires.

6. Analysis and Calculating Consequences

The purpose of analyzing is preparing oneself to make a choice that will
lead to an action. This point includes analyzing the different action impulses.
First of all, you have to figure out to what degree your options are in accordance
with your basic values, goals, and directions in life.

If you do not have clear directions and goals, you may end up arguing indef-
initely. One main reason for getting lost is that the original impulse was erased
from consciousness. The intellect takes over without any bodily awareness,
which makes it impossible to move forward in the process and makes your
decision process very difficult. The analysis has to be based on available facts.
The illusion may be that it is possible to obtain all possible information, and
this illusion will obstruct the decision process.

It is necessary to make decisions even on incomplete information, which
implies the possibility to change a decision when new evidence comes along.

This is an example of analyzing a given situation:

During a quarrel with an employer, a person has the impulse to leave the
room and slam the door. Perhaps the person limits his or her analysis to the
thought that this would not be a good idea. But he might also go through a
longer chain of reasoning: If I leave now, I cut off the contact and risk losing
my job. My impulse to leave arises because this situation reminds me of situations where I felt rejected by my father. But I know that my employer is not
my father. I also know that he is usually willing to listen to me even if this
takes time and involves him in committing to a new plan of action.

7. Choice

Choice is the point in the model where the different analyses are weighed
against each other. Many action impulses can be present at the same time,
which means that an inner dialogue—an internal weighing of the pros and
cons and taking a stand—will be going on. The decision can be made more

whole-heartedly if it is based on your basic values and norms, and these are bodily integrated. The decision causes a sensation of presence, intensity, and trust in your body, whether the choice is easy or difficult.

A factor connected with making a choice is overlooked by many, namely that a selection automatically implies a rejection. The career-oriented person, for instance, who is fully conscious that his work situation is given a very high priority (selection), can be unaware that focusing too much on your career means giving low priority to your partner and children (rejection). If the person is confronted with a choice between work and family, it may not be fully considered. Making a full choice may make the person aware of painful emotions such as sadness and shame. Keeping the feelings that arise from difficult choices away from our conscious awareness actually reduces our resourcefulness. It takes energy to maintain that denial.

One of the problems that may block the pathway from analysis to choice and action is lack of courage. There are two main roads to courage: Firstly, you have to strengthen your connection with your original action impulse. Does it still feel all right? Secondly, you may strengthen your commitment by verbalizing your decision for yourself and others.

On special occasions (very high intensity situations) your most basic values, like personal dignity and mutual connection, may overrule all other considerations. An example of this was the German officers in World War II who took on the task of assassinating Hitler. The plan was fragile. They knew it would likely go awry but they decided to try it anyway. If it went wrong they would die. If they succeeded, they might die anyhow, but die with dignity. So, the bottom line has to do with values and dignity, and toward the end you will demand something from the choice you made.

8. Getting Choice into Action and Expression

When all the previous elements are clear and not clouded by lack of awareness, the last link in the chain—the action—should be simple. However, this is not always the situation. Many examples show that when the gap in time between choice and action gets too big, the whole situation gets messy and the action may be "forgotten." Too many work-related assignments may also hinder the accomplishment. Moreover, most actions depend on negotiations with others. It is not enough to decide and carry out an action; communicating it to your partner in the matter is just as important.

It can be difficult to take action. The action can imply sharing how difficult the choice has been, and why you have to do it the way you do. Contemplating the dialogue with an employer might run like this: "When this happened I felt like leaving (impulse), because I felt rejected (personal statement). But it is important for me (personal statement) to try to solve the problem, and I am not interested (personal statement) in having the situation pushed to an extreme, which is going to happen if I leave. So I will stay and tackle the problem; I want (need) to do that, but I also need to know that you are interested in solving the problem. Otherwise I will feel stupid, so will you listen to my version of the story (action)?

In daily life, communication might seem so straightforward and uncomplicated. Why use a very deliberate model like the BodyKnot Model? It is our experience that the clarity in communication created by use of the model makes it possible to maintain a high level of contact with oneself and others, even in high intensity situations.

In real life, a lot of things described here happen simultaneously. In educational and therapeutic situations, it may even be very rewarding to watch people's usual way of using the elements: Which ones are strong, which ones do they omit? The elements that are most often omitted seem to be the reason why the communication breaks down and becomes a conflict.

At this point, the reader has viewed the complete BodyKnot Model. Now, in Step 3, we will present a more schematic analysis of the relationship dynamics involved in this model.

Step 3: Anxiety, Trust, and Levels of Contact

Communication between two people takes place in a context. The most important elements of this context are:

The anxiety level of the participants.

The level of trust among the participants.

The intensity in the communication situation.

The level of contact between the participants.

When lovers, friends, colleagues, neighbors, and partners are on good speaking terms with no conflict, or wish to change their relationship (communicate), they do not usually need a communication model. Each person speaks from the heart and the other listens with a sensitive ear. The anxiety level of the participants is low, the level of trust is high, the level of contact is excellent, and the relationship can manage high intensity discussions without falling apart.

This ideal situation seldom occurs. Over longer periods of time, conflicts are part of life and potentially lead to growth. The problem, however, is that lack of contact with oneself and the other may quickly lead to damaging situations in the communication exchange, and to conflict escalation or avoidance. This is the situation in which a conflict resolution model is needed.

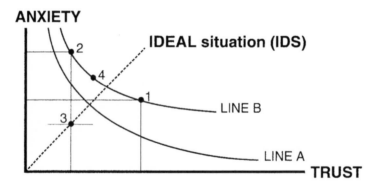

Figure 1. Anxiety chart

The relation between trust and anxiety is illustrated in Figure 1. The figure shows the relationship between trust and anxiety: In problematic situations it often happens that the higher the trust, the lower the anxiety. This is shown with the line (A). For some people, there is a tendency to place so much importance in trust that they avoid anxiety by giving their responsibility to other people they trust (safety seekers). For others, anxiety is so important that they'd rather let go of trust in order to keep the feeling of anxiety inside (risk takers).

The ideal growth-oriented relation is that both anxiety and trust increase normally (line IDS). This will also give a higher intensity in the communication relationship and in each person. The example is that when there is love in the air, intensity is higher, and it makes a person expand their trust in the other person; at the same time it expands their ability to handle higher levels of anxiety.

In Figure 1, we have placed the numbers 1-2-3 indicating an example where client M was situated in Point 1 (showing his ability to cope with the anxiety and showing his level of trust in the other, his employer). However, when he was suddenly asked to sign a paper, documenting things he did not know about, his trust in the employer fell dramatically and his anxiety raised just as dramatically (Point 2) to a level he could not handle.

The size of the rectangle (created by the location of the points) will change as one moves from one point to another. This rectangle represents the quality of life, happiness, contentment. The size of the rectangle decreased when M "moved" from Point 1 to Point 2. He then fell into depression as a survival mechanism.

Together with a therapist, the first step for the client is to create a safe space, meaning that trust has to expand (so that anxiety will lower). In terms of the diagram, he was helped to move from Point 2 to Point 3 through a mixture of support, confrontation, and teaching (skills he did not know). As a result, M was getting resources that will support him in changing a possible future situation where he might meet the anxiety level at Point 2 and change the direction rather than being blocked.

In this case, he became ready to speak with his employer again, with a different result than the first time. He was resolved to handle his own anxiety. Through the teaching, his self-esteem grew and he was able to move up to Point 4 (a little more anxiety and less trust), and from here he managed to have a satisfactory discussion with his employer recognizing his concerns.

Levels of Contact

Figure 2 illustrates the development of contact in communication. When the level of contact is already high, it takes very little to improve it even further (a smile, a small personal statement). This situation is illustrated with Line 1. Misunderstandings or irrelevant comments naturally decrease the contact, but only very slowly as illustrated with Line 2. Conversely, when the level of contact is already low, it takes a good deal of positive reinforcement to improve the situation, as illustrated with Line 3. Similarly, only a few badly placed remarks or a lifted eyebrow will have disastrous consequences, as illustrated with a very steep slope in the contact level by Line 4. Line 5 illustrates the deep freezer: the level of contact is below zero and it will take a lot of effort from both parties just to get the level of contact above zero; one bad remark will make it collapse back into deep-freeze mode. This is clearly often the situation in international conflict resolution and in long-term conflicts of marriage.

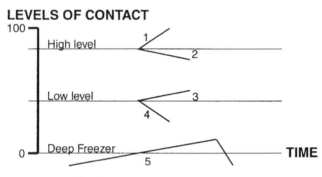

Figure 2. Levels of Contact

It is possible to improve the contact level whatever the starting point, but the lower the level of existing contact, the more a model is needed for the reestablishing of contact, communication, and conflict resolution.

Another way of explaining the same is seen in Figures 3A and 3B. In Figure 3A, when the level of contact is already high, it takes very little to improve it even further (a smile, a small personal statement). This situation is illustrated with Line A, Part Y. When the level of contact is already low, it takes a good deal of positive reinforcement to improve the situation just as much as before ($x1 = x2$), as illustrated with Line A, Part Z.

Misunderstandings or irrelevant comments naturally decrease the contact, as illustrated with Line B in Figure 3B. When the level of contact is already high, it decreases very slowly (part C), while a few badly placed remarks or a lifted eyebrow will have disastrous consequences, as illustrated with a very steep slope in the contact level by Line B, Part D. This illustrates that the same sentence ("I love you" or "you are stupid") has different impact, depending on where you are located in the "contact-diagram" when you start to notice.

The interesting question is naturally, "What makes contact increase and what makes it decline?" In other words, "Which elements in the BodyKnot Model make contact increase?"

We believe that this question may find its answer in exploring the various elements set out in the BodyKnot Model.

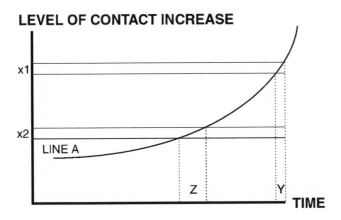

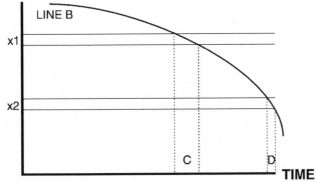

Figures 3a and 3b.

Future Considerations

We use the BodyKnot Model on a daily basis in therapy, education, and conflict resolving. The model's most prominent feature as a conceptual tool is its ability to integrate the bodily, emotional, and cognitive elements of communication.

New developmental work on the model is in progress: integration of the character structure model, the ego functions model, and the BodyKnot Model.

Addendum

The BodyKnot Model has been described previously in Erik Jarlnaes's *Body-Knot—The Art of Undoing Knots,* 1994, published by Bodynamic International, Denmark.

We want express our thanks to Kirstine Münster, Garry Friesen, and Ian Macnaughton for valuable help with the editing.

References

Rogers, Carl R. *Client Centered Therapy* (Boston: Houghton Mifflin Company, 1951)

Perls, Frederick. *Gestalt Therapy Verbatim* (Lafayette, CA; Real People Press, 1967).

Caring for Yourself While Caring for Others

—Merete Holm Brantbjerg, translated from Danish by Nille J. Bourne

.

What does it actually mean to care for oneself? Some of the first words that come to mind are personal integrity—to feel oneself and to listen to oneself.

One of the great Gestalt therapists was once asked: "Who is more important, the client or the therapist?" The answer was the therapist. It is a provocative way of seeing it, but the point is true. If the therapist does not see him/herself as the most important, it is not possible to fully help the client.

One of the deepest learning methods is *mirroring*. It is through mirroring that children learn how to be human from their parents, for better or worse. As children we repeat—*mirror*—what the grown-ups do; when they talk, eat, are angry, happy, etc. The same mechanisms are used when clients or students need help to change themselves as adults. They need new role models, new supporting people, authorities, and parent-models to learn from. And yet, once again, the deepest part of the learning happens through mirroring.

Think about it. Think it through. The client learns from who you are, no matter what technique or method you use. The client learns from you, for better and for worse. To me, it was this thought that finally made me realize that my consideration for the clients was wrong/misunderstood. I realized that the clients' chance of learning to be him or herself, feeling his or her boundaries, become familiar with feelings, find the center, find the grounding—all depended on my abilities in the same areas, together with my willingness to openly share them with the client in a session.

The Purpose of Having a Model

When I am myself, the client will learn non-verbally that the state of being oneself is a possibility in the world—something not everyone is aware of from their upbringing.

I have a practical example that illustrates this: One of my clients wanted to be able to come out more with her anger in relation to her partner, and in relation to her friends. I worked with the client on this issue for six months. I used different therapeutic methods, from stimulating hypo-tense muscles to hitting pillows, and having her talk to people she wanted to confront as if they were there. We looked at patterns from the client's upbringing, concerning how to express anger and much more. It became easier for the client to feel the world. It became easier to figure out what would be good to say when actually being angry, but she did not start using these abilities in daily life.

In the beginning, I was patient and supporting. I was busy finding new methods to help with the problem. But, slowly I got irritated—irritated that she did not make use these methods. My creativity was exhausted. I could not think of any more "clever" methods. I confronted her. I spoke my anger aloud, I expressed my irritation and my demand that she start to act *now*—that I was tired of waiting. She became angry with me. She said she could not do it. I told her it was not true, because I had seen her angry in the therapy session. I knew she could do it. The session ended in anger.

When she came to the following session, she was afraid because of what had happened. She was concerned about whether she could still be my client; she was afraid of the consequences. She discovered, through our contact, that the mutual connection was still there, and that I had not left her nor had I intended to do so. After that, she opened slowly to the possibility that anger can actually be part of contact and mutual connection. Later, she told me that she had yelled at her partner, and that he became angry, but also that things were better afterwards.

It is not always that easy, but this is a good example of how empowering it can be for a client to see, feel, or hear the possibility for action, that she is starting to reclaim—to see the possibility acted out by the therapist. Not so that she can end up showing her anger like I did, but because she needs a role model to mirror or separate from, in order to get started.

In this client's family, during her upbringing, there was never any fighting. Anger was not shown openly; you withdrew from the contact instead. She had no model of what you actually do when you get angry, and even though she learned the methods in sessions, the methods remained separated from her until she saw me become angry. She got a chance to learn—the same way children learn. The body does not believe in words alone. It only believes that something exists, when it has felt, seen, heard, smelled, or tasted it.

The purpose of this case is to illustrate the basic view, presented in this article. Taking care of yourself as therapist—to work with your own well-being in the client session/treatment situation—is necessary to avoid stress and burnout. It is also a therapeutic method and an important part of any successful treatment strategy.

The Body Supplies the Most Important Tools

It is then possible to use these tools when taking care of yourself in the therapist role. The answer in Bodynamic Analysis is that the tools are within the body. It is within the body that I can find my centering. It is sensations in the body that tell me when my boundaries are crossed or when they are respected. It is sensations in the body that tell me when to say "stop."

It is sensations in the body that tell me how good my grounding is, and it is with help from bodily and energetic tools that I can make it better.

My body is there when I sense my emotions. My stomach contracts when I am afraid. My jaw is tight when I am angry. It tickles up and down the front of my stomach and chest when I am happy or curious. To take care of myself demands closeness. Without it, I do not sense the signals with which my body tells me how I react to what is going on. I thereby lose the possibility to consciously relate to what is going on, and to choose for myself. Optimal sensation to another person is a great demand. Optimal closeness, in my opinion, means being one-hundred percent present—physically, emotionally, spiritually, and in thoughts. No one can live up to that, but we always have the possibility of relating to our own sensation, and we can learn tools that will help improve it.

In this article, I will focus on how you can increase your sensation—physically and bodily—since in our opinion, this is basis for the other sensations. The body ego is the first identity that the child develops. The young child actually thinks and experiences with the whole body. Body sensation is one with the sensation of existence—the sensation of being yourself. It is this basic bodily identity that is the foundation for the later ego development of the child. Literally speaking, the body is the shell that contains the other levels of consciousness. Without the body, the emotions have no shell to be in or to be expressed from. A person with weak contact to his or her body sensation will, therefore, become more easily overwhelmed by feelings and will lose the ability to differentiate. Something similar goes for the thoughts. Mental energy is faster and can expand almost endlessly. To maintain your body sensation while thinking gives the thoughts grounding. Without body sensation to hold and keep the thoughts, there is a risk that you will get lost in your thoughts, cannot stop thinking, or can never bring them to life.

The spiritual side of us—our essence, our soul—exists, according to my belief, no matter whether the body is there or not. But without a body there is no possibility of surviving on earth, meaning no possibility to experience, live, learn, and thereby develop the soul and expand its capacity or consciousness. Also, the soul needs the body; it needs us to accept our bodily closeness with the unique possibility it gives us to sense every cell, and the numerous possibilities of expressions that these cells give us.

What can you do to accept the possibilities of the body? Bodynamic Analysis has, over the last twenty years, developed and refined a number of methods to work with the bodily closeness (the body sensation).

A general way is to ask about body sensation. It sounds simple, but there are actually only very few people that have a developed language in which to express their sensations in the body. Because no one has heard anyone talk about it—and thereby give meaning to it—and because no one has asked about what you sense in the body, there are no models for expression. The language must therefore be rehabilitated, or it must be learned all over again if it was not there when you were a child. Curiosity and interest in bodily sensations can be awakened, and thereby it is possible to develop an increased clarity about the importance of the sensations.

The individual method is then to start asking about the bodily sensations. What are you feeling at the moment? Ask yourself, ask others, ask your clients, and notice the answers. Keep asking until the answer actually describes the bodily sensation—"my stomach contracts, I have warm hands, I am holding my breath, my neck muscles are tight and hurt," and so on. Most spontaneous answers that are given to the question, "What are you feeling at the moment in your body?" do not describe body sensations but emotions, imaginations, thoughts, impulses, etc. (For deeper insight to this, read *BodyKnot: The Art of Undoing Knots,* by Eric Jarlnaes, which is the basis for the previous article.)

Besides asking generally about the body sensation, I will describe the three most important tools in the work with bodily closeness and personal integrity:

Centering or sensation of the core;

Grounding or sensation of the connection to the ground;

Boundaries or sensation of difference between one's self and the surrounding world.

I would like to repeat: these are the *three most important tools* in relation to being able to take care of one's self as a therapist.

Finding One's Own Core

Centering is a concept used in Bodynamic Analysis, and by many others as well. The techniques used within Eastern martial arts (tai chi, karate, jiu-jitsu, etc.) teach people how to make the force from the movements come from a point in the middle of the stomach, just below the navel, on the front side of the backbone. Meditative systems talk about the *Hara-chackra* located in the same spot.

Our approach to the concept is both concrete and more abstract. The *concrete* is that people have a point of gravity, a physical point of gravity or balance, which has its place in the same mid-stomach area. This does not mean that people can always feel their point of gravity in their stomach. It can be pushed upwards or to the side. The energy can be spread out or blocked so that it can be difficult to feel anything. My experience, after teaching several groups, is that the imagination of something being a center—a core within the stomach, on the front side of the backbone—touches deep in everybody. In some, it touches deep feelings of calmness, power, being oneself; to others a recognition that they are missing contact with something within themselves—that something is missing.

To say that people have a core is also *abstract,* since we have not been able to identify a certain physical structure that would make up a core. We are still looking. Maybe our core is stored within a (fascia) center inside the stomach. Even if we cannot prove there is a physical anchoring in any other way than with gravity, we still say that people have a core. In practice, it is very useful to learn to sense the area of the body in which it lives. The feedback from people sensing their core is very different—that it can give peace, a point to return to within yourself, *grounding.* Power can feel anxious or good, all depending on how you usually see yourself—contact with deep feelings of sorrow, anger, happiness, wanting; a feeling of being me and the right to be me; contact with the essence of who I am—bodily grounding of the soul.

Concretely, it is a fact that movements with arms and legs will have increased power if you feel the core, and imagine that the movement starts there. Try it—push or pull another person who is giving you resistance. Does it make a difference whether you feel the gravity or the core? I claim that no matter what you do with the rest of your body, the action or movement will have more power without working harder, and it will feel more integrated and whole, if you have a sense of your core at the same time. The claim is based on my own and my colleagues' sensations, as well from watching hundreds of clients and students and reading their feedback forms.

So, how can you use centering in relation to taking care of yourself as a therapist? A classic error amongst therapists is to forget themselves, and get so busy understanding or helping the client that the attention moves to the other person. Centering is a tool to help break that pattern. To feel my core at the same time as I listen and watch the client is, after eighteen years as a therapist, still part of my daily training. It helps me to stay within myself. It helps me stay separated from the client and be able to differentiate the sensations coming from me and coming from the client. It helps also to sense myself in my role, to feel that I am there and that I am in some kind of mood which has something to do with my life, no matter what the work I am doing at the moment is doing to me. It means that I am keeping contact with the stream that is me. It is important to be able to do that in a job where the focus is on the other person's process. It is important so that I do not disappear in myself. And it is important for the client. The client needs me to be there, with my core and everything else.

A concrete example of centering is to ask inside the core: *How am I doing? How do I like what is happening now? Can I like it or not?* The answers that come from the core can be surprising, inspirational, difficult, and provoking, but one thing is certain—they are honest. Body sensations never lie. What you feel in your body, here and now, is not to be discussed. It *is*. The kinds of answers that this method gives are, in my opinion, a good ingredient to the decision-making process as a therapist.

How do you learn to feel your core? How do you train centering? A concrete method is to focus on the body sensations of the physical structure around the core; it means to do movements or concentration exercises around the backbone, especially in the lower back, the deep stomach muscles (*m. iliopsoas*, diaphragm, floor of the pelvis), and the outer stomach muscles. If the physical sensation of the space around the core becomes clear, it will, for most people, increase the possibility of feeling an energetic point—meaning the core.

Another part of the training is to find a language in which to describe the core. Many languages can be used. An energetic point can be described as a color, a picture, a form, a sound, a sense, or a form of movement. To find a language that fits the sensation of the core is a personal and, to some, an intimate process. The language is important. When we give language to something, we bring it within reach of the Ego. We seal it. The language is necessary in order for the centering to become a tool. One can ask oneself: How does my core feel today? Has it got a different color from yesterday? Is it smaller? Is it bigger? Is it closed on one side? Is it open on the other? It is a way in which to follow oneself, to sense one's condition. And it demands a language.

Grounding Makes It Possible To Contain

Another important tool in the work with bodily closeness is the sensation of grounding.

Sensing one's grounding has both a physical and an energetic side. The physical side is sensing one's feet and feeling the pressure against them while standing. I can then sense my physical weight—my seventy kilograms—and they are carried by the surface of my body no matter whether I stand, or sit, or lie down. Gravity works, and that is what we feel when we sense our grounding. We feel the force that keeps us on the ground.

It sounds easy, but for many people it is a matter of fear and anxiety, and may be difficult. It demands a kind of surrendering. I must let myself fall energetically toward the ground, and trust that it will actually carry me. Many people avoid this sensation by "lifting themselves away" from the ground. Even when they are on the ground, they avoid feeling it by giving up sensing the feet, by keeping busy constantly, by never standing still, or by standing up as little as possible.

The avoidance comes because the sensation of grounding would wake memories—the historical paths of life that have made it difficult or had an influence on the person's trust toward the surroundings. Literally spoken—the trust of the ground under me. Trust that it will hold me. Trust in the ground I am standing on. The willingness to sense the reality I am in. All this is created or denied during childhood in relation to the people surrounding the child. The emotional contact—the mutual connection—is what creates the ground underneath us.

Despite the problems connected to that, it is possible to revive good grounding. Fortunately, the body provides such a possibility, no matter what baggage you carry along (physical handicaps give special problems, which I will not comment on here). You are standing on your feet when standing. Gravity works. Your weight is carried by the surface. Energy can float through your body, the legs, the feet, down in the ground below you. At the same time, energy can flow upward from the ground. The postural muscles can work in your lower legs, your thighs, and your back and keep you standing—a beautiful cooperation between downwards and upwards energy. It feels like this when the grounding is in balance, and is neither held nor released, given up nor controlled—when it is just there.

What is the point of that? What can a sensation of grounding give us? It might be easiest to understand when explaining what happens when it is missing. If, for example, a person gets really frightened and cannot feel the grounding, then it is impossible to contain their fear. It is not possible to hold such a strong feeling without the sensation of grounding. The person must either suppress the emotion or be overwhelmed, destroyed, or lost in it. None of these positions contain closeness and none of these positions allow contact.

It is different if you can keep the grounding. The sensation of the grounding, the concrete sensation of the feet against the ground—that my legs and back are carrying me even though it feels like I am going to pieces—is the sensation that the ground is there (disregarding situations with earthquakes, etc.), meaning that I can see the ground and my feet can feel the pressure. All these sensations make it possible to hold the fear or any other strong emotion, if you have to live it out. What does the grounding offer? It gives balance, ground under your feet, a possibility to stand, a possibility to contain life, a possibility to be able to differ, a possibility to stay—in reality—on earth when things get hard or are very powerful.

In relation to being a therapist and taking care of oneself, it is obvious to me that good grounding is a great advantage for yourself as a therapist, as well as for the treatment and the client. As therapists, we are constantly introduced to human problems, the shadow side of life—either as physical illness/weakness or as psychological difficulties. We listen to people's problems from their past and present. We agree to see the part of reality that many people normally hide. We are there for many things. To cope with that, we need our own grounding—to feel the ground—and feel that it carries and supports us from below. I do not have to carry the load by myself; the ground is under me and allows me to feel my feet, legs, and back. This also helps to contain the reality that the client represents and to know that it is not my reality. So, I am standing here feeling my grounding, and over there is the client feeling his/her body and reality. To feel the grounding is like feeling centered—a tool to help being within yourself.

I have until now, to make things easier, described grounding only from the standing position with the feet on the ground, standing up straight. But of course, it is not only when you stand that you have access to grounding.

Gravity works no matter which position you are in. We always have a supporting surface that our weight rests upon. When we sit, the weight is transmitted through the sitting muscles and back of the thighs to the chair, and through the chair to the surface. We find grounding through the parts of the body that rest against the surface.

Depending on how our history has left traces in our body, it can be harder or easier to sense our grounding in certain positions. Some people do not feel comfortable grounding when standing, but have no trouble when sitting, or the other way around.

As a therapist, it can provide you with a good tool to stay connected if you learn your preferred grounding positions. At the same time, you learn which positions to avoid. A personal example: If I sit too long in a chair, I have a tendency to start hanging, whereby I lose my sensation—both the up-going and the down-going energy. I give up or become relaxed, and though it is not the same as "falling," I am conscious of the movement. I lose my sensation of grounding.

If I do not break this bodily pattern—if I remain sitting—then I become tired. I am not thinking clearly, and I lose control of the therapy session. The way I break the pattern is to get up and walk around the room a bit, feel my legs, and recapture my grounding when standing and walking.

What do you do to train grounding? Our methods are many. I will not mention specific exercises, but describe the principles that we focus on in the training. Firstly, we try to communicate how the optimal grounding functions bodily. But at the same time, we it make clear that you have to respect the bodily defense that humans contain, and that cannot be changed solely by grounding exercises.

Balancing leads to focusing on how the individual can obtain the best sensation of the grounding rather than focusing on whether or not the grounding is "correct."

A last comment on grounding: My description of the concept has focused on the fact that we actually have ground under our feet—that we have a solid ground to stand on. But what if you are in a boat on the water, or in a plane? Does that mean that the grounding disappears? No, you can also feel gravity work when there is water or air around you and the postural muscles are still working to keep you up. Try to sense it the next time you are in a plane: you are still connected to the planet while the engines of the plane carry you in space. As long as we are on earth, even in its atmosphere, the force we sense as grounding will work. The planet is below us and carries us. So, it would actually be sensible to call it "planet-connection."

Good Boundaries Give Clear Contact

The last tool in working with the bodily sensation that I will describe here is sensation of boundaries. Boundary setting is developed throughout several stages as we are growing up. I will briefly mention the stages that Bodynamic Analysis uses in its theory about boundary setting. The earliest boundary setting is bodily/physically. It is sensed in the skin, on the body surface. It is stimulated from the time when the embryo starts touching the side of the womb. It is stimulated a lot during birth and is nurtured through touch in the first years of living. It is a basic type of boundary setting that tells us where our bodies ends and the surrounding world begins.

The second phase in boundary setting is the development of the energetic boundary, or what we call the making of "personal space." It is the air around me that belongs to me, which I have a right to control. This boundary is made during the first few years of living. A number of psychologists, among them Margaret Mahler, have described the development from symbiosis to a gradual separation, through the rapprochement phase to the actual separation.

If this process develops normally, the child will have a sensation of his personal space, and therefore can sense an energetic separation from the mother and other closely connected adults.

The sensation of the energetic boundary setting takes place both in the physical body and with the energy. I feel in my body what is happening with my energy—whether it is respected, bothered, invaded, or met by other people. For example, heartbeat, sweaty palms, held breath, an impulse to push with my arms, or similar sensations tell me that another person is too close to me at the moment, that my personal space is being pressured or invaded. Conversely, a warm flow in my chest, a clear sensation of my feet against the floor, calmness in my stomach, or similar sensations tell me that the physical distance I have to the one I am talking to is good. In other words, my personal space is large enough for the moment.

I will only mention briefly the third and fourth phases in boundary setting. The third phase is the development of the territorial setting, where the child learns to mark her place—her home or geographical area. This process begins when the child is around three years old. The social setting is the fourth and last phase in the boundary setting in a child. This kind of limitation is about knowing who I belong to, which "we" I am part of, and how I let people know. This process runs from about seven years old and up.

In relation to taking care of oneself as a therapist, meaning taking care of oneself in fairly close proximity to another person, it is the bodily and the energetic limitation that will be most relevant.

Every person has a body and a personal space and the right to control it. It sounds simple. Unfortunately, it is not natural for all people. We are all affected by our history of patterns of relating in the family and by single trauma, which have left holes or weakness in our boundary setting, physically and energetically.

Just like with grounding, it is the body that holds the original capacity. It is hidden in muscles and tissue which have forgotten, held back, or given up. But underneath these defense reactions, the original impulses are still there: the impulse to say *stop* when I do not want to continue; the impulse to move away; impulses to state what I want; impulses in the arms to push away and pull toward; to say no and yes; the impulse to state the physical distance I want to have from another person; the impulse to fill up my body and my personal space with me.

It is training of these and similar skills that leads to a better energetic containment, and thereby an increased ability to be present with the client in a clear *I-you* contact, a contact in which it is clear which emotions, sensations, and thoughts are mine and which are yours; a contact that is based upon the respect that *you have your space and I have mine*—each having our soul energy and our own history with which to fill out the space.

Training in body sensation is important in working with physical and energetic boundaries. A focus on the sensation of the skin and the sensation of the surface of the body increases the physical limitation. Adults cannot always feel their skin. With some, it is forgotten or neglected, and needs to be rediscovered through touch, massage, nurturing with creams, rolling movements on a carpet, etc.

Training in sensing and tightening a specific group of muscles helps clarify the energetic boundary. An example of an exercise is tightening of the outer muscles in the thighs and arms. By sensing the outer limitations of the physical body more clearly, the energy around will also get clearer or more concentrated.

Taken together, **centering, grounding**, and **boundaries** are what we call the fundamental skills for contact—and therefore they are also fundamental skills that a therapist must have. They are all connected to sensations in the body. They are all extremely good tools in the project, which in my opinion must be the goal of the therapist, *to take care of oneself as a person, while taking care of your clients*.

The Therapeutic Power of Peak Experiences: Embodying Maslow's Old Concept

—Erik Jarlnaes, M.A., & Josette van Luytelaar

"In a peak experience the subject at least momentarily loses all fear, including the fear of disintegration, insanity, and death."—A. Maslow

Summary

In this article, the authors investigate the concept of peak experience and ask themselves how Bodynamic therapy can contribute to enhancing and eliciting peak experiences. Their findings are mainly based on a large number of interviews that Erik Jarlnaes conducted in his journalistic and therapeutic practice. They research the concept of "peak experience" as developed by Maslow and compare it with Csikszentmihalyi's concept of "flow." Adding from their own experience, they come to an encompassing definition and to ten core characteristics. More specifically, they pay attention to body aspects and investigate connections, differences, and similarities between shock and peak experiences. They presuppose that peak experiences contain resources of energy and ego strength. Many interviewees were not aware of utilizing resources in generating their peak experiences. Consequently, they were not able to use them to improve their daily life quality. Furthermore, they had not shared their experience with other people. This lack of awareness led the authors to explore if and how peak experiences could be involved in therapy. The authors examine different approaches of peak (and shock) experiences within the frame of Bodynamics, a somatic developmental psychotherapy system.

Since Maslow developed the concept of peak experience thirty-five years ago, it has been a continuous focus of interest for psychologists, and has been mentioned in many self-help books on personal growth. However, systematic research on the subject is still missing as well as systematic development of its qualities as a therapeutic tool. Most books on this subject tend to give only a general overview.

Erik Jarlnaes's many years of research led him to these guiding questions: "Is it possible to elicit a peak experience?" and "How can we help people develop a new peak experience?" He became interested in the subject as a journalist interviewing athletes on their peak experiences. He discovered that the interviewing process itself deepens the intensity and the quality of the interviewed person's experience. The interview helps people to get into deep contact with an essential life quality in themselves, something that they usually have not shared with another person, like a deep secret (in this case, a positive one).

Jarlnaes then decided to start more systematic research, by conducting "peak interviews" (an intense dialogue where the "peak" subject is unraveled in specific details) with a variety of people, ranging from top athletes (including gold medal holders and world champions), to leaders, managers, and therapists, but also "ordinary people." In the end, this brought him to use the peak interview as a specific therapeutic tool (we describe this in the second part of the article). He also started researching literature and developing tools and exercises for therapeutic and personal development work within the frame of the Bodynamic System (a Danish-developed body-oriented psychotherapy system that integrates psychological, social and motor development on one side and a pedagogical approach on the other).

One of the well-known top athletes that Erik Jarlnaes peak interviewed was the American track and field star Bob Beamon. When he long-jumped 8.90 meters and set an astonishing world record in Mexico City's high-altitude thin air during the 1968 Olympic Games, he had a peak experience.

Sixteen years later, at the Olympic Games in Los Angeles, Bob Beamon told Jarlnaes, "It was like jumping through a barrier, running in a tunnel, with walls of vibrant silence, time stood still, I had full access to all my muscles, to my whole body, my sensations were bright, there was a sense of joy and love …" Although the experience was still crystal clear in his mind, at first Bob Beamon did not seem to realize what had happened. Not only was he confused about what had happened to him right after the jump, but also later, when he went around asking everybody what had happened. No one could answer—no one knew. He kept searching for an answer, and one day he discovered Abraham Maslow's books. Only then he realized he had had a peak experience.

Many people, like Bob Beamon, do not seem to realize what happened to them, and are not aware of their resource qualities. This is our primary reason for exploring if and how peak experiences could be involved in therapy.

In this article we will:

- Explore Maslow's definition of peak experience and distinguish it from the concept of flow, later introduced by Csikszentmihalyi. Comparing these with Jarlnaes's research findings we will come to a more complete definition of a peak experience and an overview of peak characteristics.

- Look at differences and similarities between peak and shock and the connections between them. For this, it is necessary to explain shock trauma therapy as developed by Bodynamics.

- Throw some light upon bodily aspects of flow and peak.

- Discuss the peak interview as developed by Jarlnaes not only as an intake interview but also as an important therapeutic tool.

- Describe some therapeutic situations in which work on peak experiences, in our view, can be helpful, even essential.

1. Peak Experience and Peak Definition

In this section we will investigate the concepts of peak and flow with the following three questions as a lead:

First, can everybody have a peak experience? Or do you have to be "psychologically mature," as Maslow suggests, in order to have a peak experience?

Second, is a peak a moment or a process? Is it a state of being or a dynamic stream?

Third, is a peak something that just happens or is it possible to elicit a peak? Is it possible to repeat a peak experience? Can one foster a peak experience in therapy or in daily life? And, if yes, what are the conditions?

The following is built on the research of Maslow, Csikszentmihalyi, and Jarlnaes. With different points of view, the interview questions differ, and thus the results are difficult to compare directly, even though all are valuable to answer our questions.

Maslow: The Happiest Moment

The concept of peak experience originally came from Maslow. He was an important representative of Humanistic Psychology in which the "self-actualizing" of the individual was a core concept. According to him, a peak experience was an indissoluble part of the self-actualizing of a person. He gave the following definition of a peak in his book *Toward a Psychology of Being* (1968):

> ... an episode or sudden wave, in which all potentials of a person are flowing together in a particularly goal-oriented and intense gratifying way, in which he is more integrated and less split, is more open to experience, in which he is more coming forward with his own specific nature or disposition, is more spontaneous and expressive, more fully functioning, more creative, humoristic, ego-transcendent, less dependent on his lower instincts, etc. In these periods he becomes more really himself, more powerful in actualizing his capacities, more close to the essence of his Being, more fully human ...

In describing a peak experience, Maslow was rather broad, mainly using quotes from artists and philosophers describing their experiences in mystical or religious terms, or in terms of beauty. This creates the impression that, although in theory everyone has the possibility to have a peak, only very few people do have such experiences. Maslow identified personality traits of "peak persons," although in his later works he tended more to "secularize" the experience to everyday activities, so to be accessible to more people.

In his eighty research interviews, Maslow was focusing on the happiest moment. He was referring to a moment or a state rather than to a process, so his descriptions tend to be static.

Csikszentmihalyi: The Process of Flow

Csikszentmihalyi tends to look into the dynamics of peak experience more than Maslow. He conducted research on thousands of individuals from a variety of social and cultural backgrounds and discovered that at least thirty percent of them have peak experiences. He refers to a state of consciousness—a process as well as the peak moment. He defines peak experience, which he named randomly optimal experience, autotelic experience or flow (experience) as follows:

> *An optimal experience is the feeling that the required technical ability and the challenges are in balance with each other, in a goal-oriented rule-oriented action system that makes clear how one is performing. The concentration is so intense that one has no attention anymore for matters of lower importance or worries about problematic questions. The self-consciousness disappears and the time frame distorts.*

His concept of flow is shown in the diagram below, where challenge and skills come together in balance, and lead to a flow of high-level energy. However, if one's skills at a certain moment are "too high" in relation to the challenge present, one loses interest in the activity, and starts feeling bored; if the challenge becomes "too high" in relation to the skills, one experiences anxiety. Both conditions stimulate you to get into a flow-situation again, this time of a higher quality than the original flow-situation.

Challenge

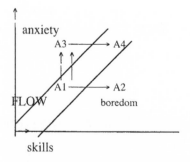

The Flow Diagram (from Csikszentmihalyi, M., 1990, p.107)

For example, A is a boy who is learning to play tennis. The diagram shows A at four different points in time. At the start (A1), he has few tennis playing skills and his only challenge is to play the ball over the net. He will enjoy this because the degree of difficulty is in balance with his limited skills. That is, he probably is in flow. When he continues exercising, he will play better tennis and start to feel bored with just the same challenge (A2). Then one day he plays against a better opponent and he discovers that tennis has more challenges than he thought. At this point (A3) he starts to be anxious because of his rather moderate performance.

Neither anxiety nor boredom are positive experiences, so A is stimulated to get into flow again: from A2 he can choose a little more advanced opponent to match his level and try to win (A4). From A3 he can increase his skills by more exercising (A4). Both A1 and A4 are flow situations. Even though both create equal enjoyment, A4 is more complex than A1.

These dynamics explain why flow activities lead to growth and discovery. The complexity and the development of the self is the essence of flow. People cannot enjoy the same thing for a long time. When we stay at the same level, we get bored or frustrated. The desire for pleasure leads to an activity that expands our capabilities, and the discovery of new ways to make this capability concrete.

Csikszentmihalyi defines flow as the moment where process and product come together: "An act is performed seemingly without effort; the goal of the stream is that it has to keep streaming." In his view such optimal experiences can happen by coincidence. However, more often they are the result of a structured activity of the individual or the ability to create flow, or both. This statement clarifies that in his view it is possible to actively do something in order to get a peak experience, or to repeat one.

The Process and the Moment

In his definition of flow, however, Csikszentmihalyi mixes the concepts of flow and peak. From the results of our peak interviews, we prefer to make a distinction between them. We define flow as the process, the working toward, or preparation for the peak moment. It is a process of coming into a state of high-level energy that increases the probability of attaining a peak experience. A peak can be prepared for, but cannot be counted on to happen as a consequence.

We agree with Csikszentmihalyi that at first sight peaks seem to happen spontaneously, but on closer investigation they often appear to be the result of a kind of preparing—a "structured activity." In our view, one can increase the probability of a peak by preparing for it (without guarantee that it will happen), both in daily life and in therapy.

Based on Erik Jarlnaes's interviews, we hypothesize that a much higher percentage of people (than Csikszentmihalyi's thirty percent score) have had peak experiences. In fact, we think nearly everyone has. The difference in results could be explained by the different methods used. Jarlnaes's initial interview question was whether a person recognized the peak qualities, while Csikszentmihalyi's did not use interviews but sampled daily experiences from his subjects by a random time schedule and then attributed flow qualities to these experiences afterwards.

We asked many people whether they recognized peak experiences. Most of them promptly answered affirmatively. However, some of them required a longer interview. Only a few people who started on the diagram with very low energy (low on skills and low on challenge) reported to have had no peak experiences at all, but they definitely had flow experiences. Like Maslow, Jarlnaes focused on the happiest moment, but added questions about the dynamics of getting into and coming back from a peak, next to the peak moment itself. Getting access to these dynamics can, in our view, help people to integrate peaks into their life and thus heighten their life quality.

Peak Experience and Peak Performance

Here are a few words here on the concepts of peak experience and peak performance, as many authors confuse them. Notably, Csikszentmihalyi makes no distinction. In our view, a peak performance is referred to mostly in sports. It is a top achievement in the realm of competition, a comparison that is measurable in quantity and in terms of winning and losing. A peak performance is a planned action with regard to strengthening skills that is focused on consciously.

A peak experience, however, is not measured in quantity but in terms of quality. It is unique in itself for each individual and not comparable with peaks of others. It refers to "being," not to "doing." This is the subject of our article.

2. Peak Characteristics

In the end we are only worthwhile because of the essential that we embody, and if we don't embody this, life is wasted—C.G. Jung

As a result of approximately three hundred interviews since 1982, Jarlnaes discovered certain characteristics that are usually present in a peak experience. He found that these common characteristics apply to a wide variety of people—world champions, Olympic Gold medal winners, Danish champions, organizational managers, military people, artists, and ordinary people—and to many different types of experiences. Combined with Maslow's and Csikszentmihalyi's peak characteristics, we can list ten core characteristics—some of them psychological ones, other ones on the body level:

1. Changed time perception, i.e., time seems to stop or to expand in the infinite—to slow down, or the opposite, to speed up.

2. Changed or distorted space perception, physical sizes or shapes change, e.g., a golf hole suddenly becomes as big as a bathtub so one cannot miss it. The experience becomes "framed," i.e., standing out from the background in a strong energy field.

3. In general, all senses become more sensitive. There are changes in all sensory perceptions, like color, smell, and sound. Colors can change and become brighter; a snow-dressed tree can "change" its color into strong green; a silence can become vibrant and a sight can become very sharp.

4. People report having had a transpersonal, transformational, or religious experience. They have a feeling of awe; they feel it as fulfilling their life goal and they express it like "if I would die right here it would be all right."

5. The body is always involved, sometimes physically, but also there can be a changed perception of the body, of body sensations and body movements. People often illustrate their peak story with movements of hands and arms in order to show an expansion—something big, bigger than they are.

6. The feeling that goes with the experience is one of softness, love, bliss, ease, wholeness, grace of the body (also indicating the lack or absence of fear). People always remember a piece of the experience very clearly, like "a spark"; at least one part stands out crystal-clear no matter how many years ago it happened.

7. A peak experience is not easily shared; usually it is experienced as something unique for a person. When they are not really seen by others in this experience, many people feel alone or isolated with it, sometimes even get stuck in it.

8. There is an inner sense of meaning, like having received a "message," sensing a life direction, or life essence; hearing a voice speaking to them.

9. The activity in which the peak is embedded is often goal-directed.

10. The experience involves a very high level of energy or a high charge.

These characteristics lead us to the following description of a peak experience:

A peak experience is the moment when a person feels everything come together, when one feels the profound joy of great achievement. It is a boundary-expanding experience, even when it does not lead to a gold medal. A peak experience is one of the greatest events of a person's lifetime, where normal perception expands so that a person can perform beyond their normal capabilities. It is an experience where time stands still, physical sizes or shapes appear to change; colors intensify. There is a feeling of softness, bliss, openness, and love; it feels like a transformation. A person may not share the details of the peak experience with anyone, but will always remember it clearly and precisely.

3. Differences and Similarities
Between Peak and Shock

Working from Bodynamic Analysis, we discovered that there are connections and some striking similarities (but also differences) between peak experiences and so-called shock experiences. We will explain the concept of shock from the viewpoint of Bodynamic shock trauma theory.

A shock is defined as a traumatic event with the following characteristics:

- The situation is actually life threatening (or experienced by the client as such).

- The situation has not been worked through or it has not been possible for the client to react to (or reexperience) the situation in an appropriate way, i.e., using the ego and the biological reflexes of orientation, fight or flight that we share with many animals.

- The client, instead, has reacted from the deep and primitive instinct pattern of paralysis.

Extrapolated from animal research we assume that people react instinctively in a sudden dangerous situation in one of three ways: fight, flight, or freeze. It is a survival reaction—and it is necessary to add that sometimes one does not survive.

Bodynamics follows Levine in the assumption that shock is in fact a kind of freezing in a situation where people have lost the possibility of moving, i.e., a fight-or-flight reaction. This is demonstrated in numbness, partially going "out-of-the-body" (dissociation) and a "holding" in specific muscles. The bodily freezing in the moment then expands into one's life; life patterns become frozen, and one gives up activity. The result is a diminished quality of life.

An example: When the ferry boat Estonia sank in the Baltic Sea in 1995, many young people sitting in the bar got numb and did not move from their chairs in the restaurant on the top deck—while others did move (flight) and escaped from the ship, and eventually survived.

Different body psychotherapies include "finishing" the frozen (or unfinished) movement to cure a shock trauma (e.g. Ogden's Sensorimotor Psychotherapy or Levine's Somatic Experiencing). Bodynamics developed a "working-with-shock recipe" where a unique running technique is practiced (in combination with working through the shock story) for the body to learn the flight reaction. The fight reflex is also relearned in the same procedure.

In addition to that, therapeutic work with peak-shock combinations showed the possibility to use peak experiences to help resolve shock. Peak and shock have many characteristics in common—like changed or distorted time and space perception. Often both are intrinsically connected: often a peak and a shock come together in the same situation and get mixed up. For example, interviews with Estonia survivors indicate that when the disaster happened time stood still, their sight got tunnel-sharp while their hearing got blurred. At the same time, they had a kind of peak seeing the beauty of the ship sinking into the waves.

Shock experiences are negative by definition. Although they have many of the same features as peak experiences, there are also features that change the whole experience into one that diminishes the quality of life. There is freezing instead of flow. The one feature that greatly diminishes the quality of life is guilt, e.g., the guilt of being a survivor, the guilt of not having helped others. It is possible to relieve the guilt and resolve the shock if one can "free" the peak part in it, or clarify its "inner message."

Containing High-Level Energy

An important aspect of a peak (and of a shock) is the state of high-level energy experienced, both psychologically and bodily (in the muscles). The Bioenergetic concept of "charge" is related to this and refers to the body energy that can be charged or de-charged. Csikszentmihalyi's diagram, where he explains that challenge and skills come together in balance and lead to a flow of ever-increasing high-level energy, is helpful here. It is conditional to get a peak experience. Some people describe this state as the air being so dense that one can nearly cut it with a knife. Others describe strong physical vibrations. High-level energy is also referred to in descriptions like, "She could not stand the intensity of the situation," "The tension was too high for him to function," or "He got cramped in his play."

People can have difficulty containing this high-level energy (or charged state) in their peak (or their shock). This often results in losing the peak or "freezing" in shock, which can cause psychological or psychosomatic problems.

Containment work therefore is the core of Bodynamic peak/shock work, where the therapist stimulates the "energy management" on the psychological level as well as the muscular level, and builds vertical channels along the spine, by physical and energy exercises.

The peak energy is built up slowly compared with the shock energy, which is more abrupt and explosive of nature. However, Bodynamic peak/shock work avoids the total energy surge. The therapist works around the core of the client's shock, looking for the location of the peak moment, and insisting on dealing first with the peak energy rather than the shock energy (especially by contact, talking, and body sensing). In fact, one works with alternately raising (charging) and containing the energy.

4. The Body in Flow and Peak

The body is involved both in the preparing (to get into the flow) and in the peak moment itself (where it changes the perception of the body, sometimes described as "moving with a kind of smoothness or grace"). Flow is about the body. Flow is like warming up, preparing the body, making it warm and strong, to get into a state of high-level energy.

Here is an example from Jarlnaes's own experience playing table tennis with a friend: "By playing, he first warms up the body, specifically the parts to be used. Then he and his friend move into flow—a steady playing rhythm. After playing like this for some time they are 'ready'; then one of them adds a 'challenge part'—something new and unexpected—and then the peak can come in."

Getting into flow is a precondition. It can even be physical hardship and requires discipline. One example is a violin player, daily practicing for many hours, in order to get into the flow. Often the peak happens unexpectedly, "suddenly there is music instead of just practicing." Another frequent example is that of athletes surpassing world records during training.

Enduring physical hardship is a way for many people to prepare for a peak.

It is a kind of "ritual." For author Josette van Luytelaar, trekking can be a peak experience. It needs the ritual to build up walking condition, to get into a certain walking rhythm (flow). The ritual presupposes that you have to suffer before there is a reward. And then suddenly the reward—the peak—can come in: "I felt I walked no longer on the earth, but above it; I felt it was not hard work; I could continue to go straight upward forever, like I had wings. The view was breathtakingly beautiful, and the color of the sand intensely red."

Stimulating the senses or sensory experiences is another commonly used way to get into the flow: seeing art works or nature, creating art, hearing or performing music, tasting haute cuisine food, moving, dancing, playing sports, and having sex.

Csikszentmihalyi also mentions the preparatory role of the body in flow. He sees many similarities between flow and eastern body-training methods like yoga and martial arts (e.g., qi gong, tai chi, judo, and aikido). Both aim for control over consciousness, for a harmonious one-point direction of the mind. Both try through intense concentration, which can be achieved by physical discipline, behavioral habits, or rituals and sensory training, to reach a state of mind where happiness or *nirvana* is experienced. A difference, however, is that flow as a Western technique tries to strengthen the self (centering), whereas yoga and other Eastern methods aim for disappearance of the self (melting into the universe).

Bodynamics developed a special technique to get the body into flow: the so-called "slow flow" movement practice, in which never-ending slow motion movements in a continuous rhythm are exercised with the help of music. It is a movement series in which there are elements of challenge, skills, and balance. It is a ritual that brings people into a state of flow by elements such as concentration, relaxation, breathing, and body centering.

5. The Peak Interview

As mentioned, Jarlnaes developed the so-called peak interview in his research. This is not just a journalistic interview, but mainly a therapeutic instrument. It is the first therapeutic intervention and its goal is to get a client's peak experiences to a conscious level; to enhance the process of resourcing; and to elicit new peak experiences. This includes an actively participating role of the therapist/ interviewer.

The interview can be introduced like this:

"Let us talk about one of your better experiences in life, no matter how old it is—an experience where you may remember something very clearly and you may have never shared it before. It will likely be characterized by a sense of 'time stops,' when your senses became very sharp, and you experienced a deep feeling of happiness."

Then, in our view, the following elements should be included:

1. To bring into consciousness elements that played a role in (getting to) the peak, in order to deepen the experience and add more energy or charge to it. This can be done by helping a person to tell the peak story in the here-and-now, and in as much detail as possible, by asking concrete questions like, "How does it feel in your body right now?" "Could you describe it in the present tense?" "What does it look like?" or "What movement is associated to it?"

2. To be in tune to awareness of the body part of the peak. Interviewing includes asking about the body sensations and body movements, in addition to the feelings and thoughts connected with the peak experience. The body aspect is important, as we have stressed before, but is sometimes easily lost because a peak can be an out-of-body experience. From the interview, the therapist elicits body statements. The next step is to ask for body movements that let the interviewee sense the sensations he/she had during the peak experience.

3. To pay attention to the peak moment, but also to add questions about the process of preparation and getting into flow, and about the "cooling down" afterwards.

4. To focus on the contact between interviewer and interviewee. This is one way of raising or charging the client's energy level, and it also helps the client to contain the high energy level.

5. To focus on the importance of sharing the experience. Usually this is the first time the peak experience is shared, and this in itself can free the client from being stuck in isolation (as in the example of Bob Beamon), and bring him/her into the flow again, sometimes into a new peak.

6. To check which peak elements are (not) integrated in the person's daily life.

7. To search for the "peak message," to pay attention to where the person feels he is in contact with the essence of his being, his life direction.

6. Therapeutic Applications

Therapists can apply work on peak experiences in different realms. Peak work is recommended in counseling or in personal growth issues, where the client's wish is to develop a higher quality of life (*resourcing from peak*).

Working on peak experiences can, in our view, be very useful, even essential, for clients suffering from shock trauma (*peak-in-shock work*).

Some people can experience a shock connected with or during the peak moment, which prevents repeating the peak experience or peak performance and integrating it in their life. They get stuck, for which they seek help. Other times it is clear that people do not try to achieve the peak-state again, either because they do not know it is possible, or because they have never thought about it, or believe they are alone with this experience. In these cases, peak work is also helpful (*shock-in-peak work*).

Below we will give examples of these different kinds of work.

Resourcing from Peak

Often people strive for the qualities inherent in peak experiences, without consciously knowing the resource elements. When people get conscious of their peak experiences, they attain the possibility to actively choose when, where, and how they can pursue and integrate these aspects in their daily life. This work is very valuable. First, the client shares—often for the first time—a peak experience with the therapist or counselor, which is often a new peak in itself, as it frees the person from his or her believed "existential loneliness." Moreover, having the elements transferred and installed in daily life, the client is able to create resources to a rich new liveliness and happiness and even enhance them.

"Resourcing" in Bodynamic terms means giving clients more options in life by putting them in contact with their ego strength, e.g., the ability to say no or stop, the ability to sense what you like to do, the ability to assert yourself.

The Window to Life Quality

A fifty-five-year-old female workshop participant had a special sunlight experience. Sitting for a written paper examination together with other students when she was eighteen years old, suddenly the sun broke through the large windows in the room and totally engulfed her. In that moment, her posture straightened with confidence, and she suddenly knew all the answers to the questions (they turned out to be correct). She then quickly finished her paper.

When asked about her working conditions, she said that her office had only small windows facing north with very little sun. However, since she was the manager, she was able to choose another room with large windows facing west. When she returned for the next workshop module, she reported that her quality of life had definitely increased, she experienced more joy, felt more present in her body and psychologically. Her colleagues picked up her changed energy, so that they also experienced more joy and became more productive.

The Message of the Body Movement

Interviewing E, a female client of forty-four, she told about a peak experience: While skiing downhill in nature, among big trunks of trees in the snow, she got into a flow. Suddenly she felt the movement opened her up, and then a feeling of total freedom, of letting go, of floating, engulfed her. During the therapy session, she was brought back to the experience by letting her consciously repeat the body movements she made spontaneously during her telling of the story. These mainly included a movement of her hands from her head down all along her body and then to the front of her. When asked to repeat and exaggerate the movement, she suddenly got the message of her peak: "This is what I have to do in my daily life more," she said, "to let go of control."

Improving a Jazz Musician's Teaching Skills

A famous jazz musician had a problem. He did not know how to teach students his method of improvising (which lead him into a peak). During our interviews, he realized that his improvisations were intuitive—not practiced or planned. He was unaware of how he attained the peak. Using knowledge of the peak-experience work, he came to understand how he prepared himself to get into the flow, and from there to the peak. He did this by conducting several rituals: by cleaning his instrument first, by doing breathing exercises before playing, and by concentrating on one particular tone. He would then exercise for some time. This gave him the insight into how he could also teach his students how to get into the flow.

Peak-in-Shock Work

Working on peak experiences can, in our view, be very useful—even essential—for clients suffering from shock trauma. There is always a connection between a peak part and a shock part in the same situation. If you can "free" the peak part or get its "inner message" clear, resolving the shock is much easier. In this sense, peak work has therapeutic value. From work with Estonia survivors and others, it shows that guilt—from surviving at the cost of other people's lives—disappears when the clients get hold of their peak quality energy, their personal dignity.

Therefore, in therapy we focus on resources in the peak part, building the bridges in the dissociation. Mainly we look for a moment of light before the shock, instead of going into the shock. Below we will give different examples of peak-in-shock work.

The Forest Worker Overcoming Shock Trauma

A forty-year-old Canadian forest worker accidentally cut off all the fingers on one hand with a chain saw. He was alone at the time of the accident, so his reaction was very important. Not only did he have to stop some of the bleeding, but he also had to decide how to survive the next hour. Should he call the local emergency station and ask them to find him, or should he take his car and drive to the station, so they could take him from there to a hospital?

This decision was taken from a "helicopter-level." His consciousness seemed to hang in the air, and from this position he could overview the whole situation. He decided that they might not be able to find him fast enough, because of lack of direction signs. He decided to drive himself, calling the emergency station and alerting his pending arrival. He survived, he lost his hand, and he later fell into a deep depression that triggered alcohol problems. These problems were the reasons for his coming to therapy.

In the moment he "hung in the air," it was as if time stood still. All senses were razor-sharp; there was a religious dimension present—all elements that indicate that a peak experience occurred in that moment. In the session the client realized, sensed, and accepted that his survival actions were based on a decision that came from a place higher than his normal Ego, a higher "me,"—the Soul—with a spiritual connection. With this experience, he also realized that the decision was to survive and make the best of it, and not to fall into a depression with alcohol. This changed his negative life script (being a failure) into a positive one (being a survivor). By staying at this particular moment, "hanging in the air," it became possible to see his action as an adequate coping mechanism. This freed him from his depression.

The work with this client started by looking for the peak element, the instinctual decision that made him survive (the best possible choice). It is in this aspect that Bodynamic therapy differs from many other approaches in working with traumatic incidents. Bodynamic shock trauma work first tries to identify the peak elements in the trauma. The next step is to let the client reexperience where these peak elements enter into the trauma story, and finally to let the person experience the unique quality from which he/she was able to act in such a way that he/she survived the traumatic situation.

The underlying goal of this approach is to free the energy frozen in the shock situation, restore the capacity to have "free floating" emotions, and let the client regain the feeling of control and choice. Another goal is to avoid entering into more fight-or-flight responses when the client reexperiences the traumatic incident in the therapy. This is important in order to develop new resources in the person that will ensure that the same kind of shock will not reoccur.

The Strength of Dissociation

A thirty-five-year-old Iranian refugee came into therapy because he "acted crazy" when he had verbal fights with his wife. He was a soldier in the war between Iran and Iraq in 1990, where the two sides had trenches that were alternately "run over" by the other side. One time his trench was run over, and all his comrades died except him.

The therapist's diagnosis was that he had developed a shock trauma from the war, which lead to dissociating and strange behavior in fight situations in his daily life, like the verbal fights with his wife.

The therapist's job was to help him understand how he survived and to accept this as a resource.

The peak moment came when a bullet hit him and his consciousness "left his body." He did it so well that the Iraqi soldiers did not want to waste another bullet on him: he was so "far out," looking "so dead" that they left him for dead. (He was saved, and later he came to Sweden, where he came into therapy with a colleague.) He described this moment as having peak characteristics, like time stood still; he suddenly experienced leaving his body and perceived it from the outside, from high up, where his soul went.

First, he had difficulty accepting that he himself had the talent and power to play dead, like being God, but he could accept the importance of Allah, who gave him that power. When this was in place, he accepted his strength in being able to leave his body whenever a situation was too intense, e.g., a fight. With this strength as a resource, it was easier to solve the specific problem, so eventually he could stay in contact with his wife during a verbal fight.

A Trapped Climber Cut Off His Own Arm to Survive

Sometimes people report this kind of work spontaneously. Recently the newspapers reported the exceptional survival of the Colorado climber Aron Ralston. Ralston was trapped by an 800-pound boulder while climbing a canyon. On the fifth day of his ordeal, he cut off his own arm with a pocketknife in order to save his life. He walked out of a remote Utah canyon alone, bloody and dehydrated. In his first public statement in a news conference, he made frequent references to prayer and spirituality. He said he felt a surge of energy on the third day, which happened to be the National Day of Prayer. "The source of the power I felt (to do the unthinkable, to cut off the arm) was the thoughts and prayers of many people, most of whom I will never know," he said in the interview. "I felt they were all praying for me." From our perspective, a more useful exploration of the peak message could be his asking himself the question: "I may never fully understand the spiritual aspects of what I experienced, but I will try." Understanding the peak in that way might help him to overcome the shock.

Shock-in-Peak Work—Bob Beamon's Shock-in-the-Peak

We end this article by continuing Bob Beamon's story:

After his world record jump, Bob Beamon had never jumped again. When he realized he had had a peak experience, the next question came to him: how to overcome this limitation and be able to jump once more. Our explanation is that he experienced a shock connected with the peak moment, which prevented his repeating the peak performance, and then he got stuck. Because he experienced the peak as coming out of the blue, not from his own effort, he became afraid. In a way he dissociated from the experience, and closed off. Here Csikszentmihalyi's diagram comes into play: When the challenge to repeat the peak performance becomes too high in relation to the skills of the person, it leads to anxiety.

It is our premise that therapeutic work could help him become aware of the fact that the peak did not happen just spontaneously, but was in fact the result of his own "structured activity," his preparation. (Partly, Bob already experienced this in the peak interview with Jarlnaes). In this way, he could regain control over the situation, regain trust in his ability, build up trust in the possibility of repeating the peak, and get into flow again.

7. Recommendation

In this article, we collected the latest findings and insights on the value of therapeutic use of peak experiences in Bodynamics. Developments are still ongoing and we can only draw tentative conclusions. Further systematic research and experimental practice is necessary.

However, we hope we have been able to transfer our enthusiasm for this approach to our readers and positively recommend the therapeutic work with peak and flow. It is very consistent with basic principles of Bodynamics, like the resource of mutual connection and emphasizing a person's positive capacities instead of (only) focusing on disabilities and dysfunction.

The authors wish to thank Tineke Dirksen for her skillful editorial advice.

References

Csikszentmihalyi, M. *Flow, the Psychology of Optimal Experience* (New York: Harper-Collins, 1990). (Referrals are from the Dutch edition, 1999.)

Jarlnaes, E. (1992). "Hvad er graenseoverskridende oplevelser?" *Tidsskrift for Idraet* 2:39–41.

Jarlnaes, E. Workshop: "Introduction Bodynamic shock trauma work." Unpublished notes of a professional workshop in the Netherlands, Bodynamic Aps, Amsterdam, 2003.

Jarlnaes, E. Workshop: "Peak, shock, and transition." Unpublished transcriptions of a professional workshop in the Netherlands, Bodynamic International Aps, Amsterdam, 1999.

Jarlnaes, E., S. Jørgensen, & L. Marcher. "Shock trauma training." Unpublished notes of a professional training in the Netherlands, Bodynamic International Aps, Amsterdam, 2001.

Jørgensen, S. (1992). "Bodynamic analytic work with shock/post traumatic stress," *Energy & Character* 23(2).

Jung, C.G. *Personality Types* (London: Routledge and Kegan Paul, 1923).

Levine, P. *Waking the Tiger: Healing Trauma* (Berkeley, CA: North Atlantic Books, 1997).

Lowen, A. *Joy: the Surrender to the Body and to Life* (New York: Arkana/Penguin, 1995).

Macnaughton, I. (Ed.). *Embodying the Mind and Minding the Body, 1st Ed.* (North Vancouver, Canada: Integral Press, 1997).

Maslow, A.H. *Religious Aspects of Peak-Experiences* (New York Harper & Row, 1970).

Maslow, A.H. *Religions, Values and Peak-Experiences* (New York: Penguin Books, 1970).

Maslow, A.H. *Toward a Psychology of Being* (New York, Litton Educational Publishing Inc., 1968).

Norretranders, T. *The User Illusion: Cutting Consciousness Down to Size* (London: Penguin Books, 1999).

Ogden, P., & K. Minton. *Sensorimotor Sequencing: One Method for Processing Traumatic Memory* (Boulder, CO: Hakomi Somatics Institute, 2001).

Ravizza, K. "Qualities of the peak experience." In J.M. Silva and R.S. Weinberg (Eds.) *Psychological Foundations of Sport* (Champaign, IL: Human Kinetics, 1984), 452–461.

Slevin, C. "Trapped climber confronts death, cuts off his own arm to survive," in the *Miami Herald*, May 8, 2003.

Face muscles generally:
Receiving impressions and
social/emotional signalling;
expressing feelings, social space,
dominance, etc.

Muscles of jaw, mouth and tongue:
Incorporation and expulsion of
physical or emotional nourishment and
response to the taste and 'digestibility'
of it. Vocal expression.

Eye and ear muscles:
Focus, orientation and
short & long term planning.

Elbow flexors:
Pulling toward oneself, holding on.

Throat Muscles
Vocal expression — talking.
Balancing head and body:
thought and feeling.

Forearm rotators:
Giving and receiving — closing
and opening to exchange.

Pectorals and serratus anterior:
Feelings of self-worth and
power in intimate and
superficial contact.

Wrist flexors, extensions, radial and ulnar flexors:
Positioning: fine control of
social and interpersonal actions,
such as modifying behavior to
suit present company.

Primary respiratory muscles:
Fullness of being —
'breathing space'.

Finger flexors, ab- and adductors:
Touching, investigating,
holding — gross and fine
adjustment in perception and
handling. Also ability to take in
and to give out. Basis of
coygnitive grasp.

Secondary respiratory muscles:
Control of heightening and
lowering energy levels — as with
emotional change or physical
exertion.

Superficial belly muscles:
Containment of feelings, visceral
streaming sensations, and
emotional and energetic
digestion.

Thumb and little finger opposers:
Refining focus and sensitivity to
minute expressions. Formation of
synthesis. Involved in reading
and writing skills.

Psoas:
Intimate bonding.
Quadratus lumborum:
Balance between acting from own
feelings and impulses or in response
to others.

Hip flexors:
Initiating forward movement
and allowing intimate/sensual
body contact.

Pelvic floor:
Sexual feelings, containment of
deep visceral and sensual/sexual
sensations.

Tensor fascia latae, fractus iliotibialis and knee extensors:
Personal boundaries in
distant and close
relationships, also
collecting oneself and
controlling forward
movement.

PSYCHOLOGICAL MUSCLE FUNCTION

*Bandinelli's Laokoon reproduced with
permission from Gabinetto Uffizi, Firenze*

Ankle and toe extensors:
Willingness to perceive
and face reality

PSYCHOLOGICAL MUSCLE FUNCTION

Neck muscles:
Holding the head up — as
in 'keeping one's head'.
Orientation, willpower, pride.

Shoulder elevators:
Carrying burdens, trying to
keep one's balance when
unsure of footing.

**Shoulder dorsal adductors
and rotators:**
Connecting core self and action.
Self-protection and ability to
receive support from others.
Creating personal space.

**Extensors, flexors, ab- and
adductors of the shoulder joint:**
Personal space and range in
interpersonal activities; when
reaching out, touching,
pushing, holding on to, etc.
Self-worth.

Spinal extensors:
Holding oneself erect —
'standing tall'. Ability to
withstand emotional and
physiological stressors.

Knee flexors:
Choice of direction, control of
forward movement.

Ankle (plantar) flexors:
Standing on one's own feet,
self-assertion, ability to jump.
Ability to take a fall.

Peronei muscles:
Personal balance in group
interaction.

Midfoot and toe flexors:
Ability to sense the ground
and take in security, support
and energy from that contact.

Some muscles respond specifically to trauma:
Pterogoids, splenius capitis, and cervicis,
sartorius, gracilis, plantaris and popliteus.
Also muscles active in the issue
and/or age level involved.

Elbow extensors:
Pushing away, throwing, holding
at a distance.

Finger extensors:
Letting go, making
fine adjustments in
boundaries,
reaching out.

Hip abductors:
Personal boundaries (breadth of
stance), sexual identity, personal
balance.

Hip rotators:
Sexual/sensual self-awareness,
boundaries and social signaling.

Hip extensors:
Strength to stand on one's own,
ability to 'forge ahead', move
powerfully forwards and also
stop forward movement.
Performance capacity and
durability. Ability to take a fall.

Hip adductors:
Intimate, sensual/sexual
contact and feelings.

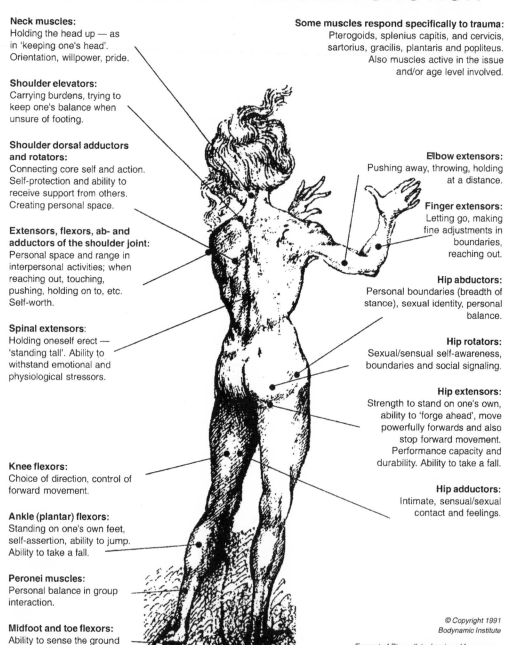

© Copyright 1991
Bodynamic Institute

*Excerpt of Pisanello's drawing of four women
reproduced with permission from the Museum
Boymans van Beuningen, Rotterdam.*

Trauma—the Bodynamic & Somatic Experiencing® Approaches

Developmental and Shock Trauma

The four articles in Part Four deepen our understanding of developmental and shock trauma. The first, "Panic, Biology, Reason: Giving the Body Its Due," by Dr. Peter Levine, is a foundational paper integrating, with numerous examples, the theory and practice of his approach to resolving traumatic experiences. Dr. Levine has created a therapeutic model for addressing trauma called Somatic Experiencing, which he currently teaches. He has developed a unique approach to Somatic Experiencing. I spent many years as client, student, and later co-teacher with Peter, admiring the brilliance of both his approach and his therapy. His exquisite attention to even the slightest shift in pulse, skin color, or eye dilation, puts him in a class by himself.

"It Won't Hurt Forever … Guiding your Child Through Trauma," by Dr. Levine and Maggie Kline, M.S., M.F.T., is a very rich exploration of various types of childhood trauma and offers many interventions that parents and clinicians can use. Kline's background as a family therapist and a school psychologist brings with it many years of exploring these issues with children and their parents.

"Using the Bodynamic Shock Trauma Model in the Everyday Practice of Physiotherapy," by Barbara Picton BSR, M.Ed. (Ons. Psych.), R.C.C., is the fifth contribution. Ms. Barbara Picton is both a physiotherapist and clinical counselor, holding degrees in both professions. She is also a Certified Bodynamic Practitioner. Here she offers her wealth of depth and experience in addressing the effects and treatment of trauma. To my knowledge, it is the first paper written encompassing physiotherapy with somatically oriented psychotherapy, and in particular the Bodynamic Analysis Model of therapy for traumatic imprints. Hence, this is a unique aid to the general reader and all those working in the helping professions.

"Character Structure and Shock" further delineates the Bodynamics theory of developmental and shock trauma. Steen Jørgesen clearly illustrates the impact that a person's character structure has on the ability to work through shock trauma.

Panic, Biology, and Reason: Giving the Body Its Due

—Peter A. Levine, Ph.D.

The Substitute Tiger

My interest in the essential role played by bodily responses in the genesis and treatment of panic anxiety began quite accidentally in 1969. A psychiatrist, knowing of my interest in "mind/body healing"—a fledgling arena at the time— had referred a young woman to see me. Nancy had been suffering from panic attacks for about two years. She had not responded to psychotherapy, while tranquilizers and antidepressant drugs gave her only minimal relief. The referring psychiatrist asked me to do some relaxation training with her. My attempts were equally unsuccessful. She resisted; I tried harder. We got nowhere. Since I knew almost nothing about panic attacks at the time, I asked her for more detailed information about the how and when of her attacks. Nancy revealed that the onset of her first attack occurred while she, along with a group of other students, was taking the Graduate Record Examination. She remembers breaking out in a cold sweat and beginning to shake. Forcing herself to complete the test, Nancy then ran out, frantically pacing the streets for hours, afraid to enter a bus or taxi. Fortunately, she met a friend who took her home. During the following two years her symptoms worsened and became more frequent. Eventually she was unable to leave her house alone and could not follow through with graduate school even though she had passed the exam and was accepted by a major university.

In our conversation, Nancy recollected the following sequence of events: Arriving early, she went to the cafeteria to have a coffee and smoke a cigarette. A group of students were already there, talking about the difficulty of the test. Nancy, overhearing this, became agitated, lit another cigarette, and gulped a second coffee. She remembered feeling quite jittery upon entering the room. She recalled that the exams and marking pencils were passed out and that she wrote vigorously. She became almost breathless at this point and quite agitated. I noticed that her carotid (neck) pulse was increasing rapidly.

I asked Nancy to lie down and I tried to get her to relax. Relaxation was not the answer. Naively, and with the best of intentions, I attempted to help her relax, and she went into a full-blown anxiety attack. Her heartbeat accelerated further to about 150 beats per minute. Her breathing and pulse rate then started to decrease. I was relieved, but only momentarily. Her pulse continued to drop, precipitously to around 50 beats per minute; she became still. Her face paled and her hands begin to tremble as she spoke, "I'm real scared ... stiff all over ... I'm dying ... I can't move ... I don't want to die ... help me ... don't let my die." She continued to stiffen, her throat becoming so tight that she could barely speak. Nancy forced the words, "Why can't I understand this ... I feel so inferior, like I'm being punished ... there's something wrong with me ... I feel like I'm going to be killed ... there's nothing ... it's just blank." Thus, we had rather unfortunately co-discovered, some years before it was reported in the literature, *relaxation-induced panic syndrome*.

The session continued as follows:

"Feel the pencil," I requested without really knowing why.

"I remember now. I remember what I thought," she replied. *My life depends on this exam.* Her heart rate increased now, moving back up into the 80s.

At this point, a "dream image" of a crouching tiger jumping through the bush flashed before me. Quite startled, a fleeting thought about a zoological article I had recently read on *tonic immobility* or *death feigning* prompted me to announce loudly: "You are being attacked by a large tiger. See the tiger as it comes at you. Run toward those rocks, climb them, and escape!"

Nancy let out a blood-curdling yell—a shout that brought in a passing policeman. (Fortunately my office partner took care of the situation—perhaps explaining that I was doing "relaxation training"). She began to tremble, shake, and sob in waves of full body convulsions. I sat with her for almost an hour while she continued to shake. She recalled terrifying images and feelings from age four. She had been held down by doctors and nurses and struggled in vain during a tonsillectomy with ether anesthesia. She left the session feeling "like she had herself again." We continued relaxation, including assertion training, for a couple more sessions. She was taken off medication, entered graduate school, and completed her doctorate in physiology without relapse.

The Body Has Its Reasons . . .

Aaron Beck and Gary Emery, in their seminal book, *Anxiety Disorders and Phobias*, make the point that to understand fear, anxiety, and panic, the person's *appraisal* of a situation is most important. In the chapter, "Turning Anxiety on Its Head," the authors consider cognitive appraisal to be a critical fulcrum in anxiety reactions. They argue that because anxiety has a strong somatic-emotional component, the subtler cognitive processing which occurs may be neglected both in theory and in clinical practice. Clearly Nancy's belief of the difficulty of the exam—based in part on the overheard conversation in the cafeteria—lead to her thought: *my life depends on this,* an unconscious threat appraisal. By focusing narrowly on the cognitive aspects of anxiety, however, Beck and Emery overlook the fundamental role played by bodily responses and sensations in the experience of anxiety. When Nancy drank the coffee and smoked the cigarette (caffeine and nicotine together can be a robust stimulant), the physiological arousal of increased heart rate—both fed into and was fed by her cognitive assessment of the "threat" from the exam, driving her heart rate sharply up. Together, both assessment and physiological activation, resonated with the 'imprinted' bodily reaction of being terrorized and overwhelmed, twenty years before during the tonsillectomy. The panic attack was triggered from that synergy.

In addition to recognizing the importance of cognitive factors, systematic study of bodily reactions and sensate experience is not only important, it is *essential*. This study needs to occur conjointly with the recognition and exploration of cognitive and perceptual factors. Appreciating the role of bodily experience illuminates the complex web called *anxiety* and connects many threads in understanding and modifying its physiological and experiential basis. In addition to turning anxiety on its head, we need also to *connect* the body with the head—recognizing the intrinsic psycho-physiological unity that welds body and mind.

Cognitive theorists believe that anxiety serves primarily to signal the brain to activate a physical response that will dispel the source of anxiety. The role of anxiety is likened in this way to that of pain. The experience of pain impels us to do something to stop it. The pain is not the disease. It is merely a symptom of fracture, appendicitis, and so forth. Similarly, according to Beck, anxiety is not the disease but only a signal: "Humans are constructed in such a way as to ascribe great significance to the experience of anxiety so that we will be impelled to take measures to reduce it." He notes that: "The most primal response depends on the generation of unpleasant subjective sensations that prompt a *volitional* intentional action designed to reduce danger. Only one experience of anxiety is necessary to do this" (italics my emphasis). As an example, Beck mentions the arousal of anxiety when a driver feels that he is not in complete control of the car, which prompts him to reduce his speed until he again feels in control. Similarly, a person approaching a high cliff retreats because of the anxiety.

What is the wisdom of an *involuntary*, primitive, global, somatic, and often immobilizing brainstem response? Is it exclusively for calling the individual's attention to making varied and specific *voluntary* responses? Such an inefficient arrangement is highly doubtful. A lack of refinement in appreciating the essential nuances played by bodily responses and sensations in the structures and experience of anxiety is typical of cognitive approaches. Beck, for example, flatly states, "A specific combination of autonomic and motor patterns will be used for escape, a different combination for freezing, and a still different pattern for fainting. However, the subjective sensation—anxiety—will be approximately the same for each strategy." In the following paragraph of this same article he adds: "An active coping set is generally associated with sympathetic nervous system dominance, whereas a passive set, triggered by what is perceived as an overwhelming threat, is often associated with parasympathetic dominance . . . as in a blood phobic. In either case the subjective experience of anxiety is similar."

Beck's statements reveal a significant glitch in the cognitive phenomenology of anxiety, highlighting its paradoxical nature. According to his reasoning, the same body signal is relayed to the brain's cognitive structures for all forms of threat. The "head" (cognitive) structures are then somehow expected to decide on an appropriate course of action. This top-heavy, Cartesian holdover goes against the basic biological requirements for an immediate, precise, and unequivocal response to threat. It is a view that is quite confusing because it requires that distinctly different kinesthetic, proprioceptive, and autonomic feedback be experienced as the same signal. We have tended, in the post-Cartesian view of the world, to identify so much with the rational mind that the wider role of instinctive, bodily responses in orchestrating and propelling behavior and consciousness has been all but ignored.

Beck's statement that "a specific combination of autonomic and motor patterns will be used for escape, a different combination for freezing, and a still different pattern for fainting" and that "the subjective sensation—anxiety—will be approximately the same for each strategy" contradicts both evolutionary imperative and subjective experience. As one working for thirty-five years in what is now called somatic psychology, these statements simply do not fit the *subjective facts* and would have had William James turning over in his grave. If you ask several anxious people at random what they are feeling, they may all *say* that they are feeling "anxiety." However, if they are then queried with the epistemological question: "How do you *know* that you are feeling anxiety," you will get several different responses. One, for example, could be, "because something bad will happen to me." Another may be that they are feeling strangulated in their throat; still another that their heart is leaping out of their chest; another that they have a knot in their gut. Other people might report that their neck, shoulders, arms, and legs are tight; others might feel ready for action; and still others that their legs feel weak or their chest collapsed. All but the first answer are specific and varied *physical* sensations. And if the person who said what he thought ("... like something bad will happen to me") was directed to a scan of her body, she would have discovered some *somatic/physical* sensation driving and directing the thought.

If we feel threatened and assess that we can escape or fight back, we will feel one set of physical sensations. If, on the other hand, we feel threatened and perceive that we cannot escape or fight back, then we feel something quite different. Now here is the key factor: Both the assessment of danger and the perception of our capacity to respond are not primarily conscious. Let's look to our distant ancestors to illuminate these questions.

Instinct in the Age of Reason

Animals possess a variety of orientation and defensive responses that allow them to respond automatically to different, potentially dangerous situations rapidly and fluidly. The sensations involving escape are profoundly different from those of freezing or collapse. I am in agreement with Beck, in describing panic and post-traumatic anxiety states as having in common "the experience of dread with the perception of inescapability." What I first gleaned from Nancy thirty-five years ago, and later confirmed by the ethological analysis of predator prey behaviors, was that the singular experience of "traumatic panic anxiety" that Beck talks about, occurs *only* where the normally varied and active defensive responses have been unsuccessful, that is, when a situation is *both* dangerous and inescapable. Anxiety, in its pathological panic form (as distinguished from so-called signal anxiety), represents a profound failure of the organism's innate defensive structures to mobilize and thus allow the individual to escape, threatening situations actively and successfully. Where escape is possible, the organism responds with an active pattern of coping. There is the *continuous experience* of danger, running, and escape. When, in an activated state, escape is successfully completed, anxiety does not occur. Rather a fluid (felt) sense of "biological competency" is experienced. Where defensive behaviors are unsuccessful in actively resolving severe threat, anxiety is generated. It is where active forms of defensive response are aborted and incomplete that anxiety states ensue. *Beneath the Monolithic label of anxiety are "camouflaged" a wealth of incomplete and identifiable somatic responses, sensations, and bodily feelings.* These body experiences represent the individual's response to past experience, but also to their "genetic potential" in the form of unrealized defensive responses. The recognition that these instinctive orientation and defensive behaviors are organized motor patterns, that is, prepared motor acts, helps to return the body to the head. Anxiety derives ultimately from a failure to complete motor acts.

Jean Genet, in his autobiographical novel, *Thief's Journal*, states this premise in bold prose: "Acts must be carried through to their completion. Whatever their point of departure, the end will be beautiful. It is (only) because an action has not been completed that it is vile." When orienting and defensive behaviors are carried out smoothly and effectively, anxiety is not generated. Instead, there is the complex and fluid sensate experience perceived as curiosity, attraction, or avoidance. It is only when these instinctive orientation and defensive resources are interfered with—thwarted—that the experience of anxiety is generated: I am not afraid of snakes or spiders, but of my inability to respond effectively to these creatures. Ultimately, we have only one fear—the fear of not being able to cope, of our own un-copability. Without active, available, defensive responses, we are unable to deal effectively with danger and so we are, proportionately, anxious.

Orientations, Defense, and Flight

A scene from an uplands meadow helps to illustrate the *motor act* concept. Suppose you are strolling leisurely in an open meadow. A shadow suddenly moves in the periphery of your vision. Instinctively all movement is arrested; reflexively you crouch in a flexed posture; perceptions are "opened" through activation of the parasympathetic autonomic nervous system. After this momentary arrest response, your head turns automatically in the direction of the shadow or sound in an attempt to localize and identify it. Your neck, back, legs, and feet muscles coordinate so that your whole body turns and then extends. Your eyes narrow somewhat while your pelvis and head shift horizontally, giving you an optimal view of the surroundings and an ability to focus panoramically. This initial two-phase action pattern is an instinctive orientation preparing you to respond flexibly to many possible contingencies. The initial arrest-crouch flexion response minimizes detection by possible predators and perhaps offers some protection from falling objects. Primarily though, it provides a convulsive jerk that interrupts any motor patterns that were already in execution and then prepares the you, through scanning, for the fine-tuned behaviors of exploration or defense.

If it had been an eagle taking flight that cast the shadow, a further orientation of tracking-pursuit occurs. Adjustment of postural and facial muscles occurs unconsciously. This new "attitude of interest," when integrated with the contour of the rising eagle image, is perceived as the feeling of excitement. This aesthetically pleasing sense, with the meaning of enjoyment, is affected by past experience, but may also be one of the many powerful, archetypal predispositions or undercurrents which each species has developed over millennia of evolutionary time. Most Native Americans, for example, have a very special, spiritual, mythic relationship with the eagle. Is this a coincidence, or is there something imprinted deep with in the structures of the brain, body, and soul of the human species that responds intrinsically to the image of eagle with correlative excitement and awe? Most organisms possess dispositions, if not specific approach/avoidance responses, to moving contours. A baby chick, without learning from its mother, for example, flees from the moving contour of a hawk. If the direction of movement of this silhouette is reversed, however, to simulate a goose, the baby chick shows no such avoidance response.

If the initial shadow in the meadow had been from a raging grizzly bear rather than from a rising eagle, a very different preparedness reaction would have been evoked—the preparation to flee. This is not because we think "bear," evaluate it as dangerous, and *then* prepare to run. It is because the contours and features of the large, looming, approaching animal cast a particular light pattern upon the retina of the eye. This stimulates a pattern of neural firing that is registered in phylogenetically primitive brain regions. This "pattern recognition" triggers preparation for defensive responding before it is registered in consciousness. These responses derive from genetic predispositions, as well as from the outcomes of previous experiences with similar large animals. Non-conscious circuits are activated, triggering preset patterns or tendencies of defensive posturing. Muscles, viscera, and autonomic nervous system activation cooperate in preparing for escape. This preparation is sensed kinesthetically and is internally joined as a gestalt to the image of the bear. *Movement and image are fused,* registered together, as the *feeling of danger.* Motivated by this feeling, we continue to scan for more information—a grove of trees, some rocks—at the same time drawing on our ancestral and personal memory banks. Probabilities are non-consciously computed, based on such encounters over millions of years of historical evolution, as well as by our own personal experiences. We prepare for the next phase in this unfolding drama. Without thinking, we orient toward a large tree with low branches. An *urge* is experienced to flee and climb. If we run, freely oriented toward the tree, it is the feeling of *directed running*. The urge to run is experienced as the feeling of danger, while successful running is experienced as *escape* (and not anxiety!).

If, on the other hand, we chance upon a starved or wounded bear, and moreover find ourselves surrounded on all sides by sheer rock walls, that is, trapped, then the defensive preparedness for flight, concomitant with the feeling of danger, is "thwarted" and will change abruptly into the fixated emotional states of anxiety. The word *fear*, interestingly enough, comes from the old English term for danger, while *anxious* derives from the Greek root *angst*, meaning to "press tight" or strangle, as conveyed in Edward Munch's riveting painting, *The Scream*. Our entire physiology and psyche become precipitously constricted in anxiety. Response is restricted to non-directed desperate flight, to rage, counterattack, or to freeze-collapse. The latter affords the possibility of diminishing the bear's urge to attack. (If it is not cornered or hurt and is able to clearly identify the approaching human being, the bear usually will not attack the intruder. It may even remain and go on with business as usual.)

In summary, when the normal orientation and defensive escape resources have failed to resolve the situation, life hangs in the balance, with non-directed flight, rage, freezing, or collapse. Rage and terror-panic are the *secondary* emotional anxiety states that are evoked when the preparatory orientation processes (feelings) of danger-orientation and preparedness to flee are not successful—when they are blocked or inhibited. It is this "thwarting" that results in freezing and anxiety-panic.

Tonic Immobility—Freezing

Anxiety has often been linked to the physiology and experience of flight. Analyses of animal distress behaviors suggest that this may be quite misleading. Ethology (the study of animals in their natural environment) points to the "thwarting" of escape as the root of distress-anxiety. When attacked by a cheetah on the African plains, an antelope will first attempt to escape through directed-oriented running. If, however, the fleeing animal is cornered so that escape is diminished, it may run blindly, without a directed orientation, or it may attempt to fight wildly and desperately against enormous odds. At the moment of physical contact, often before injury is actually inflicted, the antelope abruptly appears to go dead. It not only appears dead, but its autonomic physiology undergoes a widespread alteration and reorganization. The antelope is in fact highly activated internally, even though outward movement is almost nonexistent. Prey animals are immobilized in a sustained (cataleptic-catatonic) pattern of neuromuscular activity and high autonomic and brain wave activity. Sympathetic and parasympathetic responses are also concurrently activated, like brake and accelerator, working against each other.

Nancy, in her reexperiencing of the examination room, exhibited this pattern when her heart rate increased sharply and then plummeted abruptly to a very low rate. In tonic immobility, an animal is either frozen stiff in heightened contraction of agonist and antagonist muscle group, or in a continuously balanced, hypnotic, muscular state exhibiting what is called *wavy flexibility*. In the hypnotic state, body positions can be molded like clay, as is seen in catatonic schizophrenics. There is also *analgesic numbing*. Nancy described many of these behaviors as they were happening to her. She wasn't, however, aware of her physical sensations but rather of her self-depreciating and critical judgments about those sensations. It is as though some explanation must be found for profoundly disorganizing forces underlying one's own perceived inadequacy. Psychologist Paul G. Zimbardo has gone so far as to propose that "most mental illness represents not a cognitive impairment, but an (attempted) interpretation of discontinuous or inexplicable internal states." Tonic immobility, murderous rage, and non-directed flight are such examples.

Ethologists have found wide adaptive value in these immobility responses: Freezing makes prey less visible and non-movement in prey appears also to be a potent inhibitor of aggression in predators, often aborting attack-kill responses entirely. The park service, for example, advises campers that if they are unable to actively escape an attacking bear, they should lie prone and not move. The family cat, seemingly on to nature's game, bats a captured, frozen mouse with its paws hoping to bring it out of shock and continue in the game. Immobility can buy time for prey. The predator may drag frozen prey to its den or lair for later consumption, giving it a second chance to escape. In addition to these aggression-inhibiting responses, freezing by prey animals may provide a signaling and decoy effect, allowing con-specifics, who are farther away, a better chance for escape in certain situations. Loss of blood pressure may also help prevent bleeding when injured. An immobile prey animal is, in sum, less likely to be attacked. Further, if attacked, it is less likely to be killed and eaten, increasing its chances of escape and reproduction. In a world where most animals are both predator and prey at one time or another, analgesia is "humane" biological adaptation.

Tonic immobility demonstrates that anxiety can be both self-perpetuating and self-defeating. Freezing is the last-ditch, cul-de-sac, bodily response where active escape is not possible. Where flight and fight escape have been (or are perceived to be) unlikely, the nervous system reorganizes to tonic immobility. Both flight-or-fight and immobility are adaptive responses. Where the flight-or-fight response is appropriate, freezing will be relatively maladaptive; where freezing is appropriate, attempts to flee or fight are likely to be maladaptive. Biologically, immobility is a potent adaptive strategy where active escape is prevented. When, however, it becomes a preferred response pattern in situations of activation in general, it is profoundly debilitating. Immobility becomes the crippling, fixating experience of traumatic and panic anxiety. Underlying the freezing response, however, are the flight-or-fight and other defensive and orientation preparations that are activated just prior to the onset of freezing. The "de-potentiation" of anxiety is accomplished by precisely and sequentially restoring the latent flight-or-fight and other active defensive responses that occur at the moment(s) before escape is thwarted.

Uncoupling Fear-Potentiated Immobility: An Example

The key in treating various anxiety and post-traumatic reactions is in principle quite simple: to uncouple the normally acute, time-limited freezing response from fear reactivation. This is accomplished by progressively reestablishing the pre-traumatic defensive and orienting responses, the responses that were in execution just prior to the initiation of immobility. In practice there are many possible strategies that may be utilized to accomplish this uncoupling of the immobility-fear or panic reaction. An example of one type of reworking follows:

Marius Inuusuttoq Kristensen is a native Eskimo, born and raised in a remote village in Greenland. He is a slight, intelligent, boyish-looking young man in his mid-twenties. He is shy but open and available. As a participant in a training class in Copenhagen, Denmark, he asks to work on his tendency toward anxiety and panic, particularly when he is with a man he admires and whose approval he wants. His anxiety is experienced somatically as a weakening in his legs and a stabbing ache on the lateral midline of his right leg. There are also waves of nausea moving from his stomach to his throat, where it then becomes stuck. His head and face feel very warm and he becomes sweaty and flushed. After talking with him and using some exploratory images, he recalled an event that occurred when he was eight. While returning from a walk alone in the mountains, he was attacked by a pack of three wild dogs and bitten badly on his right leg. He remembers only feeling the bite and then waking up in the arms of a neighbor. He remembers, too, his father coming to the door and being annoyed with him. Marius still feels bitterly angry and hurt at this rejection. He remembers, particularly, that his new pants were ripped and covered with blood. When he describes this, he is visibly upset. I ask him to tell me more about the pants. He tells me that they were a surprise from his mother that morning; she had made them especially for him. He is in a transparent moment, experiencing pleasure, pride, and excitement similar to that day seventeen years ago. Marius holds his arms in front of himself feeling the fur and feasting on his "magic" polar bear fur pants.

"I feel like I want to jump up and down."

"Marius, are these the same kind of pants that the men of the village, the hunters, wear?"

"Yes," he responds.

"Do they wear them when they go out to hunt?"

"Yes." Marius becomes more excited. He describes seeing the pants with clear detail and aliveness. I have him feel the pants now with his hand.

"Now, Marius," I ask, "can you feel your legs inside the pants?"

"Yes, I can feel my legs. They feel very strong, like the men when they are hunting." (I am beginning to build, as a resource, a somatic bridge utilizing neuromuscular patterns of the leg.) Marius's walk into the mountains the day of the attack was an initiation, a rite of passage for him; his pants were power objects on this "walkabout." I have him describe the sensations and images of walking up into the mountains. His descriptions are bright, embodied with awareness of detail. The experience he describes is clearly authentic and present. He is also aware of being in a group of students, though without self-consciousness. I would call his state of being primarily a state of presence and 'retrogression' rather than regression. As images and kinesthetic perceptions unfold he sees an expanse of rocks. I ask him to feel his pants and then look at the rocks again.

"My legs want to jump; they feel light, not tight like they usually do. They are like springs, light and strong." He reports seeing a long stick that is lying by a rock and picks it up.

"What is it?" I ask.

"A spear."

"What is it for? What do the men do when they see bear tracks?" (I am hoping that this "play in dream time" will stimulate predatory and counter-attack behaviors which were thwarted in being overwhelmed by the attacking dogs. This successive bridging helps to prime required defensive responses that could eventually neutralize the tonic immobility-freeze and collapse which occurred at the time of the attack.)

He goes on, "I am following a large polar bear. I am with the men, but I will make the kill." Micro-flexor extensor movements can be seen in his thigh, pelvic, and trunk muscles as he imagines jumping from rock to rock in following the trail.

"I see him now. I stop and aim my spear."

"Yes, feel that in your whole body, feel your feet on the rocks, the strength in your legs, and the arching in your back and arms. Feel all that power!"

"I see the spear flying," he says. Again micro-postural adjustments can readily be seen in Marius's body; he is trembling lightly now in his legs and arms. I encourage him to feel these sensations. He reports waves of excitement and pleasure.

"I did it. I hit him with my spear!"

"What do the men do now?" I ask.

"They cut the belly open and take out the insides and then cut the fur off ... to ... make pants and coats. The other men will carry the meat down for the village."

"Feel your pants, Marius, with your hands, and on your legs." Tears form in his eyes. "Can you do this?" I ask.

"I don't know ... I'm scared."

"Feel your legs, feel your pants."

"... Yes, I cut the belly open; there is lots of blood ... I take out the insides. Now I cut the skin. I rip it off, there is glistening and shimmering. It is a beautiful fur, thick and soft. It will be very warm." Marius's body is shaking and tremoring with excitement, strength, and conquest. The activation/arousal is quite intense.

"How do you feel, Marius?"

"I'm a little scared ... I don't know if I've ever felt this much strong feeling ... I think it's okay ... really I feel very powerful and filled with an energy. I think I can trust this ... I don't know ... it's strong."

"Feel your legs. Feel your feet. Touch the pants with your hands."

"Yes, I feel calmer now, not so much rush ... it's more like strength now."

"Okay, yes, good. Now start walking down, back toward the village." A few minutes pass, then Marius's trunk flexes and his movements hold as in still-frame arrest. His heart rate accelerates, and his face reddens.

"I see the dogs ... they're coming at me."

"Feel your legs, Marius! Touch your pants," I sharply demand. "Feel your legs and look! What is happening?"

"I am turning, running away. I see the dogs. I see a pole, an electricity pole. I am turning toward it. I didn't know that I remembered this." Marius's pulse starts to drop; he turns pale. "I'm getting weak," he responds.

"Feel the pants, Marius!" I command. "Feel the pants with your hands!"

"I'm running." His heart rate increases. "I can feel my legs ... they're strong, like on the rocks ..." Again he pales. He yells out, "Agh ... my leg, it burns like fire ... I can't move, I'm trying, but I can't move ... I can't move ... I can't move! It's numb now ... my leg is numb. I can't feel it."

"Turn, Marius. Turn to the dog. Look at it."

This is the critical point. I hand Marius a roll of paper towels. If Marius freezes now he will be re-traumatized. (This would occur if somatic bridges were not organized and in place.) He grabs the roll and "strangles" it. The group members, myself included, look on with utter amazement at his strength as he twists it and tears it in two. (I have asked weightlifting friends to replicate this and only a few have been able to do so.)

"Now the other one, look right at it." This time he lets out screams of rage and triumph. I have him settle with his bodily sensations for a few minutes, integrating this intensity. Then I ask him again to look.

"What do you see?"

"I see them ... they're all bloody and dead."

"Okay, look in the other direction. What do you see?"

"I see the pole ... there are bolts in it."

"Okay, feel your legs, feel your pants." I am about to say, "Run!" (in order to complete the running response). Before I do, he reports, "I am running ... I can feel my legs, they are strong like springs." Rhythmic extensor-flexor undulations are now visible through his pants, and his entire body is trembling and vibrating.

"I'm climbing ... climbing ... I see them below ... they're dead and I'm safe." He starts to sob softly and we wait a few minutes.

"What do you experience now?"

"It feels like I'm being carried by big arms. He's carrying me in his arms. I feel safe." Marius now reports a series of images of fences and houses in the village. Again, he softly and gently sobs. "He's knocking at the door of my family's house. The door opens ... my father ... he's very upset, he runs to get a towel ... my leg is bleeding very badly ... he's very upset ... he's not mad at me. He's worried. It hurts, the soap hurts."

Marius sobs now in waves. "It hurts but I'm crying 'cause he's not angry at me. I can see he was upset and scared."

"What do you feel in your body now?"

"I feel very peaceful now; I feel vibration and tingling all over. It is even and warm. He loves me." Again Marius begins to sob and I ask what happens if he feels that in his body, if he feels that his father loves him. There is a silence.

"I feel warm, very warm and peaceful. I don't need to cry now. I'm okay and he was just scared. It's not that he doesn't love me."

In reviewing the session, recall that initially the only image or memory of the event Marius had was the bloody pants, torn flesh, and his father's rejection. Yet here also was the positive seed of the emerging healing nucleus, the "magic pants." The experience of the pants is the thread by which the altered states, related to the traumatic event, were experienced and progressively renegotiated. In working with over a thousand clients, I have never found an instance where there was not this dual aspect of a critical image. Within an initial image are the first stirrings of the motoric plan that a person will develop. The renegotiation processes occur stepwise, from periphery to center, toward a de-structuring of the particular anxiety response or thwarting pattern, and restructuring of the underlying defensive and orienting responses.

The image of the ripped and bloodied pants was arousing to Marius, but so was the happiness (his legs wanting to jump for joy) he experienced when he saw the same pants for the first time earlier that morning. He was joyful when presented with this first possibility of manhood. In wanting, literally, to "jump for joy," Marius activated motor patterns that were essential in the eventual renegotiation of his freezing response. It is necessary to build just such adaptive motor patterns successively with increasing activation. In moving from the periphery of the experience to the freezing "shock" core, one moves away from maladaptive neuromuscular patterns. The latter are neutralized by adaptive, flexible patterns at similar levels of activation.

As I encouraged Marius to track the initial positive pants experience gradually toward the traumatic, freezing shock core, the joyful extensor-dominated pants experience became linked to support, aggression, and competency. That is, when in somatic experiencing, Marius sees the image of the rock field, the seed begins to sprout. In jumping from rock to rock and finding and picking up the stick, Marius's dynamic body-unconscious propels the motor plan sharply ahead. He is now prepared to meet the impending challenge. He takes the offensive and moves toward mastery of the previously thwarted situation. Like the hunters, he tracks the polar bear as I track his autonomic and motoric responses. Supported by the magical pants and the village men, he makes the find and the kill in a crescendo of high activation, approaching ecstasy.

In the next sequence of events, the true test will be made. Empowered and triumphant, he heads back down toward the village. There is expansion and awareness. For the first time, he sees and describes the road and the dogs. (Previously, these images were constricted as in amnesia.) He senses orientation movements away from the attacking dogs and toward the electric pole. Because he now senses his legs moving, the inhibitory freezing response is no longer the exclusive channel of response. The ecstatic trembling for the kill is now bridged into running. This action is, however, only partial; he begins to run but does not escape! I ask him to turn and face his attackers so as not to have him fall back into immobility. This time he counterattacks, first momentarily with rage, and then with the same triumph that he experienced in the previous sequence of killing and eviscerating the bear. The motor plan has succeeded. Marius is now victorious; he is no longer the defeated victim.

The event, however, is still not complete. As the sensations and autonomic responses shift from highly activated sympathetic to parasympathetic resolution, the more primary orienting responses can come into play. Marius not only sees the pole, he orients toward the pole and prepares to run. He had begun this maneuver years ago, but until this moment, it had not been executed and completed. He consummates this preparation now with the act of running. Since he has already killed his attackers this may not make "left brain" linear sense, but it is completely logical in the biological, reptilian (body-brain) language of preparation, defense, and orientation. It is that sequence of activity (somatic experiencing) that alters the basic patterns of an individual's adaptive responses. When I returned to Denmark a year later, I learned that Marius's anxiety reactions were no longer a problem.

Jody—In a Fraction of a Second

(Another example of resolving anxiety states through completing innate defensive responses)

Twenty-five years ago, Jody's life was shattered. While walking in the woods near her boyfriend's house, a hunter came up to her and began a conversation. It was mid-September. There was a chill in the air. Her boyfriend and others thought nothing when they saw someone apparently chopping wood. A madman, however, was smashing Jody's head again and again with his rifle. The police found Jody unconscious. Chips from the butt of the rifle lay nearby where they had broken off in the violent attack.

The only recollection Jody had of the event was scant and confused. She vaguely remembered meeting the man and then waking up in the hospital some days later. Jody had been suffering from anxiety, migraines, concentration and memory problems, depression, chronic fatigue and chronic pain of the head, back, and neck regions (diagnosed as fibromyalgia). She had been treated by physical therapists, chiropractors, and various physicians.

Jody, like so many head-injured and traumatized individuals, grasped desperately and obsessively in an attempt to retrieve memories of her trauma. When I suggested to Jody that it was possible to experience healing without having to remember the event, I saw a flicker of hope and a momentary look of relief pass across her face. We talked for a while, reviewing her history and struggle to function. Focusing on body sensations, Jody slowly became aware of various tension patterns in her head and neck region. With this focus, she began to notice a particular urge to turn and retract her neck. By following this urge in slow gradual "micro movements," she experienced a momentary fear, followed by a strong tingling sensation. Through following these movements, Jody began a journey through the trauma of her assault. In learning to move between flexible control and surrender to these involuntary movements, she began to experience gentle shaking and trembling throughout her body. Thus began, ever so gently, the discharge of her trauma.

In later sessions, Jody experienced other spontaneous movements, as well as sounds and impulses to run, bare her teeth and claw at her assailant. By completing these biological defensive responses, Jody was able to construct a sense of how her body prepared to react in that fraction of a second when the hunter raised the rifle butt to strike her. In allowing these movements and sounds to be expressed, Jody began to experience a deep organic discharge along with the *experience* of her body's innate capacity to defend and protect itself.

Jody, through her felt sense, was able to follow her body's intentional movement. Intentional movement is non-conscious. It is experienced as if the body is moving of its own volition. Through completing the life preserving actions that her body had prepared for at the time of her attack, she released that bound energy and realized that she had, in fact, attempted to defend herself. Gradually, as more defensive and orienting responses reinstated, her panic anxiety progressively decreased.

In Somatic Experiencing, traumatic reactions are addressed by a wide variety of strategies. What unifies them is that they are all used in the service of de-structuring the thwarted anxiety response and restoring defensive and orienting resources. The overall picture shows how each individual's needs and resources call forth a unique, creatively adaptive solution.

References

Ahsen, Akhter. *Basic Concepts in Eidetic Psychotherapy* (New York: Brandon House, 1972).

Beck, Aaron "Theoretical Perspectives on Clinical Anxiety." In A. Hussain Tuma & Jack D. Maser (Eds.) *Anxiety and the Anxiety Disorders* (New Jersey: Lawrence Erlbaum Associated Publishers, 1985), 188.

Beck, Aaron, & Gary Emery. *Anxiety Disorders and Phobias: A Cognitive Perspective* (New York: Basic Books, 1985), 188.

Gallup, G. Gordon, & Jack Maser. "Human Catalepsy and Catatonia." In Jack D. Maser & Martin E.P. Seligman (Eds.) *Pyschopathology: Experimental Models* (San Francisco: W.H. Freeman, 1977), 334–357.

Gendlin, Eugene T. "On Emotion In Therapy." In J.D. Safran & L.S. Greenberg (Eds.) *Emotions and the Process of Therapeutic Change* (New York: Academic Press, 1988).

Gelhorn, Ernst. *Autonomic-Somatic Integrations: Physiological Basis and Clinical Implications* (Minneapolis: University of Minnesota Press, 1967).

Levine, Peter. "Stress." In Michael G.H. Coles, Emanual Donchin, & Stephen Porges (Eds.) *Psychophysiology* (New York: Guilford Press, 1986), 331–354.

Levine, Peter A. *Waking the Tiger: Healing Trauma* (Berkeley: North Atlantic Books, 1997).

Morris, Desmond. *Primate Ethology* (London: Weidenfield & Nicholson, 1969).

Porges, Stephen. (1995). Article in *Psychophysiology* 32:301–318.

Salzen, A. Eric. (1967). "Social Attachment and a Sense of Security." *Social Sciences Information* 12:555–627.

Zimbardo, Paul G. "Understanding Madness: A Cognitive-Social Model of Psychopathology," invited address at the annual meeting of the Canadian Psychological Association, Vancouver, B.C., June, 1977.

Using the Bodynamic Shock Trauma Model in the Everyday Practice of Physiotherapy

—Barbara Picton, B.S.R., M.Ed. (Cns. Psch.), R.C.C.

Currently I work in parallel practices of physiotherapy and clinical counseling/psychotherapy.

In both practices I work with clients post trauma. In the physiotherapy practice the traumatic incident may be a traffic accident, a fall (including sports injuries), an assault, or an acute onset of spinal pain that suddenly removes the client from their normal activities.

Trauma (an extraordinary event in a person's life) evokes both a psychological and a biological response. People react with a personal shock reflex—flight, fight, or freeze (paralysis), and feeling distressed, overwhelmed, and vulnerable are normal reactions. At intake, the physiotherapist may find their client emotional with behavior ranging from being withdrawn and non-communicative (freeze), to hyper-vigilant and quick, to attack (fight). Common symptoms clients report include disturbed sleep, poor concentration, confusion, and irritability.

The majority of people will naturally heal and resolve their stress over a few weeks but it is not uncommon for the physiotherapist to work with clients who fail to negotiate the transition phase between their shock reactions and "landing" back into normal daily life. These clients may develop prolonged physical and emotional symptoms that become the foundation of diagnoses such as chronic pain, chronic fatigue, or fibromyalgia. Unresolved emotional and/or psychological issues may present as a failure to resume life—the client develops anxiety toward driving, an insurmountable fear of falling, persistent confusion, or difficulty in returning with confidence to activities and roles in their lives.

While the physiotherapist primarily sees the patient for their physical problems, such as pain and restricted function following such an incident, he or she is in a good position to support and guide the client through resolution of the shock response and help minimize ongoing problems.

Within the general education of the physiotherapist, there is no model to guide the therapist in assisting clients to heal from the emotional/psychological aspect of trauma. However, the Bodynamic System has a model of resolving shock and trauma, parts of which can very easily be incorporated into everyday practice of the physiotherapist or massage therapist.

The Bodynamic System is a broad and in-depth developmental somatic psychology and psychotherapy that has been developed over the past thirty years by a core group of therapists in Denmark. It is now taught to body-therapists and psychotherapists worldwide. Bodynamic therapists understand the healthy potential lying in the muscles of the body and have developed methods to use this knowledge to build resources in clients.

My intention in this article is to outline both the traditional physiotherapy treatment plan for the post trauma patient and the Bodynamic System's model for shock and trauma. I wish to show how physiotherapy treatment can be augmented with simple techniques and a consciousness that will assist clients to resolve emotional and psychological issues associated with the trauma more effectively.

Outline of Physiotherapy Treatment of the Post-Trauma Client

Clients seek physiotherapy to find relief from pain and to restore physical functioning.

The physiotherapy treatment is planned to augment the body's physiological response to healing. Factors influencing the degree of physical trauma sustained include:

- the force and direction of the trauma;
- the tissues affected (a fractured bone will require a different approach than a soft tissue injury);

- whether there has been previous history; and
- the client's level of health and fitness at the time of injury.

The client's culture and personality also influence the planning of a treatment protocol and are taken into consideration.

When the client comes for physiotherapy, a history is taken—including what happened during the incident itself, any previous history, general health issues, functional limitations, and location and pattern of pain. A physical assessment is then completed, looking at the limitations of function in the affected location and how this impacts the whole body, including range of joint motion, flexibility and strength of muscles, nerve conductivity, and imbalances in the mechanics of the musculoskeletal system.

Typically, the client's focus is on pain relief and various treatments can be given to reduce inflammation, muscle spasm, and pain including: various modalities (heat/ice, therapeutic machines); manual therapy techniques; exercises; and education in resting positions, good posture, and self-care. Gradually the client's exercises and activities are increased until as full function as possible is gained and the client has been rehabilitated back to, or close to, their pre-incident life style. Sometimes the client takes this as an opportunity to "get in shape" and aims to even exceed their prior activity level.

Outline of the Bodynamic Model for Working with Shock Trauma

Two theories inform this Bodynamic model. One is Cullberg's crisis resolution model where crisis is defined as what happens in the aftermath of the traumatic incident—the "rings on the water." There are four stages of healing following the traumatic incident: *Acute,* lasting hours or days, where reality is not yet grasped; *Reaction,* lasting one to six weeks where the client is still experiencing healthy emotional release and has not yet regained a cognitive container around the events; *Reparation,* lasting one to six months where the client is integrating understanding of the traumatic incident but remains focused on it even though they are able to see how their life has been impacted;

and *New Orienting Phase,* which continues after six months. In this last stage, the client makes the necessary choices to move on in their life and move beyond the incident.

The other approach is that researched by van der Kolk and his colleagues, who consider physiological response, pre-existing personality structure, previous experiences, and the degree of social support as factors in a person's ultimate response to trauma. This person-based approach differs from the DSM categorization that defines the trauma response as an anxiety disorder based on the incident. It does not explain why some people resolve their trauma response within the allotted three-month time frame and others do not, thus being diagnosed with post-traumatic stress disorder (PTSD). We have all met the clients who walk away from a major accident with no lasting effect and those who are severely impacted and have difficulty resuming their life following a minor incident.

In many body therapies, such as those using deep tissue release and breath work, the aim is to release body memories and stored emotions and clear those energies from the body, often through catharsis. Many clients report difficulty integrating their experience following these sessions and feel more traumatized and ungrounded. Bessel van der Kolk, discussing approaches to the treatment of PTSD, writes, ". . . the goal of treatment is to find a way in which people can acknowledge the reality of what has happened without having to reexperience the trauma all over again. For this to occur, merely uncovering memories is not enough: they need to be modified and transformed, i.e. placed in their proper context and reconstructed into neutral or meaningful narratives."

The ideal response to a traumatic incident is to find the personal resources necessary to move through the process. Failure to do so leaves the client with symptoms of PTSD; reexperiencing the event through flashbacks or nightmares, autonomic hyper-arousal seen as hyper-vigilance and exaggerated startle response, emotional numbing (including depression), emotional irritability, sleep difficulties, difficulty concentrating and learning from experience, memory disturbances, and psychosomatic reactions.

The goal of Bodynamic shock work is the creation of a new imprint of the old event, replacing unsuccessful outcomes to situations with successful ones.

Firstly, Bodynamic therapists work to build resources (expanding the client's capacity for coping) through the careful building of body awareness. This serves to reestablish or develop healthy ego skills of centering, grounding, boundaries, containment, and balance; develop the ability to use the arms to negotiate appropriate contact by pushing away and pulling toward; and develop the capacity for the client to handle the high energy of the trauma response.

Secondly, the therapist helps the client release the shock reflexes of fight, flight, and freeze, allowing them to cycle to completion. Following sensations and motor patterns until they are fully resolved, ensures successful integration of experience. Clients are thus helped to "renegotiate" neuromuscular patterns to attain a new "imprint" of somatic, emotional, and psychological resources. For example:

- Reestablishing orientation reflexes enables us to recognize a threat and initiate the fight-or-flight reflex;
- Reacting to the fight-or-flight reflex allows us to protect ourselves and reach a state of safety;
- Establishing a deep somatic experience of safety secures our ability to find deep relaxation and peace; and
- Being at peace permits us to establish a sense of a boundary between our self and the world. By keeping boundaries and being present we may become influenced by the situation, but it will not take over our reality.

The stages of Bodynamic shock work are:

1. Assessing the client's presenting symptoms and how they affect daily life and teaching the client strategies for coping, including:
   - Teaching the client the body's natural physiological response to trauma;
   - Teaching the client to build body resources (coping skills) such as centering, grounding, boundaries, containment, balance, and the ability to say "no" or "stop";
   - Helping the client to recognize, or build if necessary, a support system or personal network—a group of family and/or friends and work colleagues who are willing to help out at this present time;

- Helping the client to define a physical safe place with safe people in the client's life at the current time; and
- Teaching the client to be gentle with themselves. Strategies may include "cocooning," taking relaxing baths, receiving a massage, walking, eating favorite foods, and playing music.

2. Exploring the crisis of the shock:
   - Looking at how the client's life has continued since the incident and defining the issues that remain unresolved.

3. Exploring the power in the shock defense:
   - Teaching and supporting the client to sense and experience the power in the fact that they survived. Finding dignity in that whatever they did was the perfect thing for them to do at the time and owning their own creativity.

4. Working with the peak experience found in the strategies used to cope with the shock:
   - In shock, a very high energy state is elicited and a "bigger part of me" is evoked and challenged. This expanded consciousness is similar to that experienced during a peak experience. Working with the peak experience in the shock response helps clients find the qualities that ensured survival. In peak experiences there is a state of bliss—a higher kind of joy. It certainly is a conflict to think that intense fear or horror can be present at the same time as bliss, but it is true. Working with this enables the client to find dignity and strength in the difficult experience. Culturally we have no rituals to help us deal with shock. Shock itself often becomes for us an initiation for knowing a greater reality and a sense of greater or larger self. Bodynamic therapists work in such a way to explore this initiation and find hope.

5. Working with the core of the shock:
   - The Bodynamic model of processing shock trauma includes an opportunity for the client to tell their story of the event as seen in a slow-motion video—frame by frame—and escape to safety as they need. The client lies on a mat and physically "runs" to the safe place from

the scene of the incident (visualizing the route as they run) and is met by their safe people. As the client tells their story, there will be points where they will sense their anxiety/fear rising and they run to safety, increasing the heart and respiratory rates. Arriving safely, they are able to take in a deep physical sense of being safe and in contact with other people. Physiologically, as their system settles, they move further along the continuum toward the relaxation response. In this way the flight aspect of the flight/fight/freeze response is modulated. There are also techniques to assist the client resolve anger/deep rage (the fight) and the dissociation (freeze) in this process. Getting in touch with the impulses that may not have been completed at the time of the incident and following them through to completion restores a sense of personal power and the normal, healthy fight-or-flight response. Completion of this stage of the trauma work is for the client to own their experience and the strategies they used for survival, and integrate the event both emotionally and cognitively.

6. Completion and Integration:
   - To fully resolve the trauma response the individual must find ways to connect to the larger community. Some cultures have established rituals and others do not, seen for example in their response to death and the ritual of the funeral. In our culture, the survivor will often take up a cause related to the traumatic incident and use their experience to benefit others, such as working for a charity or raising social consciousness. This is a necessary part of the healing.

Two other models developed in the Bodynamic System and used in shock work are useful for the physiotherapist to understand:

1. Four Aspects of Ego

Bodynamic therapists understand the development of the Ego in overlapping, or nesting, developmental stages, which can be represented in a simple form in the table below. The physical body supports the Individual Ego—the sense of "I," which then supports "me" in the roles I have in the world. The observing ego provides a vantage point to review and reflect on behaviors done and choices made. Besides these Ego states is the ME.

ME is personal power—instincts, the body's reflex system, gene knowledge, and autonomic behavior (the behavior that is learned through experience and used without thought). The higher ME is spiritual intuition. In a high-stress situation we find ourselves operating from this reflex system and making decisions for our survival. Bodynamic teaching confirms that half a second before something happens we already have the awareness of it. This half-second can mean the difference between life and death. This moment is when we have access to our resources, our ME, and we need to trust and act on them. It is not a place of ego, even though some may have called it such; responses from ego and consciousness are too slow.

The challenge is that some of the things we did, or the decisions we made, may be surprising to us when we return to our individual and role ego states— our "ordinary knowledge"—and we may feel ashamed or guilty of our behavior. For example: "I can't believe I got out of the car and swore so loudly at that stupid driver. I feel so embarrassed! Whatever must he have thought of me?" However, in shock there is no conflict in consciousness. When we are out of shock, consciousness starts to question and doubt and ego cannot deal with that. Something inside a person does have a greater knowledge and this

Schematic View of the Bodynamic Aspects of Ego Showing the Ages of Development

ME
_____

BODY EGO
_____
conception   4 years

        INDIVIDUAL EGO
        _____
        2.5 years   10 years

          ROLE EGO
          _____
          3 years   14 years   21 years

             OBSERVING EGO
             _____
             4 years

needs to be acknowledged and accepted. We must trust that decisions were made from a place of deeper knowing and that the right action was taken to ensure survival at that time. The important thing to remember following any traumatic event is, "I survived!"—whatever the shame, whatever the event— "I made it!" Trusting in the process that got you through, gaining personal trust and self-respect brings you to a place of greater choice for the things you want in your life.

Body Ego

In this stage of development we find meaning through our physical body. As young infants we know our world from how it fits into our mouths and how our bodily needs are taken care of. We learn to sense threat through our body and this ability stays with us through our life.

Individual Ego

As we learn to individuate, we start to know ourselves as, "I am some-body." We develop our individual ego, also knowing it in our bodies and gain-ing a sense of personal space, feelings, thoughts, and emotions.

Role Ego

Our role ego develops as we find our place in the world in relation to oth-ers. It has a lot to do with understanding where we come from, our norms and values and social background. Part of the struggle of being a teenager (fourteen to twenty-one) is in reevaluating these constructs and making new choices that individuate us from our upbringing. Ideally, in this ego state there is a bodily sense of "me" and a broader sense of an individual ready to step out into dif-ferent roles. The ability to express 'the essence of me' in these roles is necessary to be able to function in society.

Observing Ego

The observing ego is the viewpoint we gain to see "the bigger picture." We can observe our behaviors and hear our inner voice.

2. Functions of Ego

The Bodynamic System groups certain muscles together and links them with eleven particular skill sets known as Functions of Ego. The five defined here are addressed when working with trauma response.

Centering

Being centered is having sensation of the core, an ability to fill our self out from the inside and hold feelings of self-worth. When we are centered we are less judgmental—things are what they are. We are better able to maintain our boundaries—our ability to recognize where our physical, personal, and energetic spaces end and those of the other person begin. Centering muscles include the rhomboids, erector spinae, gluteals and deep hip rotators, pectorals and iliopsoas. The ability to center can be strengthened through visualization, breathing, developing body awareness, and core stabilizing exercises.

Grounding and Reality Testing

Developing skills in grounding means enhancing our ability to sense the physical ground and the support provided by our feet, legs, and back. Being grounded equates with knowing our personal reality. Grounding muscles include those in the sole of the foot, the long toe flexors and extensors, erector spinae, supraspinatus, and muscles in the anterior neck and face.

Boundaries

Boundaries are related to self-definition at an energetic, body, and psychological level in the realm of human contact. A boundary is the felt energetic experience of contact, where one individual ends and engagement with another begins. Boundaries are a tool to help distinguish us from the outer world; every person has a body and a personal space and the right to control them. The skin is a physical boundary and boundary muscles include deltoid and quadriceps.

Containment (Energy Management)

From a physical standpoint, the pelvic floor, back, buttock, abdominal muscles, and diaphragm make a container around our center. Using these muscle consciously leads to a better energetic containment—an increased ability to be present with others in a clear "I-you" contact. In this level of contact it is clear which emotions, sensations, and thoughts are mine and which are yours. Containment muscles help us manage our emotions and stress and provide us with feelings of self-containment and being "backed up." They include breathing muscles, core stabilizers, tensor fascia lata, trapezeii, latissimus dorsi, and muscles of the anterior neck and jaw.

Social Balances

We are constantly balancing many things in our social interactions, including our own feelings and desires against other's expectations, managing stress and resolving it, and pulling our self together and letting go as necessary. The main muscles involved in managing stress and pulling ourselves together are gracilis, sartorius, popliteus, plantaris, vastus medialis, TFL, and ITB.

Integrating Bodynamic Theory into Physiotherapy

Shock impacts the client physically, emotionally, and psychologically—and healing will occur on these levels. While it is not the intent here to train the physiotherapist in strategies of psychotherapy, many of the routine physical therapy approaches have a profound effect in providing social support, a cognitive frame, and building and strengthening the body resources the client needs.

Safe Place/Safe Person

Coming to the physiotherapy office for the first visit following a traumatic injury can provide a safe place and safe person for the client, especially if the client has had previous positive experiences with the therapist and front office staff. A trusted family physician may have provided a referral, further consolidating a supportive network of caring professionals. Following a traumatic event, reality is challenged and the client may be confused and forgetful. They will need help to think clearly and organize, so help them with the details—write things down, (appointments and exercises), help them contact insurance adjusters, call them with reminders for appointments if necessary.

The physiotherapist's initial focus with any new client is to build the therapeutic relationship through empathetic listening, open communication, expressing human kindness, and providing support and education without colluding with the client. Accept the facts as you hear them and refrain from passing judgments on the client's experiences. The client's experience was true for them at the time and whatever they did was the right thing for them to do in the stress of the moment.

Telling the Story

The client is then encouraged to tell their story: "Tell me what happened to you at the time of the accident." The physiotherapist is interested in fact-finding and does not usually encourage the expression of emotion—and this serves the client well. Telling and retelling their story helps the client to orient and find support and safety in an empathetic listener. Over several sessions the physiotherapist can ask for more details. In the retelling the client will often recall something they had not remembered, which helps to both fill out the story and strengthen their reality. Often clients will say they appreciate being able to talk to the physiotherapist and are encouraged to do so. The appointment times are longer than the doctor's and being touched builds intimacy. The physiotherapist, of course, must be aware of their own sense of self and of maintaining their professional boundaries within this relationship.

Acknowledging Reality

During the physical assessment the physiotherapist acknowledges the injury, pain, and its affect on the client's life. Often the client feels validated when the physiotherapist finds a stiff joint or muscle in spasm and can genuinely understand the discomfort they are in—even bursting into tears and saying, "You can feel it? You know I'm not making it up!" Touch is very healing in itself and a trained physiotherapist who is used to working with a boundaried touch can provide much reassurance to the client, aside from relieving physical tension through manual therapy techniques. The therapist's professional expertise further strengthens the "safe place, safe person" concept.

Education: Strengthening Cognitive Understanding

During treatment the physiotherapist is an educator, teaching the client the body's normal response to injury, the resolution of the inflammatory response, and what the client can expect over the next few weeks or months. At the same time the physiotherapist has the knowledge to describe the workings of the autonomic nervous system and the flight/fight/freeze or stress reflex. A helpful example is to ask the client to remember a movie where there was a scary scene. The audience jumps, people gasp, startle, and hold their breath, the heart rates speed up. Then as the situation resolves, people start to laugh nervously, shuffle in their seats, the energy starts to settle and the body's physiological response returns to normal. People will turn and whisper to each other, "Oh, that was scary!" This is the normal sympathetic/parasympathetic response: startle, orient, respond, settle. In an unresolved situation, the body remains caught in the fright (the aroused sympathetic response) and the client must learn and practice ways to stimulate the relaxation (parasympathetic) side of the equation.

Education provides the client with a cognitive frame—understanding—which will help further to normalize their experience and provide a level of reassurance that somebody knows what is happening, even if they don't like the idea that it may take several more weeks/months to resolve.

Physiotherapists also teach strategies for pain management—helping the client develop necessary "self-soothing" coping skills. Teaching relaxation techniques is within the physiotherapist's breadth of practice. Introducing the concepts of centering and grounding makes a lot of sense to the client who talks of being "knocked off my center" or "feeling like my legs have been kicked out from under me!" As the client lies on the table in a warm, supported position, they can be guided to imagine they are on a lovely soft white sandy beach and to let their body gently form an imprint in the sand. An alternate image to use is the deep, spongy, mossy forest floor where they can slowly sink into the support under the shade of an ancient growth fir; glimpsing the sky and the sunshine falling gently dappled through the leaves . . .

Guide the client to breathe easily with a slight emphasis on the exhale. Helping the client settle within their own body in this way is very helpful to them "coming home," building a safe place within their body. Guide them to let the imprint deepen with each breath, deeply sensing the skin contact, noticing how it feels—the areas where there is more or less support, warmth, coolness, pressure. Ask them to sense how it feels deep inside their body to be supported in this way. They may say a few words like, "relaxed" and "warm," telling you of their body sensations or "peaceful" and "safe," talking of their body experience. As they follow their breath, the flow of air in and out of the body, they deepen the breath, sensing the lower ribs moving into deeper contact with the table—gradually becoming aware of the rise and fall of the abdomen. Resting their hands on the belly (thumbs in the umbilicus) they can both feel the effect of the breath and become aware of the warmth/coolness of their hands in contact, letting the sensations sink deeper inside the body until they settle into the center.

The physical and energetic center of the body lies just in front of the sacrum about two-thirds from the front of the body and one-third from the back. Guide the client to sense the anterior aspect of the spinal column and estimate the size of the bones, front to back. The lumbar spine is about four and a half inches in depth, and this fact can be quite surprising to somebody who is feeling vulnerable and not coping well. Grasping a sense of a sturdy spine lets the client know they have internal support and this often can be a turning point.

Guide the client to stay connected to this center and notice if there is a colour, light or shape forming. If so, this energy can be expanded with the inhale and allowed to flow through the body on the exhale. Slowly it will fill every space and every cell, gently and calmly with healing energy, clearing stress and unwanted tensions from the tissues which can be released from the body with the exhale.

At the end of this exercise the client is asked to bring their focus back to their breathing, back to their contact on the table, to the support they feel—and gradually bring their awareness back to the room and into contact with the physiotherapist.

This is an exercise to practice at home. Besides helping the client to relax and self soothe their system, it also is very helpful for strengthening the abilities of body sensing—regaining a sense of safety, centering, and grounding.

The Psychology of Physiotherapy Exercises

In the Bodynamic System, from decades of research and testing, a psychological content and developmental age has been attributed to most of the muscles in the body. Bodynamic therapists know that working with muscles affects character structure (personality) and functions of ego. The functions that are most important to regain in a shock situation are centering, grounding, boundaries, containment, balance, and also the body ego.

Some of the most important exercises the physiotherapist teaches are core stabilizations. These exercises bring the client's attention to the pelvic floor and the deep transversus abdominal muscle that are container muscles for the center—the self. Other muscles that help the client contain their sense of self, emotions, thoughts, and feelings are the breathing muscles, trapezeii, latissimus dorsi, tensor fascia lata, and deltoid. Latissimus also gives a sense of "being backed" (supported) and the TFL and deltoid help define the edges of the body giving a sense of "this is my space" and strengthening boundaries.

Exercises given on a piece of exercise equipment such as a Shuttle can be very helpful as the first step toward activation. As the client is lying in a well-supported position they can sense their spine being supported and their feet in contact with the footrest. Pulling the arm straps with correct technique activates the latissimus/abdominal muscle sling and the pelvic floor. Arm exercises are also psychologically empowering. Being able to push and pull allows us to regulate contact, which is self-defining and builds boundaries. As exercises are progressed through sitting and standing, further trunk strengthening is developed along with grounding and balancing.

Instruct the client to be mindful of the muscle activity—to feel the energy building and sense the support within the muscle tissues. As the muscle relaxes, ask the client to hold onto the memory of the contraction for a little longer, reinforcing the emotional sense of building energy within the body. Traditionally one exhales when contracting muscle but some people may feel as if they are letting go of their energy. Experiment and ask the client to inhale when contracting notice if they feel any different inside.

In our colloquial language we talk of "going weak at the knees" in a shock situation and any exercise that uses the legs to push, if done mindfully will help regain the client's sense of being grounded and dissipate the effects of the shock. Three simple exercises to help the client regain contact with their legs and the ground are:

- In standing, shift the weight to one leg. Bend the knee and hip as deeply as possible. Notice your breathing. As tension builds in the leg muscles to the point of being too much, slowly push up and stand equally on both legs. Sense how your body is feeling. Sense your contact with the ground. Repeat on the other leg.

- Standing with your feet slightly apart, sense the muscles along your outer thigh and lower leg as you push your feet both into the ground and outward. Inhale and exhale. Keep the muscles energized so that they do not collapse on the exhale.

- Integrate the sensation of grounding by walking with purpose. As you walk, lead with your big toe and notice the butt muscles as they contract. Sense both the push off and contact with the ground and how your body feels in motion.

Physio ball work and balance exercises will also help the client regain a sense of center and grounding, as well as stimulating and reorganizing orienting and balance reflexes. Stretching exercises affecting fascia will also help reorganize the reflex system; take the stretch lightly but for an extended period of time. Three minutes per stretch will allow time enough for the fascial system to respond. A parasympathetic state is also aided by "slow flow," a staple in the Bodynamic repertoire. This is like a slow moving tai chi: As the person moves through space they extend arms and legs, trying to go off balance but staying in balance; finding the edge; moving around center.

Asking clients to sense physical support behind their back and under their buttocks as they sit, as well as feeling the feet in contact with the ground, is grounding. Finding this connection with the world around them is very calming and validating and helps rebuild a sense of self. Consequently, it is important to teach the client to sense their posture as they prepare for an exercise; making sure they are grounded on the floor, their back or seat before they exercise muscles and maintaining this grounding while they perform the activity.

Aspects of Ego

By the age of five we have ideally developed all levels of our ego but this is dependent on our upbringing and early childhood experiences. Many people lack a solid ego development and this shows up in how they handle their injuries and physiotherapy treatment. Clients may have little sense of their body ego or individual ego and carry their sense of self in their roles, usually related to their family, work, or hobbies. Loss of ability to work may compound the disorientation of self a client feels, besides precipitating fear and insecurity due to loss of income. This stress cycles back increasing fear, increasing muscle tension, increasing the pain/spasm cycle. Similarly with the loss of ability to play sports, which for so many people impacts deeply into their social life and personal support system. As they become more isolated from their daily life they start to fear permanent injury and fear for their future and their psyche collapses.

Trauma deeply impacts all levels of the ego and for the client who does not have strong resources, the effects can be quite disabling. As seen above, the physiotherapist is in the ideal position to help the client fill in some of the gaps, starting with building body resources and developing an external structure of goals and guidelines; holding the possibility of the client's return to what is meaningful for them.

Conclusion

The trauma response is both a psychological and a biological process underpinned by developmental issues, the client's personality, coping skills, and their personal support system. All of these factors impact the ways people view themselves and how they make their way forward in the world. People who learn to move through difficult times in their lives well are better resourced for future events. We all take knowledge and combine it into something new to increase our coping abilities.

While healing from trauma is a multi-layered and highly complex process, the physiotherapist is well positioned to assist clients resolve the normal trauma response by providing support, guidance, education and teaching exercises to strengthen body resources. Both body skills and a safe place are necessary to process the trauma response.

The physiotherapist can provide the client with a safe place and a cognitive frame in which to normalize their experience. Building an external structure through regularity of therapy sessions, establishing progressive achievable goals, exercise, and homework activities helps to settle the client's internal structure and personal organization. Building body resources is key and it is important for every post-trauma client to work on core stabilization and balance exercises, not just those with low back problems. Additionally, a routine of simple stretch and strengthening exercises, executed mindfully, for the whole body—and especially for latissimus dorsi, trapezeii, deltoid, TFL, and the quadriceps—will assist the client to move through their trauma and enhance their psyche as well as soma.

References

American Psychiatric Association. *DSM-IV Diagnostic and Statistical Manual of Mental Disorders Fourth Edition* (Washington, D.C.: American Psychiatric Association, 1994).

Bodynamic International ApS. "Handouts and articles for Bodynamic shock training." (Copenhagen: Kreatic Press, 2003).

Cullberg, J. *Kris och utveckling* (Stockholm: Natur och Kultur, 1975).

Jarlnaes, E. "The Bodynamic Analysis guidelines for working with the core of a shock-trauma. The Bodynamic shock-trauma 'recipe'." (Denmark: Bodynamic Institute, March 2000).

Van der Kolk, B.A., A.C. McFarlane, & L. Weisaeth, Eds. *Traumatic Stress. The Effects of Overwhelming Experience on Mind, Body and Society* (New York: The Guiford Press, 1996).

Van der Kolk, B.A., O. van der Hart, & J. Burbridge. "Approaches to the Treatment of PTSD." (Bookline, MA: Trauma Clinic, undated).

Personal notes from training in Bodynamic Analysis with Lisbeth Marcher, Merete Holm Brantbjerg, Ditte Marcher, & Erik Jarlnaes.

It Won't Hurt Forever ... Guiding Your Child Through Trauma

—Peter A. Levine, Ph.D., & Maggie Kline, M.S., M.F.T.

Lisa cried hysterically every time the family prepared to get into their car.

Carlos doubled over in his chair as he sat with his head in his hands in the school psychologist's office. He is a painfully shy fifteen-year-old and chronically truant. "I just don't want to be here. I don't want to feel scared all the time anymore ... all I want is to feel normal."

Sarah, on the other hand, reported dutifully to her second-grade class on time everyday. Inevitably by 11:00 AM, she could be found in the nurse's office complaining of stomachaches. No medical reason could be found for her symptoms.

Curtis, a popular, good-natured middle school youngster, told his mom that he felt like kicking someone ... anyone. He had no idea where this urge was coming from, and had never felt this way before. Two weeks later, he started behaving aggressively toward his little brother.

The pediatrician referred three-year-old Kevin for a special education preschool assessment. His "autistic-like" play was becoming of increasing concern to his parents. Lying on the floor, he stiffened his body pretending he was dying and slowly coming back to life saying, "Save me!" repeating the same scenario over and over.

What do Lisa, Kevin, Carlos, Sarah, and Curtis have in common? And why do their symptoms persist? Will they disappear on their own or grow worse over time? Let's take a deeper look at these children's histories:

What Do These Youngsters Have in Common?

- Lisa was strapped into her car seat when the family's station wagon was rear-ended in a "fender-bender" at about fifteen miles per hour with no physical injuries.

- Carlos had been intimidated for five years by an emotionally disturbed adult stepbrother when his mother remarried when he was six years old.

- Sarah was told abruptly and unexpectedly that her parents were getting divorced and her father would be moving out during her first month of second grade.

- Curtis witnessed a drive-by shooting that left the victim dead on the sidewalk while waiting for his early morning school bus to arrive.

- Kevin was delivered by emergency C-section due to fetal distress and had a life-saving surgery within twenty-four hours of his birth.

Although each youngster is a different age with different symptoms and circumstances, a common thread unites them: They have all experienced overwhelming life events. And, although the events are over, they continue to experience life as if they are not! These children are all suffering from traumatic stress that has not gone away on its own.

Children Can Be Traumatized by Things That May Not Seem Traumatic to You

By now, it is common knowledge that traumatic reactions can develop in anyone, regardless of age. Those at greatest risk, however, are infants and children. Childhood abuse and neglect, the all-too-frequent witnessing of violence, war, auto accidents, and natural disasters such as earthquakes, tornadoes, fires, and floods are now being recognized as potentially traumatic. You may not be surprised to learn that being witness to a murder has affected Curtis; but what about the others? You may not have considered that symptoms can also have roots in what are generally thought to be "common" occurrences like fender benders, medical procedures, divorce, chronic bullying, and even falling off a bicycle!

From the Story of Dory:
On her last birthday, this girl's dream came true
She got a new bike that was bright shiny blue
She jumped on the bike and rode down the block
Faster and faster, then the bike hit a rock.

She felt the wheels skid, and she flew off the seat
And then she landed real hard on the street.
She hit the pavement with a big thud.
Then she noticed her knees were covered with blood.

She started to cry, but the sound wouldn't come
She couldn't breathe, and her body went numb
When she saw all that blood on her knees . . .
Like Oscar Opossum (refer to animal stories), she started to freeze.

The good news is that, while the events themselves may be an inevitable part of growing up, traumatic symptoms are often preventable and, if they cannot be prevented, can be healed. We shall see both *why* and *how* as we explore ordinary and extraordinary common sources of potential overwhelm for children.

Common Causes of Childhood Trauma

- Animal attack (such as a dog or snake bite)
- Physical injuries from accidents and falls (bicycle, auto, stairs, etc.)
- Life-threatening illnesses and high fevers
- Being lost (at the mall, in a strange neighborhood, etc.); prolonged separation
- Natural disasters (fires, floods, tornadoes, hurricanes, and earthquakes)
- Medical and dental procedures and surgeries

- Exposure to extremes of temperature, particularly when left alone
- Sudden loss (death or divorce)
- Near drowning (pool, ocean, pond, or bathtub)

Note: Events that may not be traumatizing to an adult may be overwhelming to a child.

What Exactly Is Trauma?

Drawing on thirty years of Dr. Levine's research and experience, he asserts that the basis of trauma is physiological rather than "psychological." Because there is no time to think when facing threat, our primary responses are instinctual. In other words, we're born with them. At the root of a traumatic reaction is the 280 million-year-old heritage that we share with nearly every living creature on earth ... a heritage that resides in the most primitive parts of the brain, known as the reptilian brain. When the reptilian brain perceives danger, it automatically activates an extraordinary amount of energy ... just like an adrenaline rush that allows a 120-pound mother to lift and pull her child out from under a Chevrolet! This, in turn, triggers a pounding heart and numerous other bodily changes, designed to give our bodies every advantage it needs to defend itself or protect its loved ones. The catch is that to avoid being traumatized, *all of that excess energy must be used up to deal with the threat and emerge victorious.* When excess energy is not discharged, it does not simply go away; instead, it stays trapped, creating the potential for traumatic symptoms to occur. The younger the child, the fewer resources she has to defend and protect herself, resulting in a greater amount of undischarged energy. The likelihood of the onset of future traumatic reactions is directly proportional to the amount of mobilized energy that was ready to fight, flee, or protect, but had no place to go.

Jack:

I treated Jack, an eleven-year-old Boy Scout and straight-A student, who had sudden onset school phobia following a minor earthquake. The incident was so inconsequential by California standards that it might be more apropos to call it a minor tremor. What could possibly have made Jack's experience so traumatic as to keep him home from school, a place he truly enjoyed? When Jack first felt the tremor, he was unable to predict the accurate level of danger … the only thing that registered in his reptilian brain was the "red flag" of threat. Jack's nervous system responded to the perceived danger with full-on alert … like it was supposed to. However, Jack continued to feel panicky well after the event. The severity of this response became understandable, as I came to find out that as a small child Jack had been confined to a body cast following a surgery. He had to lie in bed for several weeks. It was a terrifying experience for Jack. Frightened by the procedure and then trapped and immobilized by the cast, was he powerless to move or respond to the dangers he perceived lurking all around him—as small children do after such a scary event. Feeling the intense energetic impulse to flee, and yet coming up against the hard confines of his cast, he collapsed into fearful resignation, which is what any healthy animal does in a situation where escape is impossible. Just like in the story illustrated below with Oscar Opossum, Jack "rolled up in a ball," and had "all of his energy boiling inside." Unfortunately, even after removal of the cast, the undischarged energy remained present in his nervous system. And then some years later, Jack was again lying in his bed when the small tremor occurred just before it was time to get up for school. His body "remembered" the old helplessness and responded to the present danger as though he was still confined in the cast. He feared that he would be unable to protect himself out in the world and became panicky. What looked like school phobia was really a fear of his own internal sensations and loss of trust in his bodily responses instilled many years before.

Children like Jack can be helped through simple rhymes and images like the ones below. Since animals are non-judgmental and instinctual, they can be powerful resources to help children connect directly with their own innate healing process, without getting distracted by the more typical human judgments of shame and blame.

Lessons from the Animal World

The link between wild animal behavior and the field of human trauma was made by Dr. Levine in the late 1960s when he observed that prey animals in the wild, through threatened routinely, are rarely traumatized. Further research led to the discovery that animals have a built-in ability to rebound from a steady diet of danger. They literally "shake off" the residual energy left behind before going about their business. This can be observed as trembling, rapid eye movements, shaking, panting, and taking a deep spontaneous breath as the body returns to equilibrium. Without a well-developed cerebral cortex, they do not have words to pass judgment on their feelings and sensations. Instead they do what comes naturally. There is no shame or blame ... just the primitive language of the instinctual reptilian brain ... the language of sensation. The "emotional first aid" presented here is intended to provide a journey into the inner world of a child's bodily sensations as a way of fostering resilience to the challenges and stresses that all children face.

From Oscar Opossum:

Oscar escapes, you see, by lying quite still
Not like the rabbit who runs up the hill
Oscar has all his energy BOILING inside
From holding his breath to pretend that he died.

Can you pretend that you're Oscar rolled up in a ball?
You're barely breathing, and you feel very small
It's cold and it's lonely as you hold on tight
Hoping coyote will not take a bite!

Oscar Opossum has to lie low
But inside his body, he's ready to blow
When Charlie Coyote finally takes off
Oscar Opossum gets up and shakes off.

See Oscar tremble, see Oscar shake
Just like the ground in a little earthquake.
After he trembles and shakes for awhile
He feels good as new, and walks off with a smile.

Different Sensations That Help Your Child Heal

Children need their caregivers to make ample time for them to experience, through bodily sensations, specific elements that relate to their recovery from things that have overwhelmed them. These include sensations of empowerment, such as strength and grounding.

Verses from The Magic in Me:
We're going to play, but before we begin,
I want you to find your own magic within.
Just take some time to feel and to see
All the great things that your body can be.

Pretend you're a tree with your branches so high
That you can reach up and tickle the sky.
What's it like to be strong like a big old oak tree?
With roots in your feet and your leaves waving free?

Giving Appropriate Support to an Overwhelmed Child

In order to prevent or minimize trauma, it is important to make sure that you're not overwrought by your child's mishap. It may be easier to remain calm with the knowledge that children are both resilient and malleable. Children, when supported appropriately, are usually able to rebound from stressful events. In fact, as they begin to triumph over life's shocks and losses, they grow into more competent and vibrant beings. Because the capacity to heal is innate, your role as an adult is simple: to help the little ones access this capacity. This is similar in many ways to the function of a band-aid or a splint. The band-aid or splint doesn't heal the wound, but protects and supports the body as it restores itself. The suggestions provided here are meant to enable you to be a good "band-aid" for your child.

So how can adults give appropriate support? First of all, it is important to let your child know that any powerful emotions that she/he may be having (e.g., sadness, anger, rage, fear, and pain) are not only okay—they are normal under the circumstances. (We will see later there may be exceptions; for example, in needing to calm your child for a medical procedure.) Children are comforted and empowered by the knowledge that their pain is time-limited, that it won't last forever, but that whatever they are feeling now is accepted. Children will move through their feelings rather quickly when they are not rushed. Having the patience to attune your pace to your child's rhythm gives him/her permission to be authentic. This acceptance and respect sets the conditions for the child, in his or her own time, to rebound to a healthy sense of well-being. Often children react the way their parents think they should, in order to please them. They will act "strong" and "brave," overriding their own feelings only to end up with trauma symptoms that could have averted. Countless adults in therapy have reported stifling their feelings as children to protect their parents from "feeling bad."

Be alert to this pitfall and circumvent it by paying close attention to your child's expression. When there is shock, it is common for them to not feel much at first, as the chemicals released for fight-or-flight also serve as a kind of natural anesthesia. For example, if they are cut, they may not notice it until they see the blood, as the pain is usually delayed until the shock begins to wear off. The child may seem dazed and pale but act as if nothing really happened. On the other hand, they may be crying hysterically. Validate your child's emotional and physical pain in a calming voice assuring them that you will stay with them to do whatever needs to be done. Children benefit most from the sense that there is a calm, centered adult in charge, who is accepting, knows what to do, and is able to keep him/her safe.

Your Calmness Is Essential

The importance of the adult's calmness cannot be overemphasized. When a child has been hurt or frightened, it is normal for the adult to feel shocked or scared. Because of your own fears and protective instincts, it is not uncommon to respond initially with anger, which can further frighten the child. The goal is to minimize—not compound—feelings of fright, shame, embarrassment, and guilt the child is likely to be experiencing already. The best antidote is to tend to your own reactions first. Allow time for your own bodily responses to settle rather than scolding or running anxiously toward your child. Experiences with our clients in therapy confirm that often the most frightening part of the experience for the child was their parents' reaction! The younger the child, the more they "read" the facial expression of their caregivers as a barometer of how serious the danger or injury.

Emotional First Aid for an Overwhelmed Child

After paying close attention to your child's bodily responses, support these reactions by not interrupting their natural cycle for coming out of shock. If you have an infant or young child, hold her/him safely on your lap. If it's an older child, you can place one hand on their shoulder, arm or middle of the back. Be careful not to hold your child too tightly or in such a way as to stop the natural discharge that will follow. You will most likely observe shaking, trembling, tears, chills, or heat. Help your child to remain calm with a reassuring voice and a few words, such as, "That's okay"; "It's all right to feel ..."; "Just let the shaking happen." After the trembling, tears, etc. stop, validate your child's emotional responses. Let him/her know that whatever they are feeling is okay and you will stay with them to listen. Resist the temptation to "talk them out" of fear, sadness, anger, embarrassment, guilt, or shame to avoid your own discomfort. Trust that your child will move through these feelings when supported. An exception would be when the parent needs to actively calm and distract their child when preparing them for a medical procedure like surgery. A parent's ingenuity would take precedence here as they help their youngster to relax.

The Reptilian Brain Speaks Not in Words, but Rather in the Language of Sensation

The language of sensation is, to many, a relatively foreign language. There is a world of sensation and feeling inside of us that exists whether we are aware of it of not. Fortunately, it is easy to learn … and as essential when traveling the "road to recovery" as learning some survival phrases when traveling abroad. It is a good idea to get acquainted with your own inner landscape first. All it takes is some unhurried time set aside, without distractions, to pay attention to how your body feels. Sensations can range from pressure or temperature changes on our skin to vibrations, gurgles, muscular tension, constrictions or spaciousness and temperature changes deep within. This is the language of the primitive brain that acts on our behalf when in danger. It ensures our survival. It is the wise adult who begins to know this deep instinctual consciousness. Before an emergency comes up, spend some quiet time sitting and learning this language. Or you can sit with a partner as witness to what you are experiencing—to "stand guard" as animals in nature do for an added feeling of safety. As with any new language, it helps to develop a vocabulary. The box below will get you started. Your child and you can have fun adding to the list and watching it grow as you explore your depths!

Sensation Vocabulary Box

cold/warm/hot/chilly	twitchy/butterflies	sharp/dull/itchy
shaky/trembly/tingly	hard/soft/stuck	jittery/icy/weak
relaxed/calm/peaceful	flowing/spreading	strong/tight/tense
dizzy/fuzzy/blurry	numb/prickly/jumpy	owie/tearful/goose bumpy

---

*Note that sensations are different than emotions. They describe the physical way the body feels. Non-verbal children can be invited to point to where in their bodies it might feel shaky, numb, or calm, etc.

How To Tell if Your Child Has Been Traumatized

Common indications of trauma after a stressful event are withdrawal, fearfulness, irritability, clinging, trouble sleeping, emotional outbursts, nightmares, excessive shyness, and aggression. Other symptoms are an exaggerated startle response and regression to earlier behaviors such as bedwetting and thumb sucking. Some children become avoidant to the point of developing phobias. These can be specific, such as a phobia of dogs if bitten, or more general like in the example of Jack who developed a school phobia after the earthquake. Physical symptoms are also common, such as tummy and headaches, nausea, vomiting, diarrhea or constipation, and sometimes even fevers. Several of these symptoms may also be caused, of course, by an illness like the flu. If they are due to flu, they should pass in a day or so; phobias and other symptoms usually do not. In fact they often get more complex over time.

First Aid for Accidents and Falls

1. Attend to Your Responses First

Take time to notice your own level of fear or concern. Next, take a full deep breath, and as you exhale slowly, sense the feelings in your own body until you are settled enough to respond calmly. An overly emotional or smothering adult may frighten the child as much as the accident.

2. Keep Your Child Still and Quiet

If injuries require that they be picked up or moved, make sure they are supported properly. Do not allow them to move on their own—remember they are probably in shock and do not realize the extent of the injury. Keep the child comfortably warm by draping a sweater or blanket over them.

3. Encourage Plenty of Time for Safety and Rest

4. Assess the Situation

If your child shows signs of shock (glazed eyes, pale skin, rapid or shallow breathing, disorientation, overly emotional, overly tranquil, or acting like nothing has happened), do not allow them to jump up and return to play. You might say something like, "We're going to sit (or lie) still together for awhile and wait until the shock wears off." A calm confident voice communicates to the child that you know what's best.

5. As the Shock Wears Off, Guide Your Child's Attention to Her Sensations

The language of recovery is the language of the reptilian brain—which is the language of sensations. Softly ask your child how she feels "in her body." Repeat her answer as a question, "You feel okay in your body?" and wait for a nod or other response. Be more specific with the next question: "How do you feel in your tummy (head, arm, leg, etc.)?" If she mentions a distinct sensation, gently ask about its location, size, shape, color, or weight. Keep guiding your child to stay with the present moment with questions such as, "How does the rock (sharpness, lump, 'owie,' sting) feel now?" If they are too young or too startled to talk, have them point to where it hurts.

6. Allow a Minute or Two of Silence between Questions

This may be the hardest part for the adult, but it's the most important part for the child. This allows any cycle that may be moving through to release the excess energy to completion. Be alert for cues that let you know a cycle has finished. These cues include a deep, relaxed, spontaneous breath; the cessation of crying or trembling; a stretch; a yawn; a smile; or the making or breaking of eye contact. Wait to see if another cycle begins or if there is a sense of enough for now.

7. Encourage Your Child to Rest Even if They Don't Want To

Deep discharges generally continue during rest and sleep. Do not stir up discussion about the mishap by asking questions. Later on, the child may want to tell a story about it, draw a picture, or play it through. If a lot of energy was mobilized, the release will continue. The next cycle may be too subtle for you to notice, but the rest promotes a fuller recovery, allowing the body to gently vibrate, give off heat, and go through skin color changes, etc., as the nervous system returns to relaxation. In addition, dream activity can help move the body through the necessary physiological changes. These changes happen naturally. All you have to do is provide the calm, quiet environment. (Caution: Of course, if your child has had a head injury, you want them to rest but NOT sleep until your doctor declares it safe.)

8. Continue To Validate Your Child's Physical Responses

Resist impulse to stop your child's tears or trembling, but keep contact with them, reminding them that whatever has happened is over. In order to return to equilibrium, your child's distress needs to continue until it stops on its own. This part usually takes from one to several minutes. Studies have shown that children who are able to cry and tremble after an accident have fewer problems recovering from it. Your job is to use a calm voice and reassuring hand to let the child know that "It's good to let the scary stuff shake right out of you." The key is to avoid interrupting or distracting your child, holding her too tightly, or moving too far away.

9. Attend to Your Child's Emotional Responses

Later, when your child is rested and calm—even the next day—set aside some time to talk about his feelings and what he experienced. Children often feel anger or shame. Help your child to know that those feelings are normal and that you understand. You might then share a similar experience that you or someone you know had, if you feel it would help. Or, additional help through stories and poems like the ones shown here, together with your child's artwork, illustrations, and play can be very helpful.

Helping Your Traumatized Child Heal Through Play

If the first aid guidelines minimized the traumatic effect but did not prevent it altogether, or if your child is suffering from symptoms caused by an earlier event, you can still help them be in touch with their sensations and move through them. Children show adults what parts of the overwhelming experience are unresolved through their drawings and play. The effects of trauma, regardless of the cause, can be healed. Trauma is a fact of life but doesn't have to be life sentence. Parents and others, such as teachers and medical personnel who work with children are routinely confronted with reenactments of the traumatic event. These situations often surface during playtime. The question is, what can be done to help resolve the feelings of shame, injustice and betrayal that usually underlie the compulsion to reenact an experience? Let's take a look at an example of a typical youngster named Sammy to see what can happen when a relatively common incident goes awry, and how, through play and appropriate guidance, a successful outcome can be achieved.

The Story of Sammy

Sammy has been spending the weekend with his grandparents where I am their guest. He is being an impossible tyrant, aggressively and relentless trying to control his new environment. Nothing pleases him; he is in a foul temper every waking moment. When he is asleep, he tosses and turns as if wrestling with his bedclothes. This behavior is not entirely unexpected from a two-and-a-half-year-old whose parents have gone away for the weekend—children with separation anxiety often act it out. Sammy, however, has always enjoyed visiting his grandparents and this behavior seems extreme to them.

They confide in me that six months earlier, Sammy fell off of his high chair and split his chin open. Bleeding heavily, he was taken to the local emergency room. When the nurse came to take his temperature and blood pressure, he was so frightened that she was unable to record his vital signs. The two-year-old child was then strapped down in a "pediatric papoose" (a board with flaps and Velcro straps). With his torso and legs immobilized, the only part of his body he could move was his head and neck; which naturally, he did as energetically as he could. The doctors responded by tightening the restraint and immobilizing his head with their hands in order to suture his chin. After this upsetting experience, his mom and dad took Sammy out for a hamburger and then to the playground. His mother was very attentive and carefully validated his experience of being scared and hurt, and all seemed forgotten. However, the boy's overbearing attitude began shortly after this event. Could Sammy's tantrums and over-controlling behavior be related to his perceived helplessness from this trauma?

I discovered that Sammy had been to the emergency room several times with various injuries, though he had never displayed this degree of terror and panic. When the parents returned, we agreed to explore whether there might be a traumatic charge still associated with this recent experience.

We all gathered in the cabin where I was staying. With parents, grandparents, and Sammy watching, I placed his stuffed Pooh Bear on the edge of a chair in such a way that it immediately fell to the floor. We decided that it was hurt and had to be taken to the hospital. Sammy shrieked, bolted for the door, and ran across a footbridge and down a narrow path to the creek. Our suspicions were confirmed. His most recent visit to the hospital was neither harmless nor forgotten. Sammy's behavior told us that this game was potentially overwhelming for him.

Sammy's parents brought him back from the creek. He clung frantically to his mother as we prepared for another game. We reassured him that we would all be there to help protect Pooh Bear. Again he ran—but this time only into the next room. We followed him in there and waited to see what would happen next. Sammy ran to the bed and hit it with both arms while looking at me expectantly.

"Mad, huh?" I said. He gave me a look that confirmed my question. Interpreting his expression as a go-ahead sign, I put Pooh Bear under a blanket and placed Sammy on the bed next to him.

"Sammy, let's all help Pooh Bear."

I held Pooh Bear under the blanket, and asked everyone to help. Sammy watched with interest, but soon got up and ran to his mother. With his arms held tightly around her legs, he said, "Mommy, I'm scared."

Without pressuring him, we waited until Sammy was ready and willing to play the game again. The next time, his grandma and Pooh Bear were held down together and Sammy actively participated in their rescue. When Pooh Bear was freed, Sammy ran to his mother, clinging even more tightly than before. He began to tremble and shake in fear, and then his chest opened up in a growing sense of excitement, triumph, and pride. The next time he held on to his mommy, there was less clinging and more excited jumping. We waited until Sammy was ready to play again. Everyone except Sammy took a turn being rescued with Pooh. Each time, Sammy became more vigorous as he pulled off the blanket and escaped into the safety of his mother's arms.

When it was Sammy's turn to be held under the blanket with Pooh Bear, he became quite agitated and fearful. He ran back to his mother's arms several times before he was able to accept the ultimate challenge. Bravely, he climbed under the blankets with Pooh while I held the blanket gently down. I watched his eyes grow wide with fear, but only for a moment. Then he grabbed Pooh Bear, shoved the blanket away and flung himself into his mother's arms. Sobbing and trembling, he screamed, "Mommy, get me out of here. Mommy, get this thing off of me." His startled father told me that these were the same words Sammy screamed while imprisoned in the papoose at the hospital. He remembered this clearly because he had been quite surprised by his son's ability to make such a direct, well-spoken demand at two-plus years of age.

We went through the escape several more times. Each time, Sammy exhibited more power and more triumph. Instead of running fearfully to his mother, he jumped excitedly up and down. With every successful escape, we all clapped and danced together, cheering, "Yeah for Sammy, yeah, yeah. Sammy saved Pooh Bear." Two-and-a-half-year-old Sammy had achieved mastery over the experience that had shattered him a few months earlier.

If he hadn't received help, might Sammy have become more anxious, hyperactive, clinging, and controlling? Would his trauma have resulted in bedwetting or in restricted and less healthy behaviors later? Might he have violently reenacted the event as a teenager or young adult? Or would he have developed symptoms like tummy aches, migraines, and anxiety attacks without knowing why? All of these scenarios are possible, and equally impossible to pin down. We cannot know how, when, or even whether a child's traumatic experience will invade his or her life in another form. However, we can help protect our children from these possibilities through prevention. This "ounce of prevention" will help them develop into surer, more spontaneous adults.

Children like Sammy rarely get the help they need immediately following an incident such as this one. Youngsters can most easily be supported at this critical time while they literally shake and tremble through the immobility, shame, loss, and rage. This process will enable them to safely discharge the intense energy mobilized to defend themselves. If this does not happen, then the healing impact of therapy that focuses on the "story" of what happened is severely limited.

Falls

When working with falls, big soft pillows can be helpful in giving your child the opportunity to practice falling safely. With your hands to support them securely, gently guide a slow fall, pausing it when they seem to stiffen or startle. It's often best to start with them sitting and gently rock them first from side to side and then forward and backward. Then they can "fall," a little at a time, into your supporting arms and onto the pillows when standing. All of this helps to develop good protective reflexes and restores confidence. You can use a doll or stuffed animal like we did with Sammy. Be sure to watch your child's responses closely. Always leave them with a sense that they can succeed, giving them only as much support as they need.

Desensitizing After an Automobile Accident

Often the adult needs to tell the story of what (they believe) happened, and then invite the child to add their version. Sometimes it is best to use a different name for the child in the story. This may help initially to give needed distance from the event. You may also want to reintroduce your child to ordinary objects or experiences that remain "charged" because they in some way remind the child of the incident that overwhelmed them.

After an automobile accident, for example, the infant or toddler's car seat could be brought into the living room. Holding the infant in your arms, or gently walking with the toddler, you can gradually move toward it together and eventually place the child in the seat. The key here is to take "baby" steps, watching and waiting for responses such as stiffening, turning away, holding their breath and heart rate changes, for example. With each gentle approach to the avoided or fear-provoking encounter, the procedure outlined above can, again, be used as a guide. The idea is to make sure that your pacing is in tune with your child's needs so that not too much energy or emotion is released at once. You can tell if this is occurring when the child seems to be getting more "wound up." Calm them by offering gentle reassurance, touching, holding, rocking, etc.

Preparing Your Child for Surgery and Other Medical Procedures

One common and frequently overlooked source of traumatization in children is routine or emergency medical procedures. Armed with knowledge, parents can work together as a team with clinic and hospital personnel to reduce unnecessary overwhelm from invasive medical and surgical procedures. But before giving you tips on how to do this, I'd like to tell you a story that may surprise you about a boy named Teddy ...

"Daddy, daddy, let it go, let it go ... Please don't kill it ... Let it go."

These are the terrified screams uttered by ten-year-old Teddy as he bolts from the room like a frightened jackrabbit. Puzzled, his father holds a motionless tree shrew in the palm of his hand, one that he found in the back yard and brought to his son. He thought it an excellent and scientific way to teach Teddy how animals "play possum" in order to survive. Startled by the boy's reaction to his seemingly harmless gesture, Teddy's father is unaware of the connection that his son has just made to a long-forgotten event. It was an "ordinary" event, similar to one that millions of us have experienced.

On Teddy's fifth birthday, the family pediatrician and lifelong friend came for a visit. The whole clan gathered around the doctor as he proudly showed them a photograph he had taken at the local hospital, depicting baby Teddy at age nine months. The boy took a brief look at the picture, and then ran wildly from the room, screaming in rage and terror. How many parents, teachers, babysitters, and health care providers have witnessed similar mysterious reactions in children?

At nine months of age, Teddy developed a severe rash that covered his whole body. He was taken to the local hospital and strapped down to a pediatric examination table. While being poked and prodded by a team of specialists, the immobilized child screamed in terror under the glaring lights. Following the examination, he was placed in isolation for seven days. When his mother, who had not been allowed to see him for over a week, arrived at the hospital to bring him home, Teddy did not recognize her. She claims that the boy never again connected with her or any other family member. He did not bond with other children, grew increasingly isolated, and began living in a world of his own. Though by no means the only factor, the hospital trauma experienced by nine-month-old Teddy was an important, possibly critical, component in the shaping of Theodore Kazcinski, the convicted Unabomber.

Without appropriate support, children do not have the inner resources to comprehend the blinding lights, physical restraints, surgical instruments, masked monsters speaking in garbled language, and drug-induced altered states of consciousness. Nor are they able to make sense of waking up alone in a recovery room to their own moans of pain, the eerie tones of electronic monitoring equipment, and the random visitations of strangers. For infants and young children, events such as these can be as terrifying and traumatizing as being abducted and tortured by revolting alien giants. Ted Kazcinski's crusade against the dehumanization of technology begins to make sense when we learn about his overwhelming and dehumanizing experience as an infant.

Other parents have witnessed the disconnection, isolation, despair, and bizarre behavior of their children following hospitalization and surgery. The evidence has pointed to the possibility that these long-term behavioral changes were connected to traumatic reactions resulting from "routine" medical procedures. But, is this possible? The answer is yes.

Does this mean that if your child has been traumatized by a medical procedure he or she will become a serial killer? Not likely. Most traumatized children do not "act out" their traumas. Instead, events like these become internalized in a process we call "acting in," which may later show up as anxiety, inability to concentrate, or aches and pains. Let's look at a more ordinary story from the pages of Reader's Digest entitled *Everything is not Okay*, a father describes his son Robbie's "minor" knee surgery:

The doctor tells me that everything is okay. The knee is fine, but everything is not okay for the boy ... waking up in a drug induced nightmare, thrashing around on his hospital bed ... a sweet boy who never hurt anybody ... staring out from his anesthetic haze with the eyes of a wild animal, striking the nurse, screaming, "Am I alive?" and forcing me to grab his arms ... staring right into my eyes and not knowing who I am.

Stories like this are commonplace events, often leading to the formation of tragic psychic scars. In 1946, Dr. David Levy presented extensive evidence that children in hospitals for routine reasons often experience the same "nightmarish" symptoms as shell-shocked soldiers. Fifty years later, our medical establishment is just beginning to recognize this vital information. If properly used, this knowledge could prevent the unnecessary traumatization of millions of children annually.

What Can You Do?

Fortunately, you do not have to wait for our medical care system to change. You can be proactive.

If you select a doctor and hospital wisely, you've won half the battle. Medical personnel frequently don't want parents to be partners on the team—for good reason. An emotional, demanding parent would interfere with safety and efficiency, to say nothing about upsetting the child. If you remain calm with a helpful presence, the staff is more likely to allow you to push the limits a bit in terms of how much you can be with your child. It is important to educate not dictate!

Guidelines When Preparing Your Child for Surgery

All kids want a parent to be with them during treatment. Your presence can be helpful if you are not anxious yourself. During the procedure, the parent needs to reassure and comfort—at times, even distract the child. Don't make the situation worse. If you feel like you are going to break down in tears, you may encourage your child to cry. However, during the procedure, this is not what is needed (though right after the child is injured—before medical procedures are begun—crying can help allowing the child to discharge the fear and shock).

When the Medical Procedure Is an Emergency

1. Once the imminent danger is over and, for example, you are riding with your child in the ambulance, take time to observe and assess your own reactions. Allow time to stop, remind yourself that you have tools now to help, allow time to settle your own shakiness, and wait for your own breath to come before proceeding. A sense of relative calm is essential. Just like the stewardess who informs the adults in an emergency to put their own oxygen mask on before assisting their children, your own physiological and emotional responses must be attended to first.

2. Reassure the child that it will be okay, that the doctor will help make them better, stop hurting, etc.

3. Distracting your child right before the medical procedure can be helpful. Retell their favorite story, bring their favorite toy, or talk about their favorite place … like the park, making plans, perhaps, to go there when they are better. If your child is in pain, you can have them clap, sing, or tap themselves to lessen the pain. Or, you can ask them to tell you a place in their body that feels okay or has less pain, and direct them to focus on that body part.

4. If they are old enough to understand, tell them what will happen at the hospital or doctor's office. For example, "The doctor will sew up the cut so it will stop bleeding," or, "The nurse will give you either a pill or a needle with medicine to stop the pain, and make you feel better."

Practical Steps in Preparing Your Child for Scheduled Surgeries and Procedures

It is extremely common for children to be traumatized by surgeries and other medical interventions. Two procedures that can be particularly terrifying are being strapped down to an examining table and being put under anesthesia without being properly prepared. Be proactive in the following ways:

Before surgery:

1. Choose a doctor and hospital that are sensitive to children's needs. Not all facilities are created equal. Some hospitals even have social workers with specially designed programs using story and role-play with children beforehand. Sometimes doctors aren't aware of these programs, so investigate on your own and find a user-friendly team that will listen to what you have to say. Remember, you are the consumer!

2. Prepare your child for what will happen. Tell them the truth without unnecessary details. Children do better when they know what to expect. If you tell them it won't hurt when it will, you have betrayed their trust. They will come to fear the worst when they cannot rely on you to tell the truth.

3. Arrange with the doctors (especially the surgeon and anesthesiologist) to meet your child beforehand in her ordinary doctor attire before dressing in surgical garb and mask. It is important for your child to see that the doctor is a human being who will be helping her ... not some monster. Perhaps your youngster can put on a doctor's costume, too! If that's not possible, she can put a disposable surgical mask on herself, or on a doll or favorite stuffed animal.

4. If the hospital does not have a program to prepare children, or even if they do, you can have your child dress up in a white gown, or dress puppets, dolls, or stuffed animals up in medical attire and play "operation" at home, going through all the steps including riding on a gurney, getting injections, and preparing for anesthesia. Have a dress rehearsal. Most toy stores have play figurines and medical kits for children.

During surgery:

1. Be with your child as much as possible before and after the operation. Ask to be with your child during administration of pre-operative drugs, and remain until your child transitions from waking consciousness to a "twilight" state.

2. A child should *never* be strapped down to an examining table or put under anesthesia in a terrified state. This leaves an imprint deep in their psyches and nervous systems. Your child should be soothed until calmed. Ask the doctor if you can hold your child. If the child must be strapped down, explain this to your child and remain with him until comforted and supported enough to go on. Fear coupled with the inability to move, puts a child in a terrified shock reaction—a recipe for trauma!

3. Ideally, be in the post-operative room when your child is waking up. The child should never awaken in the recovery room alone. Without a familiar adult to comfort them, many youngsters wake up disoriented and panicked. Their state is so altered that they may believe they have died … or that something horrific has happened to them. It is important that you talk with the hospital personal and request strongly that there be a nurse or someone there to make soothing contact when the child awakes.

After surgery:

1. Rest speeds recovery. All of your child's energy needs to first go into healing physically.

2. If your child is in pain, have them describe the pain and then find a part of the body that is pain-free, or at least less painful. As you sit with your child, have them alternate awareness between the part that hurts and the part that doesn't hurt so much. Often, this can alleviate the pain. You can also distract your child through the tough places by humming with them, or have them clap or tap a part of their body. The image of differently colored balloons taking the pain into the sky can be useful.

3. If your child appears fearful, assist them by using storytelling. Use another child's name or make the story up about their favorite stuffed animal. Begin it with "I know a little child named Jake who…" Watch your child's body language. Slow down and work with the parts that seem to be stuck by using the tools listed under First Aid at the beginning of this article. The main idea is to help your child through any "frozen" or shocked states into the shaking and trembling of discharge and finally to calming and resolution.

4. And remember to monitor your own level of calmness ... your calmness and confidence is contagious!

A Word about Elective Surgeries

Unnecessary surgeries could easily be the topic of another article. Without going into depth, suffice it to say that there are two procedures that are administered routinely that you would be wise to question their health benefits. These are circumcision and Caesarean Section. Weigh the advantages and disadvantages by reading as much as you can and talking to professionals on both sides of the controversy.

If you choose to circumcise for religious or other reasons, at least make sure that a local anesthetic is given and that your baby is calmed. Do not allow your infant to cry and scream until exhausted.

Of course, in the case of C-sections, they are often performed in an emergency to save lives. But if your C-section is an elective one that was suggested by your doctor for convenience, take some time to explore the options. You can also check the hospital's records to see if C-sections are almost a standard operating procedure. It is better for infants, when safety is not an issue, to work their way into the world, fully engaged in the process of their own birth. Many operations that were once considered routine, such as tonsillectomies and operations for "lazy eyes," have now come into question. Always seek second and third opinions to assess if a surgery is really necessary.

A Final Note

If your child develops trauma symptoms and these symptoms persist, or if you suspect that your child has been sexually molested or physically abused, it is important to seek the help of a professional therapist who specializes in working with traumatized children. Ask for referrals from your local school, pediatrician, or friends that have had good experiences with a child therapist. Interview the therapist about his/her training and experience in working with children.

No matter what the event, if after trying these exercises and first aid suggestions, your child is still having symptoms or problems, again, seek professional help. Do not wait for symptoms to become full-blown. Taking advantage of the help offered by a competent professional could be the wisest investment in your family's health that you will ever make.

Our New Reality

On September 11, 2001, our collective reality was shattered. We were left with profound unanswered questions and fears about what might happen next, and what to tell our children. In fact, what is most important is not so much the tragic event, but rather how to speak with them about such horrible things, and how we listen to their feelings and their concerns.

Children take more from the feelings of their parents than from their words. Their needs have less to do with information and more with security. Children need to know that they are protected and loved. The words: "I love you and will protect you"—spoken from the heart—mean more than any kind of explanation. Young children need to receive communication through physical contact—through holding, rocking, and touch. In families where both parents work, it is important to take time to phone your young child so that they know you are still there. Predictability and routine are important for children of all ages. The making of plans—to give them a sense that life will go on and that will have fun again—is another important thing we can do with our children.

Because the media use graphic fear as a selling point, it is important to minimize TV news exposure—particularly during dinner. Of course, it's best to watch the news after they are asleep. Kids, three to five years old, may ask questions about things that they have heard or seen on TV. At these ages, children are beginning to put feelings into words and you can let them know that it is okay to have these feelings. Drawing pictures and talking about what they have drawn and how it makes them feel (see article for more specific information) can be helpful, as can the telling of stories where the hero/heroine has overcome difficult situations, and been made stronger by meeting and mastering their ordeals. Then for older children, six to twelve, more direct discussions can be added. It may be important to find out where they got their information, and what their specific fears are. It is important to tell them that the government is doing everything to catch and stop these people, and suggest things that they can do to help people who have been affected, such as sending letters and collecting money.

Below is a guide to post on your refrigerator or medicine chest as a summary of the valuable tools you have just learned. Remember, trauma is a fact of life, but not a life sentence. "It doesn't have to hurt forever."

First Aid for Accidents and Falls

A Quick Reference Guide

1. Attend to your responses until relatively calm.

2. Keep your child still, quiet, and warm.

3. Encourage plenty of time for safety and rest.

4. Assess the situation.

5. As the shock wears off, guide attention to sensations.

6. Allow a full minute or two of silence, observing cues.

7. Encourage your child to rest before talking about event.

8. Continue to validate your child's physical responses.

9. Finally, attend to your child's emotional responses.

Character Structure and Shock

—Steen Jørgensen, Cand. Psych.,
translated by Kathryn Mahaffy

In Bodynamic Analysis, we distinguish between two factors affecting the development of the personality, and thereby a person's ability to cope with the difficulties he encounters in his life.

The first factor is developmental traumas. The child's interaction with parents, siblings, and other key figures of his early childhood; and later, his interaction with adults outside the family, with peers and with institutions; leads to the development of certain patterns of experience and behavior—character structures. A developmental trauma occurs when the child is met with adverse responses from his environment. He will then become restricted to use some of the character structures—and often to use the early or late positions in them—in his interaction with others.

The experience and behavior of the adult is influenced by the character structures. Some people are primarily influenced by a few character structures, others by many different character structures. The rigid and unconscious use of these character structures adds to many of the difficulties we encounter in our contact with others. The Bodynamic Analytic Psychotherapeutic way of working with the developmental traumas is directed toward the character structures.

The second factor is life-crisis traumas and shock traumas. During childhood, adolescence, and adult life, people are affected by many kinds of events that lead to changes in their life. We say that the person involved goes through a life-crisis. In many cases, the life-crisis is resolved; e.g., the central experiences are dealt with and integrated. In other cases, only partial resolution and integration of the crisis takes place, and the reactions and decisions related to the experience continue to influence the person and his behavior, even though the original event occurred many years previously. We term this a *life-crisis trauma.* A result of this is that the person has some degree of residual stress in the system. Depending on the degree of stress, the resulting state of this is either unnoticed or diagnosed as post-traumatic stress disorder (PTSD).

A special form for life-crisis trauma occurs when a person has a shock reaction under a life-crisis, or the life-crisis in fact is started because of a traumatic event where the person has a shock reaction.

We term it a *shock trauma* when a person has had a shock reaction to a traumatic event:

- that is actually life threatening (or experienced by the client as such).
- that hasn't been worked through, or where there hasn't been a possibility for the use of the ego and the biological reflexes of orientation, fight, or flight.
- where the client, instead, has reacted from the deep and primitive instinct patterns (paralysis and other biological reactions that lack the cerebrum's assistance) that we share with many other animals (Jørgensen, 1992).

A result of a shock trauma is always that the person has some degree of residual stress after the experience. In the Psychiatric Diagnostic System, shock traumas are included under PTSD (American Psychiatric Association, 1987). A shock trauma often includes a life-crisis trauma, but it is important to differentiate between life-crisis traumas (without attendant shock traumas) and shock traumas, because in our experience, they should be treated with different psychotherapeutic procedures.

When a client enters Bodynamic Analysis, he presents his difficulties and problems as they appear in his life at present. We initiate the therapeutic relationship with an interview that reveals the client's present and past. A physical diagnostic test is then carried out which measures muscular response to palpation. This response is registered in nine categories (four degrees of muscular hyper-response, a neutral response, and four degrees of muscular hypo-response). The test result is entered on a diagram of the human body, on which each muscular response is represented in the appropriate anatomical position by a system of variously coloured lines and dots; this is called a Bodymap (Rothschild, 1989).

Assisted by the interview, the Bodymap, and the client's description of his problems, the Bodynamic analyst forms a hypothesis about past and present sources of the client's problems and of his present resources. The past sources are to be found in the person's character development and in incompletely resolved life-crisis traumas and shock traumas.

The following sections concern the guidelines of Bodynamic Analysis for work with character structures (developmental traumas), life-crisis traumas, and shock traumas. In describing the general considerations for these procedures, I risk giving the impression that Bodynamic analytic treatment is very technical. This is far from true in most cases. Any therapeutic work takes place in a framework of personal interaction between the therapist and the client, where a transference occurs. At the same time, it is important for the therapist to maintain (and admit to) guidance of the therapy, based on diagnostic considerations and a therapeutic model for the optimum treatment of various difficulties.

Work with Character Structures

In Bodynamic Analysis, we describe personal development in seven stages, each characterized by a central vital theme.

A person develops and manifests certain personality traits at each stage of development. We call the patterns of experience and behavior typical of each stage character structures. In the course of development, a person will be characterized by one of three positions at each stage of development: an *early* position, marked by resignation; a *late* position, marked by restraint; and a *healthy* position, in which the various experiential and behavioral patterns connected with the stage's vital theme are integrated. The Bodynamic Analysis model of character structures is outlined on page 203 (Bentzen, Jørgensen, & Marcher, 1989).

In the course of a healthy and ideal personality development, a person would go through all three positions of all seven developmental stages, so that all of the various character structures that are met with adverse responses from his personalities are developed optimally. If a person is met with adverse responses from his environment, he will become (unconsciously) restricted to the use of certain character structures at the expense of others, which then do not develop fully. Consequently people are most usually influenced by certain character structures, which they typically apply to their contact with others.

A character structure includes patterns of experience and behavior that are used in one's contact with oneself and others, including defense patterns. The corresponding physical pattern of tensions is seen in the form of hyper-responses and hypo-responses in the muscles.

In Bodynamic Analysis, we view character structures as an integrated part of the personality structure. In our view, the goal of psychotherapy is to enable the client to choose freely which of his character structures to employ, not to make him abandon all character structures.

In working with character structures, we often start with concrete situations in the client's past involving interaction between parents and child. Work with single experiences is an important element in our form of psychotherapy. The most important change, however, takes place when the client recognizes and resolves his character structures as they appear in his everyday life and in his transference relationship to the therapist. Psychotherapy for characterological problems, especially in the case of the first five structures, birth to six years old, requires the establishment of a relationship of contact with the therapist in which transference can occur, and in which it is possible to work on the relationship to the therapist while also working on the historical sources of the personality structure.

During the past ten years, Bodynamic analysts have formulated some guidelines for work with the various character structures. I will present some of the most significant of these in the following; I will concern myself only with the *early* position (marked by resignation), and the *later* position (marked by restraint), in each character structure. (There is obviously no point in "treating" the healthy position in each character structure, but it will of course be included as resources, which the clients will be helped to use when they are working with their issues.)

Existence—Second Trimester to Three Months Old

The two positions in the *existence structure* are the most diametrically opposed of any, and therefore, the methods of working with these two positions also differ greatly. Common for work with both positions is the importance of improving the client's body awareness. This helps to enlarge the client's capacity for energy, feelings, emotions, and cognitive awareness.

In working with the early position, the *mental existence structure*, it is important that the client gradually learn to feel emotions, to be in emotional contact, and to be able to cope with the anxiety that this initially involves. The therapist accepts the client's thoughts and concepts, and on this basis, gradually builds the possibility of experiencing meaningful emotions and emotional contact.

Conversely, in working with the later position, the *emotional existence structure*, it is important that the client gradually learn to understand cause and effect, and to cope with separation-anxiety. The therapist meets the client's strong feelings and reactions in such a way that the client feels seen and experienced; mental understanding often has little immediate significance for someone who experiences and acts on an emotional basis. On the basis of this contact, the therapist works for the development of understanding and insight in the client's interaction with people who have a strong emotional effect on him.

Need—One Month to One-and-a-Half Years Old

A common characteristic of both early and late positions in the *need structure* is the inability of clients to be aware of their bodies (they also frequently have little physical or mental energy). Physical exercises involving resistance against pressure are often used in such cases to anchor the client in his body.

In working with the *despairing need structure*, the client needs to accumulate experiences of receiving something from others—of accepting it and feeling what it means to him. When this ability has been built up, he will be able to begin to ask and make demands for himself. Often, he will have to practice doing this with the therapist before he can manage it elsewhere. He won't be able to feel the pain and the anger of not getting what he wanted until he has experienced that it is possible to receive something and appreciate its significance.

The opposite is true of the *distrustful need structure*. A client who is locked into this position will not be able to absorb something from another person until he has resolved some of the massive bitterness, anger, and sorrow he feels at not automatically receiving what he wants without having to ask for it. Clients with this position have a massive aversion to asking for anything for themselves, based on experiences of unfulfilled needs. At the same time, the deadlock inherent in this position prevents this person from accepting anything he hasn't asked for himself. If someone else offers something that doesn't precisely meet his needs, it feels like getting the wrong thing again as usual, and of course, the chances of guessing his exact needs are slight. If another person did happen to guess right, the chances are that the client would not realize it or accept the gift.

Autonomy—Eight Months to Two-and-a-Half Years Old

For both positions in the *autonomy structure*, it is important to retain the experience of being in charge of oneself and one's own life. For this reason, open or hidden conflicts concerning control often arise between the therapist and clients in these positions. At the same time, therapeutic change is only possible for these clients if they are willing to examine and come to terms with their conscious or unconscious insistence upon leading and controlling every circumstance of their lives. In both cases, it is important to have a crystal clear agreement concerning the framework, content, and goals of the therapeutic process, and not to engage in power struggles with the client.

The *non-verbal activity changing structure* avoids approaching unpleasant experiences and memories, e.g., going blank. This blankness is at the same time real and a way of escaping from the ongoing activity—the structure was developed when the child depended on external stimuli to activate him, and before his speech was fully developed or much differentiated. It is thus important for the therapist, according to a clear agreement, to explore this emptiness together with the client. It is often necessary to offer suggestions as to what might exist in the blank spots, and ask the client whether these possibilities feel right.

It is also important to support the client in his initial attempts to feel, express, and contain his emotions, and in experiencing these emotions as his own. It is important that he hold on to these emotions and be responsible for them, independent of the reactions of others. The client does not connect what happens in therapy with everyday life, so it is important that the therapist help him with this, for instance, by assigning "homework," and being sure to ask the client what important things have happened since the last session. Clients with this character position find it hard to become attached to others, and this of course will also affect their contact with and transference to the therapist.

In the *verbal activity changing structure,* the client avoids feeling and recognizing his own emotions by actively and verbally changing the subject. He finds it dangerous to commit himself—asking for help also feels dangerous and threatening, and there is a strong conscious or unconscious resistance to manipulation. This accounts for the fact that people with strong patterns from this position seldom enter psychotherapy, unless by "force," or at least not with this issue.

It is a challenge for the therapist in that clients in this position change the subject as soon as unpleasant feelings begin to surface in their awareness. It is essential in working with this pattern that the client be made conscious of it, and in the beginning it is the therapist who must point it out, and keep the client working on the issue. Doing this without engaging in struggles for control with the client is the main therapeutic task in working with this position.

Setting up the therapeutic contract and choosing work themes are central issues in a therapeutic process with the autonomy structure. If the therapist asks the client what he wants to work on today, the client will often suggest two possibilities without choosing between them. If the therapist then chooses to focus on one of these possibilities, the client has avoided committing himself, and need not participate wholeheartedly in the therapy. Often, one choice leads to the next: If the therapist manages to get the client to commit himself to one of the two alternatives initially suggested, he will often present two possible ways of approaching the issue he has chosen, and so on. Continually establishing agreements and making choices may seem like constantly approaching therapy without actually working, but this is not the case. Working with agreements and choices is, in fact, essential for this position.

Will—Two to Four Years Old

Clients acting under the influence of the *will structure* find difficulty in using their own efforts and power together with others. Therefore it is an essential therapeutic element with both positions in this structure to work with expressing oneself energetically—both verbally and physically—in the presence of others.

A client with a *self-sacrificing will structure* has trouble acting for himself in accordance with his own wishes, and must be encouraged to do so by the therapist. He has difficulty making choices and is not good at planning ahead—he needs guidance in the principles of planning. He needs help in accepting that choice involves choosing something as well as rejecting something. It is difficult for him to cope with opposing or ambivalent emotions; he needs help in learning how to handle them. This position is established at an age when the child's ability to distinguish between fantasy and reality is developing; his ability to distinguish between thoughts and actions, and between "you" and "me," are likewise not fully developed at this stage. Developing awareness in this area is important for this position. To assist us with this work, we use our special communication model, which we call BodyKnot (breakdown of communication is most often experienced as knots in the body). This model systematizes a somatically based awareness of self, and is due to undue punishment or over-protection in their upbringing. It is therefore important that the client resolve his relationships to key figures in his childhood.

A client with a *judging will structure* seems much better able to act upon his own wishes. His problem is, however, that although he can take action independently, he cannot cope with carrying out his own intentions in the presence of others. In this case, it is important that the therapist can meet the client's strength of purpose with strength of his own, thus letting the client experience that a sense of contact and solidarity can be maintained even while actively carrying out one's own wishes. Clients influenced by this position tend characteristically to indicate their dissatisfaction indirectly—often by sarcasm or snide remarks—rather than clearly telling other people what they would prefer. An essential task for the therapist is to confront the client with this pattern, and to support him in stating his wishes directly and energetically.

Love/Sexuality Balance—Three to Six Years Old

Clients with a *love/sexuality structure* have difficulties with romance, sexuality, and contact. Here especially, the therapist must be personally well-defined—securely rooted in his own sexuality, and must maintain an unambiguous sexual boundary between himself and the client. Sexual contact between therapist and client will lock the client deeper into this structure. It must *not* happen. The client needs to be met by the therapist as his parents should originally have met their child: accepting his love and sexuality, and at the same time setting and keeping clear sexual boundaries. It is essential to work toward an awareness of the difference between neutral and sexualized contact, as clients with problems in this structure are confused about this distinction and its implications.

If the client experiences and acts from the *romantic position* in this structure, he will fall in love with the therapist in the course of therapy. The client needs to be met by the therapist's clearly defined boundaries, and to be made aware of his own more or less unconscious flirting. Work with this position involves both the transference-relationship to the therapist and the client's relationship to his/her father and mother (as well as to other central figures who have influenced the development of this position).

If the client is primarily locked into the *seductive position* in the structure, he/she will try to seduce the therapist in order to make contact. Failure on the therapist's part to maintain clear sexual boundaries will be disastrous—all the more so since many clients in whom this structure is dominant have often experienced molestation, sexual abuse, or massively incestuous behavior on the part of one or both parents. Work with the therapeutic transference and with the client's relationship with his mother and father are the essential elements in this therapeutic process.

Opinion—Five to Eight Years Old

Clients with an *opinion-forming structure* have had problems with inter-action and contact at an age when the child is engaged in formulating and expressing his opinions, learning about rules, and discovering how there can be similarities and differences in various forms of community: his own family, other families, school, and peer groups. It is therefore important that the therapist support the client in expressing his opinions, while helping him learn how to get along with others despite varying opinions, and how to cope with necessary mutual rules for interaction without losing his own integrity.

Clients locked into the patterns of the *sullen opinion-forming structure* do not openly express their dissatisfaction to the therapist. Instead, they sabotage the interaction and the process by indirect means: withdrawing from contact, or violating the therapeutic framework and rules in devious ways. The thera-pist's task is to make the client aware of this in such a way that the client is encouraged to stand up for his views, while the therapist maintains his own views, and also maintains the necessary limits and rules of the therapeutic process. Working with this structure also involves work with the client's feel-ings about opinions and rules, but we have found that this pattern can only be dealt with by allowing the opinions themselves, and the exchange of opin-ion to be meaningful and real. As far as we have seen, it is impossible to resolve this position, if one focuses exclusively on the "emotional-release" aspect inher-ent in therapy.

Clients locked into the *opinionated opinion-forming structure* usually engage open conflict and struggles with the therapist regarding opinions, rules, and the framework of the therapy. Their pattern is to confront the therapist, attempt to convince him that they are right; and if they don't succeed, to leave, slamming the door behind them. Here the challenge to the therapist is to meet the client on the strength of his expressed opinions, while still retaining his own opinions and the necessary rules and framework of the therapy.

Both the *sullen* and the *opinionated* positions are in part developed in relation to parental figures and other figures of authority, and in part in relation to peer groups. Because of this, it is often necessary for clients with this structure to work through some of their problems in group therapy. It is seldom possible to alter in individual therapy those aspects of the pattern that arose in a group context.

Solidarity/Performance Balance—Seven to Twelve Years Old

The final character structure, the *solidarity/performance structure*, is even more difficult to approach through individual therapy, since it is primarily developed in relation to playmates and schoolmates, and manifests itself in the client's attitude to groups. Therefore, working through the patterns belonging to this structure often requires participation in group therapy.

Clients locked into the *leveling position* must be supported in daring to achieve on their own, and daring to own up to their personal qualities, skills, and abilities. The therapist can, of course, encourage the client in these attempts during individual therapy, but unless the client is able to go out and change the pattern in his everyday life, it will be necessary to work on breaking it in a constructive group situation.

Clients locked into the *competitive position* attempt to "achieve their way out" of their difficulties. They often try to be the good client, working away at their therapy, even when the therapeutic process requires that they let go and feel how certain events and experiences have affected them. Some aspects of this pattern can be dealt with in individual therapy, especially when it is rooted in performing in order to be accepted by the parents, but just as in the early position, supplementary group therapy is usually indicated for a thorough resolution of the pattern.

The above-mentioned character structures are a result of a continuing interaction over a considerable period of time—unlike life-crisis traumas and shock traumas, in which a change in the life situation or a special event has had a massive effect on the client's personality development. In the following section, I will discuss the psychotherapeutic difficulties in working with life-crisis traumas and shock traumas.

Work with Life-Crisis Traumas and Shock Traumas

Work with life-crisis traumas includes recalling and reliving the experiences, emotions, and decisions that are bound up with the crisis. It often becomes evident that a client has made vital decisions during a crisis, or that his concept of reality—and his options of feeling and acting—have been biased during the crisis.

In some life-crisis traumas, the client has reacted with a shock reaction. A shock reaction is a normal reaction to overwhelming traumatic events. Everyone has experienced shock reactions, although some people have had more than others. This may be due to circumstances beyond the individual's control, such as natural disasters or war, or the fact that unresolved shock reactions have reduced that person's alertness and orientation abilities, thus making him vulnerable to further shocks. When a shock reaction has not been worked through and integrated fully, the client is having a shock trauma.

Working with shock traumas can be a very simple process, but it is often very complex psychotherapeutic work. This is because seemingly simple and uncomplicated shock traumas may activate other hidden shock traumas. Also, the experiences and decisions connected with the shock events often tend to intensify the person's established character structures. These factors complicate the therapeutic task.

Life-crisis traumas and shock traumas have this in common: In both cases, one is dealing with events that the client has not resolved and integrated. This is because the client, at the time, lacked the help, support, security, and contact necessary for working through and integrating trauma and shock. Therefore, the therapist must provide secure and safe surroundings in which the client—

with the help and support of the therapist—can re-live and resolve his more or less unacknowledged experiences, emotions, and decisions. Psychotherapy for life-crisis traumas and shock traumas has this method in common: The therapist helps the client to remember what happened—what physiological reactions (sensations, feelings, emotions) the client had in the situation—in order to scrutinize the absent or truncated feelings and actions inherent in the situation, and to become aware of what the event meant, and still means, for the client.

When we work with life-crisis trauma through Bodynamic Analytic psychotherapy, we generally begin with the client's memories of the important events in the crisis. We ask the client to recall the situations vividly, both visually and physically. We ask him at the same time to reexperience, register, and describe the motor and tension patterns he connects with the events. Next, we work through the events chronologically, letting the client express uncompleted reactions and experiences verbally and physically, and encouraging him to integrate his experiences in an appropriate way.

During the verbal and emotional work, we help the client to resolve the tension patterns (in the form of hyper- and hypo-muscular response) connected with the crisis. Some patterns of tension are normalized as the client gives expression to experiences, feelings, and impulses that were withheld in the traumatic situation. In other cases, the client must learn consciously to release his tension patterns after he has gained an insight into their sources.

The psychotherapy often begins with the client's memories of an important event during the original crisis, but it is also possible to begin working with somatic movement patterns or blocks, where the connection with the traumatic event and its implications in the crisis first come to light in the course of therapy.

In the case of shock traumas, the above-mentioned method does not lead to a simple or easy process, and if used without insight into the complicated nature of shock reactions, the method may reactivate the original shock reaction, leaving the client in a worse state than he was before entering therapy.

It is therefore vital to be able to diagnose shock traumas, and also to recognize signs of a client approaching a state of shock. Certain disturbances in interactional behavior and certain psychosomatic reactions indicate the occurrence of shock traumas in the client's past. Changes in his behavior, when the client talks about or approaches a traumatic incident, indicate whether or not the client is going into a shock reaction (Jørgensen, 1993).

In the course of the last ten years, we have developed psychotherapeutic guidelines for work with shock traumas (Jørgensen, 1992). Before we begin working with a shock trauma, we work on increasing the client's body awareness. We support him in widening and intensifying his social network, if it is meagre. We work on the contact between therapist and client, so that the client trusts the therapist and is in rapport with him before starting work on a specific shock trauma. We interview the client about events in his past history, which may have involved shock reactions; we observe his behavior for signs of shock reactions, and compare these with the information we have gained from the interpretation of his Bodymap concerning character structure and shock traumas. On this basis, we form a hypothesis as to what kinds of shock traumas and chains of shock traumas the client has experienced, and consider whether the client's personality structure (if for example the client has a late autonomy character structure) will require special consideration during therapy.

After this initial preparation, Bodynamic Analytic therapy for shock traumas proceeds along the following six steps:

1. **The therapist and client together choose which shock trauma they want to work on.**

   It is very unusual for a client to have had only one shock trauma—most people have had several. A shock trauma is generally connected with other shock traumas with a common theme or a related emotional significance.

   If the client is relatively healthy, it is most appropriate to start with a shock trauma from early in life. This will release some of the shock energy, and make it easier to work with subsequent shock traumas.

   If the client's observing ego is not functioning well, and if he has little awareness of his own characterological patterns, it is better to start with a more recent shock trauma. This is also indicated when working with clients whose boundaries or sense of self are weak, or clients with borderline disorders.

2. **The therapist explains the therapeutic framework, and outlines the guiding rules that the client must follow.**

The reason that many people are affected by unresolved or partially resolved shock traumas is that they don't work through the shock traumas they have undergone in appropriate circumstances; i.e., in contact with other people, in secure surroundings, where they can react emotionally and receive help and support in resolving and integrating what they have experienced. Ideally, a person should take refuge with his nearest and dearest after a shock reaction has occurred, and work through the shock reaction in their presence. Bodynamic therapists create a therapeutic equivalent of this situation in their work with shock traumas, and this may involve that the client bring their friends along.

In the therapy room, where the client feels safe, he is asked to lie on a mat. Nearby sits the therapist and whatever helpers are taking part in the therapy. We ask the client to shift between being present in the actual situation, where it is possible to work through the shock trauma with the therapist's support, and vividly imagining himself back in the traumatic situation which brought on the shock reaction. When the client enters into this imagined reality, a bodily memory of the posture and tension patterns connected with the traumatic event is activated.

When the client shows signs of going into a shock reaction, we ask him to "run" on the mattress in order to break the rigidity ("freezing") that results from the shock reaction. We ask the client to picture that he is running away from the original traumatic situation to a safe and secure place. This technique is very efficacious in cases in which the client has not resolved his shock trauma in the company of other people.

We explain the technique to the client, and make sure of his cooperation. In our experience, working with shock traumas arouses so much resistance in the client that he will use all his defense mechanisms in order to halt the course of the therapy. It is not unusual for clients in the middle of an intense shock trauma psychotherapy to urge us to work on something quite different instead. Working with shock traumas activates not only defense mechanisms, but also powerful reactions from the autonomic nervous system. It is therefore necessary that the client consent to work with the shock trauma until it is resolved. If the work is interrupted, the client may be left in an unbalanced physiological state of stress, vulnerable to psychosomatic sickness and new shock traumas.

3. **The client relates what he remembers from before and after the shock reaction.**

In working with a shock trauma, which the client can remember, we approach it gradually, starting with what the client remembers of the time immediately preceding the shock reaction. Resources are thus made available to the client, so that he can assimilate and contain the energy of the shock reaction. This enables him to work through the core of the shock trauma without going into a shock reaction again.

4. **The client practices running, and establishes the ability to relate and resolve the shock trauma in a safe place.**

As a client approaches the central experience in a shock trauma, he must actively will himself to run, so that he can get out of the state of immobility that is the core of a shock reaction. To be able to mobilize his will power, the client must have practiced running to the safe place before undertaking work on a shock incident. He must also be sure that the therapy room, with the therapist and helpers in it, is itself a safe place, where he is met with attentive contact and care.

5. **The client gradually works around and through the shock incident.**

The following elements are contained in working through a shock trauma—their relative importance changes according to the type of shock trauma involved:

- In the course of the psychotherapy, it becomes possible for the client to recall and re-live the traumatic course of events in its entirety. Vital emotions, experiences, and decisions during shock reaction are either forgotten or have never been consciously felt, as cerebral connection is reduced during acute shock reaction. Memories and feelings of which the client was completely unaware often emerge during therapy. If the client became unconscious during the shock incident, it is not possible for him to recall the whole sequence. This does not, however, seem to hinder a complete resolution of the shock trauma.

- In the course of therapy, we help the client to reestablish the orientation reflex which is often frustrated during a shock reaction. We bring him out of the tonic immobility, which is a central feature of shock reaction, and encourage him to recall, re-live, and resolve the fight-or-flight reflexes that were activated by the shock incident.

- Shock traumas that are not completely resolved leave the body in a state of tension. We help the client to overcome this by reconstructing his movements in the traumatic situation, and by providing physical resistance to the motions that he would have made, but which froze in the shock reaction. In working with clients who have shock traumas, it is not appropriate to use somatic techniques involving energy charge, as these increase the risk of reactivating the shock reaction. We therefore work primarily to relax tension patterns after powerful feelings connected with the shock trauma are resolved, and our work with the physical expression of action impulses connected with shock trauma is highly structured.

- Most people make important decisions in relation to shock traumas. Such decisions will typically reinforce certain aspects of the client's character structures, and restrict him even more in his use of them. Therefore, the therapist must help the client verbalize and alter the hampering decisions he made under the shock trauma.

- Most people have parapsychological experiences—principally "out of body" experiences—in connection with shock traumas. Sometimes the client remembers such experiences and relates them prior to psychotherapy. In other cases, they come to light while the client is recalling and assimilating the traumatic incident. The client usually remembers central episodes of the incident as seen from above, or from some place other than where he actually was while it was happening. We consider this to be the result of an out of body experience. The therapist must understand and accept the existence of such phenomena, and master techniques for dealing with them. If not, it will be impossible for the therapist to help the client resolve and integrate the shock trauma completely. Parapsychological experiences usually occur when the client is immobilized by the shock reaction. The experience is frightening for people who are not used to such experiences. It can become necessary to "teach" the client to leave the body and return again, and to help him develop a cognitive understanding and acceptance of these phenomena. If the client's religious beliefs deny the existence of such occurrences, it will be difficult to work with his experience of them.

6. **The shock trauma is resolved when the client is able to recall the whole sequence of the original shock trauma without going into a shock reaction, and when the traumatic experience is integrated in the client's life and self-understanding.**

In Bodynamic Analysis, psychotherapy for shock traumas follows this pattern. However, we are always working with clients who have developed character structures in the course of their lives, and who tend to use certain structures whenever they feel threatened. Therefore, we have to take a client's character structures into consideration when working with his life-crisis traumas and shock traumas.

Character Structures Are Reinforced by Life-Crisis Traumas and Shock Traumas

When a person undergoes a life-crisis trauma or a shock trauma, he attempts to save himself by intensifying the defense mechanisms he already uses. His typical character structures become more inflexible and immutable (rigid) if he has undergone unresolved life-crisis traumas and/or shock traumas. Simultaneously, it becomes ever harder for him to relax his rigid use of character structures, because such a relaxation would bring the unresolved life-crisis trauma and/or shock trauma closer to the surface.

Shock trauma, and most life-crisis trauma, is experienced as threatening—a threat to life, independence, freedom of action, or other themes of character development. Therefore, shock trauma often results in a reenforcement and solidifying of the character structures and the defense mechanisms connected with existence, autonomy, and will.

Most life-crisis traumas and all shock traumas pose a threat to a person's existence. Therefore, the existence structure will usually become more dominant after life-crisis traumas and shock traumas. The person may withdraw from the world and shun contact with others (as seen in the mental existence structure), or he may cling to the tangible world and insist upon contact (as seen in the emotional existence structure).

The autonomy structure and/or the will structure always tend to become reinforced and inflexible as a result of life-crisis trauma and shock trauma. It is with these character structures that a person seeks to maintain his personal integrity and freedom of action when faced with a threatening situation. Work with life-crisis trauma and shock trauma will vary according to whether the person primarily uses the autonomy structure or the will structure in his attempts to retain control of his world in the face of traumatic events.

Traumatic events may also lead to a intensification of the other character structures. A person may develop a more rigid opinion forming structure, so that he either expresses very rigid opinions and viewpoints, or else has quite given up having opinions and viewpoints. This can be seen as a defense against experiencing the traumatic event and the feelings it evokes. People may also seek to achieve in order to avoid new traumatic situations. This achievement may be manifested in social relations or in individual competitiveness, as seen in the two positions in the solidarity/performance structure. This is, however, most common in cases where the traumatic situation had to do with achievement or social interaction.

The following two character structures generally become rigid when the traumatic experience is connected with the central theme in the character structure. Life-crisis trauma and shock trauma, in connection with sexuality, will often lock the person into either the romantic or the seductive position of the love/sexuality structure, and a life-crisis trauma or shock trauma connected with personal needs may lock the person into the despairing or the distrustful positions of the need structure.

Aside from these considerations, it is important in working with shock traumas to notice how the client handles his own personal boundaries. In many forms of shock traumas, the client has undergone a violation of his boundaries, and this affects the client's ability to set and maintain his own boundaries. This ability is normally developed in the course of the child's first three years of life, together with the developing character structures. An extreme expression of difficulties with boundaries is seen in narcissistic and borderline disorders, but less radical tendencies are also often evident in an ordinary personality development. It is important to be aware of any signs of boundary diffusion in the client (which finds its extreme expression in a borderline personality structure) or boundary-provoking behavior (which finds its extreme expression in narcissistic personality disorder). If the client has strong tendencies in either of these directions, it will be necessary to work with boundary problems side-by-side with the client's shock traumas. This is especially true when working with clients who have been violated as children (in the form of incest or other physical abuse). These clients have a personality structure in which reactive patterns resulting from shock traumas are intrinsically woven together with character structures (Ollars, 1995). Such clients can change, if work with boundary problems, character structure, and shock traumas is integrated within the framework of a long-term transference relationship.

The Significance of Character Structures in Therapeutic Work with Life-Crisis Traumas and Shock Traumas

Before beginning work with a client's life-crisis and shock traumas, it is important to determine whether the client's personality is influenced by an autonomy structure and/or a will structure.

If the client has a marked autonomy structure, it will be difficult to work with life-crisis trauma and shock trauma until this has been resolved. If the client operates with a non-verbal autonomy structure, he will often go completely blank when he approaches a life-crisis trauma or shock trauma. If he operates with a marked verbal autonomy structure, he will vacillate from issue to issue during therapy to avoid focusing on traumatic events.

In either case, it may be virtually impossible to keep him on track long enough to effect a resolution.

If the client is influenced by a will structure, it is possible to work with life-crisis trauma and shock trauma, but it requires considerable effort on the therapist's part to keep the client working on the experiences in an appropriate way. Clients with a self-sacrificing will structure find it difficult to imagine acting in any other way than they did originally, and it takes time for them to develop new possibilities of action. Clients with a judging will structure find it difficult to trust the therapist, or to believe in the possibility of sympathetic support in resolving their difficulties. They are convinced that they must manage everything by themselves. It may therefore be necessary to work with the client's will structure before working directly on his life-crisis trauma or shock trauma.

Consideration must be taken for the client's existence structure in working with life-crisis trauma and shock trauma. If the client is influenced by a mental existence structure, it will be difficult for him to feel and express certain emotions related to the traumatic events—the client can usually feel fear, but has difficulty feeling anger. If the client is influenced by an emotional existence structure, he will often be overwhelmed by emotions and experiences; as a rule he feels anger easily, but often finds it difficult to feel his own fear. In addition, it often takes time for a client with an emotional existence structure to develop and integrate a cognitive understanding of events and their significance.

Strong patterns from the other character structures will of course also influence therapeutic work with life crisis trauma and shock trauma. These must also be considered, but generally speaking, it is the influence of the client's existence structure, autonomy structure, and will structure which have the strongest effect on the therapeutic resolution of life-crisis trauma and shock trauma.

References

American Psychiatric Association. *DSM-IV Diagnostic and Statistical Manual of Mental Disorders Fourth Edition* (Washington, D.C.: American Psychiatric Association, 1994).

Bentzen, M., S. Jørgensen, & L. Marcher. (1989). "The Bodynamic Character Structure Model." *Energy & Character* 20(1). Corrections in Vol. 21(1).

Bernhardt, P. (1992). "Individuation, Mutual Connection, and the Body's Resources: An Interview with Lisbeth Marcher." *Pre and Peri-Natal Psychology Journal* 6(4). See also pp. 93–106 in this book.

Jørgensen, S. (1992). "Bodynamic Analytic Work with Shock/Post-Traumatic Stress." *Energy & Character* 23(2).

Jørgensen, S. *Chok/Posttraumatisk stress.* Symptomer og arsager.

Jørgensen, S. *Forlosning af choktraumer.* Ed: Forlaget Kreatik (Kobenhavn: 1994).

Ollars, L. (1995). "Bodynamic Analytic Work with Assault and Abuse." *Energy & Character* 25(1).

Rothschild, B. (1989). "Filling One of Psychology's Gaps," *Energy & Character* 20(1).

Part Five

Breathing Interventions

There is much interest in both the mind-body and psychological-spiritual therapeutic and meditative communities regarding the use of breathing patterns to affect psychological and spiritual explorations.

This section extends Parts Three and Four by illustrating approaches to working with breathing patterns in psychological, traumatic issues, and spiritual development.

The first article, "The Bioenergy System" (written 1981, revised 1983), describes Reichian vegetotherapy, which was a major part of my early practice. Beginning in 1983, I combined it then with other such modalities as Gestalt therapy, hypnosis, and cognitive approaches.

After beginning my studies of somatic developmental psychology (Bodynamics) in 1988, I changed my approach to working with people. During these studies, Peter Levine (also a student of Bodynamics at that time) and I decided to write a revised article on breathwork, entitled "Breath and Consciousness," integrating the Bodynamics model and character structure into our breathwork therapeutic interventions.

The Bioenergy System: Restoring the Wisdom of the Body through Reichian Breathing Therapy

—*Ian Macnaughton, Ph.D.*

Reichian Therapy is a method of working directly with the body to harmonize and balance the bioenergy system. The objective of this approach is to enhance a person's physical, emotional, and spiritual sense of well-being, and to reclaim the capacity of personal knowing. Reichian Therapy was invented by Wilhelm Reich, M.D., around 1920 in Europe.

Reich was a psychiatrist who initially was a student of Freud. When he found himself perplexed that various patients did not respond favorably to treatment, he began to notice more of their non-verbal body language, how they presented themselves, how they held their musculature and breathing patterns. Curious, he began experimenting with allowing movements, muscles, and breathing to loosen up in the direction to more full and natural expression. The results were encouraging and he explored further, developing a whole therapeutic model of optimal health, and with it, the restoring of the wisdom of the body to be self-regulating. In his work, he saw that the body operated as an energy system, and to the degree that system operated well, the person reported that they felt better and more functional. Reich postulated that human beings are part of a vast energy field, which he called the Life Force. To Reich, the human dilemma was in learning how to yield to this Life Force and to allow it to flow freely through the human organism—or rather, not to block its free flow. He theorized that problems of individual health, whether physical, mental, or emotional, are caused by the blocking of this energy flow. Higgins and Raphael (1970) quote Reich's explanation:

> *If you have a stream, a natural stream, you must let it stream. If you dam it up somewhere, it goes over the banks, that's all. Now, when the natural*

streaming of the bioenergy is dammed up, it also spills over, resulting in irrationality, perversions, neuroses, and so on. What do we have to do to correct this? You must get the stream back into its normal bed and let it flow again ...

Reich felt that we have armored ourselves physically and psychically from experiencing the deep feelings of connection to that flow of the Life Force through our bodies. In fact, he felt that this comfortable, pleasant sensation of feeling—the soft pulsation of energy within oneself—has become so foreign to us that we are frightened to feel it again. In other words, pleasure and ease has become alien to us, and what is now felt to be more familiar is tension, anger, sadness, depression, and pain. This state of disease has become so usual within us that it becomes the "normal" feeling tone, and all other experiences are considered unusual and are considered threatening.

Often when talking to people, I will notice their eyes growing wet with feeling. Upon discussing this with them, I will find that they are not sad, but touched deep inside—that the feeling is wonderful, "but almost too much." Often, they initially mistake the feeling for sadness and break down—rather than melting, fullness, and opening up.

Reich felt that until we came to terms with this dilemma and restored our biological ease—this capacity to be comfortable with our own sensations, feelings, and emotions—there could be no outer peace or harmony in our social interactions because there is no inner harmony. He felt that we project out into the world that which we are, and the social system in turn feeds and controls the individual to continue the oppression of him/herself. I would change this slightly to say that we are part of an interactive system that we adapt to our environment, and that our environment accommodates to us. Thus, we can influence the total system through changing how we adapt and thus influence the feedback.

Reich believed that the internal blocking of this energy flow was the repression of natural feeling at an early stage of life, particularly natural sexual feelings. He felt that the holding onto and denial of these normal feelings and sensations resulted in a blocking of our biological capacity to feel our own natural energy flow. Certain basic feelings then had to be controlled and put out of awareness, and to do this different muscle groups had to be tightened against experiencing those feelings. Soon those muscles became locked in the tightened and numbed pattern of holding against the natural energy flow. He viewed sexual functioning as a method of regulating the accumulation of stresses in the body. I hasten to add that many people have misunderstood what Reich meant when he talked about healthy sexuality. He was *not* talking about rather compulsive and strained sexual relations. Rather, he was speaking of an experience that had love and yielding as its natural component rather than what many think of as "sex." Reich felt that the act of sexual union provided each partner with a bonding with another and release of accumulated stresses—blocks to a broader and fuller self. Healthy sexuality then would become a move toward restoring the harmony of the Life Force pulsation. Such matters as holding in emotional expression and becoming largely unaware, out of contact with the normal sensations of the body, resulted from this sexual suppression. We then are no longer a dynamic self-regulating energy system, but rather an awkward and constrained person at war with ourselves.

Current theorists in this field have expanded this view. Each accent one area or another of human functioning as the primary cause, but all agree with Reich's basic premise *that disharmony is created by a blocking of the natural biological energy flow and that this leads to mental, emotional, and eventually to physical disease.* One researcher, Dr. Levine, a medical biophysics specialist, has done considerable work to understand how overwhelming stresses experienced early in a person's life, including intrauterine and birth stress, reduce the adaptive capacity of the organism to handle subsequent stresses. He is particularly interested in developing treatment methods that restore this capacity for self-regulation of the autonomic nervous system and the entire organism. He suggests use of Reichian breathing as one way to restore that capacity, and while the treatment is more complicated than that presented here, for practical purposes, an outline will be given of a typical treatment session.

In the treatment session, we are seeking to bring the person up to their usual limits in dealing with biological stress, to allow them to experience the possibility of being more comfortable with intense sensations of feelings, and to have this prove to be a pleasurable, relaxed experience. Generally, we all avoid tension beyond a certain threshold point. After that point, tension becomes stressful and can result in us becoming physically tight and nervous, frightened or angry. All of these feelings are very uncomfortable and are indications that we have built up a high degree of nervous system "charge." We have activated the sympathetic response of the autonomic nervous system—the fight-or-flight response. The person is now approaching a state which if maintained for a long time with no release (such as may be the case in birth and intrauterine stresses), the nervous system becomes set in that response—that is to say, a pattern of high activation of the fight-or-flight response, anger and fear, and tied into that feeling a behavioral pattern of not being able to release from the overwhelming feeling by appropriate action. If we can safely navigate a similar stressful pattern, and make the appropriate response, the sympathetic alarm response is peaked and the relaxation parasympathetic response is enhanced. The nervous system discharges, and this leads to a feeling of relief and of well-being.

Each successful navigation of this charging and discharging cycle will enhance the person's potential for tolerating increased biological excitation and its natural release when appropriate; i.e., to be able to fully embrace a stressful situation, complete the appropriate behavior, and return to a relaxed, resting state. I want to emphasize that it would be an error to *just* go through charging and discharging phases without addressing the overall pattern of what is occurring within the person's total life, their behavior, their beliefs about themselves. With that reservation, let's continue.

A typical breathing session is done with the person lying on their back on a bed with their knees bent pointing upward and the feet flat on the bed. This bent-knee position assists the energy to be discharged through the pelvis and down the legs. Most of the breathing patterns are done through the mouth—the therapist guiding the client through various breathing patterns, according to his/her sense of what is appropriate for the client.

The client is then asked to begin noticing his breathing, giving him time to become aware of what his breathing pattern feels like to him, and what areas of his body seem open and what areas seem tight or blocked. This will give him a sense of a beginning point. He is then asked to begin to slightly exaggerate his breathing. As he breathes through his mouth, he is asked to exaggerate slightly on the exhale. Each person has his/her inner individual breathing pattern, the way he/she usually breathes. Examples of various patterns are: breathing into the chest but not the abdomen—or the reverse; very shallow breathing in either the chest or abdomen or both; a tentative, cautious type of breathing or a determined pushing pattern. There are many other variations and while the list could be extensive, a mechanical list is a poor replacement for the therapist's own feelings and for his/her own sense of the client's breathing pattern. As the breathing continues, there is increased biological excitation, and at this state the person's individual *Stress Response Pattern* will emerge.

The next phase, generally, is to request the client to breathe more completely, more fully using both the chest and abdomen, and encouraging her to include the parts where breath seems limited. Once this breathing pattern is done for a period of time, using full breathing (but not highly stressed hyperventilation), different breathing patterns are introduced. Each pattern will begin to be difficult to continue with as the client begins to reach her limit in developing charge with it; that is, she will usually just seem to lose the ability to concentrate on the pattern or begin to tighten up. The skill of the therapist then is to know which new breath pattern to use to build the excitement (energy) further, beyond the amount the client would usually allow. This is usually done by some combination of chest panting in rhythms—sometimes having the client make sounds while the therapist might use his hands to manipulate the tight areas. In many cases, it will now become obvious what the client's Stress Response Pattern is. She may begin to breathe faster and begin to lose ability to concentrate, or start to squirm around or want to talk. The task of the therapist at this point is to raise the Bioenergetic charge to the level that an overall sympathetic response is activated. This can be observed by noticing skin color, the type of sounds and subtle movements the client makes, and primarily sensations the therapist feels inside his own body. This becomes a very crucial point in the session as just "pushing" the person on the breathing is not the answer.

For a successful session, the charge build-up must be gradual and not reinforce existing limitation patterns by pushing too hard. *Just creating intense breathing patterns and experiences may often do the client a disservice by covering over various stages of unfolding that need to be integrated if the client is to experience a sense of full well-being and a restoration of the organism's capacity for self-regulation.* The energy build-up can be felt by the therapist in her own body and is used to judge (along with external clues given by the client) the appropriate point to allow the client to discharge. In this phase, the client has moved from an excitement state into a tension state.

By successfully navigating this tension phase, the client can move into discharge. This may occur spontaneously with the client suddenly peaking the sympathetic charge and experiencing subtle-to-intense autonomic sensations felt as longitudinal streamings or pulsations. It may also be necessary to assist this phase by having the patient bounce on the bed, hit the bed to raise the charge quickly, and promote a peaking out of the sympathetic charge. The therapist may also manipulate the muscles (sometimes quite intensely, other times almost imperceptibly) to promote the release. Sometimes emotional feelings will be released at this point—the main ones being anger, sadness, or fear, as repressed feeling states emerge.

The last phase is relaxation. Once the nervous system has begun to discharge, feelings of relaxation, pulsation, and soft autonomic streaming may occur throughout the client's body. A feeling of peace and well-being will be experienced. Ordinarily, I encourage the client to rest a few minutes to allow the process of release and rebalancing to continue and the necessary integration of the experience to occur.

To summarize what has occurred in this session, the person has been encouraged to breathe more fully throughout more parts of her body, freeing the chest to more letting go and allowing the breath movements to include the whole body. The stiff, awkward, jerky movements change to more spontaneous, fluid ones as the involuntary nervous system becomes more heightened. The energy that had been held and locked in the muscles of the body has been released to some degree, and the person has a more felt sense of well-being and personal knowing about themselves. Reich called this his four-beat formula: *tension - charge - discharge - relaxation.*

It again bears repeating that this approach is not just a technique. I concur with Jan Franklin, who writes in his article, "The Search Part II:"

> *I respect very much the philosophy of homeopathy that says that since every human being has his own individuality, every disease has an individual character as well. As a consequence, every therapy, if it is rightly applied, is individual. "Technique," however, assumes that different people can be treated in the same way ...*

To guide someone through a session primarily requires a degree of awareness of one's own sensations—one's own biological energy system. It is very important that the therapist experience considerable therapy of this kind so that the appropriate steps can be taken at the right times. It is not enough to know the "technique" or to just push people with exaggerated breathing under the naive belief that all will eventually be well. Reich himself was very cautious about how one could be said to be qualified to be a Reichian Therapist, and, even after years at work both as a client and as a therapist, I must admit I find myself at times lacking in the sensitivity I need to feel excellent in my own work in a consistent way. David Boadella in *Wilhelm Reich, The Evolution of His Work*, states:

> *For this reason, no attempt will be made here to describe vegeto-therapeutic techniques in greater detail. The indispensable prerequisite for whatever methods the therapist uses to release the emotions held in the musculature is that he is in touch with his own sensations and be able to empathize fully with the patient and to feel in his own body the effect of the particular constrictions on the patient's energies.*

In general, for those people who wish to explore this type of breathing without the aid of a Reichian therapist, there are a few guidelines. The first would be to have a friend with you when doing it. This will aid in giving the experimenter someone to talk to should uncomfortable emotional feelings or intense sensations occur. The second would be to lie down as described, and just commence full and relatively easy breathing, allowing breath to fill both the abdominal and chest cavities. It is best not to strain the breathing; if it feels like a strain point has been reached, just rest and pay attention to the sensations, feelings, and sense of that limit. Often people feel a tendency to push through the limit. Many times that is because they cannot stay with the sensation of being limited. When they do stay with that sensation, images, memories, and connections occur that allow the limit to be resolved. By not pushing through, you may resolve and transform old patterns. The unwillingness to stay with the limitation and explore it, the compulsive need to push and act out, may just reinforce the existing limitation, driving it deeper into the body, and making it less accessible. At such a stress level, there is much to be learned about the characteristics of the biological, emotional, and cognitive stress response pattern. If pulsation and streaming do occur, then it is best to yield to them and rest, giving in to the experience.

Working with the breath to expand consciousness and well-being has been a part of many cultures. Walt Anderson, in his book *Open Secrets: A Westerner's Guide to Tibetan Buddhism*, relates one such exercise:

> *A simple but powerful breathing exercise in the Tibetan system is useful either for self-healing or when working with someone else. It is a "deep-roll" breath, somewhat similar to breathing techniques employed in hatha yoga and Reichian therapy. To do it, you should be lying comfortably on your back, either on a bed or on a floor with a pad. The precise details of the position are not too important, but since the exercise involves diaphragmatic breathing, it is usually advisable for people who have not practiced similar exercises to keep one hand lightly on the stomach. The inhalation is in three parts: You begin by raising the belly so that the air flows into the lower part of the lungs. In the second part of the inhalation, which flows smoothly form the first, fill the middle part of the lung cavity, above the stomach. In the final part of the inhalation, the upper chest cavity is filled, and there may be a slight raising of the shoulders. Then the breath is slowly and smoothly exhaled, releasing first the upper chest, then the middle, and finally the lower section of the lungs; you should feel your belly lowering under your hand as the final part of the breath is expelled. This exercise should ideally be performed for at least twenty minutes, to allow it to do*

its work. You will find that it tends to bring up feelings, to make you aware of what is going on in the physical/emotional centers of your being. Sometimes strong feelings of grief or anger may surface, and for this reason it can be helpful to have someone else present; sometimes it will put you in touch with areas of physical tension, and when this happens, massage or self-massage can be helpful. Basically it is a clearing process, a way of allowing feelings to come up and move out, a release for stored blocks in the nervous system.

This sounds rather similar in many ways to our description and cautions about Reichian Therapy!

It is important to realize that much good expansion, growth, and self-healing can be done with this approach on one's own. Equally important is to realize that the bioenergy forces are extremely powerful and that if breathing approaches are used intensely without an experienced guide, there is a possibility of causing oneself psychic, emotional, and physical distress.

References

Anderson, Walt. *Open Secrets: A Westerner's Guide to Tibetan Buddhism* (New York: Viking Press, 1979).

Boadella, David. *Wilhelm Reich, The Evolution of His Work* (Chicago: Henry Regency Company, 1974).

Higgins, M., & C.M. Raphael. *Reich Speaks of Freud* (New York: Noonday Press, 1967).

Franken, Jan. (1979). "The Journal of Bioenergetic Research." *Energy & Character.*

Breath and Consciousness: Reconsidering the Viability of Breathwork in Psychological and Spiritual Interventions in Human Development

—*Peter A. Levine, Ph.D., & Ian Macnaughton, Ph.D.*

Summary

This paper offers a conceptual framework and guidelines for using breathing techniques as a tool in psychospiritual development. It is intended to expand the field of theory and practice for therapists who utilize attention to the body, and specifically breathing patterns, in the course of psychotherapy. The relationship between respiration and consciousness is explored, and two main patterns or styles of breathing response are identified. The paper discusses the wisdom of attending to the respiratory pattern of an individual, and parameters are given for assessing the patterns and following through with intervention. Guidelines for appropriate intervention are given for therapists working with both developmental and traumatic shock issues. This includes any contraindications and cautions that may be necessary if breathing interventions are used with clients who have various medical, psychological, and spiritual concerns.

The information contained in this article should not lead the reader to assume that a therapist should use breathing techniques as the approach of choice. It is primarily intended to outline some of the parameters for a therapist to consider if they should choose to work in this way.

Introduction

Our world is undergoing rapid and complex change in its social, economic, and political activities. Human affairs are becoming increasingly turbulent and uncertain, and we need to learn new ways of managing this uncertainty to keep pace with the growing rate of change. Thus, each of us is faced with the challenge of making appropriate adjustments to maintain some degree of stability in the world.

Some theorists are alarmed by society's seeming inability to cope with the flood of new information, technologies, socioeconomic forces, and political issues at local, national, and even global levels. Since change, in itself, demands adjustment, we must respond in fresh and new ways that are outside our personal and societal experience. This, in turn, requires innovation and flexibility, and we must develop the ability to think in terms of complex relationships associated with the change process.

Not only is change challenging in its own right, but the rate of change itself is also on the increase. In his 1971 book, *Future Shock,* Alvin Toffler points out that it is absolutely necessary to develop both capability and organizational capacities to deal with change if we are to address its increasing rate successfully. According to Toffler, "Future shock is the dizzying disorientation brought about by the premature arrival of the future. It may well be the most important disease of tomorrow."

The challenge to be proactive in developing our capacity to cope effectively with these changes is great, and many have speculated about our ability to do so. Russell identified the exponential increase in the amount of information we must confront, and Campbell "wonders if we must soon fumble through another age of darkness."

As individuals we need to find new ways of coping with this rate of change, and develop collective methods for transforming the challenge, it presents into opportunities to improve the human condition—locally, nationally, and globally. Breathwork is one important response to the challenge.

Section 1: Breath and Consciousness

For thousands of years, attention to breathing has been a significant focus in many psychological and spiritual practices. Many of the Eastern systems relating to human development are actually developmental psychologies that begin where Western psychologies leave off. Eastern and shamanic systems use breathing for both psychological development and spiritual growth, and they do not make a clear differentiation between the two as the Western system does.

In Eastern cultures, there are two main approaches to working with breath. The first uses an awareness of breath to develop a focus and mindfulness, and the second uses over-breathing or hyperventilation as a way of generating transformational experiences, as in Kundalini or other yogas. In Eastern and shamanic cultures, it usually takes years of training, meditation, control, and awareness, under the strict guidance of a teacher, shaman, master, or guru, before an individual is able to utilize the breath and energy of the body (bio-energy) for personal transformation.

In the West, there are a number of new approaches to working with breath. One of the latest involves the use of "high energy" hyperventilation, often described as the use of Eastern methodologies translated into Western terms. Examples of this include the Grof Holothrophic Breathwork, some types of rebirthing, and certain Western versions of shamanic practices.

The authors of this paper have some concerns about such kind of "high energy" hyperventilation. "High energy" breathing is usually conducted without the extensive preparation and guidance that is a part of the eastern and shamanic traditions of consciousness exploration. When we attempt to import Eastern techniques into our culture, we need to address the context in which they were developed, since human beings function in a way consistent with society and context. Our challenge is to develop breathwork techniques that are congruent with Western culture.

Traditionally, athletic activities form the basis for the Western way of working with breath and body. This gladiator or warrior model emphasizes the physical aspects of breathing—of being really alive in one's body. In this context, Westerners run the risk of using a "high energy" breathing approach without an overall sense of the larger framework. The use of culturally appropriate breathing methods for psychospiritual development is at an evolutionary stage in the West. We believe it is important to go beyond thinking of it as a technique, and argue for a conservative approach in the use of breath for transforming consciousness.

In order to decide which approaches are appropriate, therapists need to understand the process of personal transformation, and recognize when there are significant shifts of perception. It is important for them to recognize the effects of various breathwork approaches, such as hyperventilation, on our functioning as organisms, whether it is within a specific cultural context or because we possess a certain psychophysiology.

The origins of Western psychology are relatively recent compared with the various systems in use worldwide that explain, control, and affect the human condition. The first Western psychologist to look at respiration and its effect on consciousness was Freud. In his later life, he developed a rudimentary awareness of respiratory changes occurring in the nervous system, and of vegetative (autonomic) changes experienced by his patients during what he believed to be birth regressions.

It was Wilhelm Reich, a student of Freud, who became the main researcher in the field of breath. Reich used more active breathing patterns and provocation of muscle to dissolve what he termed *character armor*. His theory was that the person's neurosis was interwoven with a tendency to create armoring as a defense against feeling a fuller sense of a healthy self. This armoring took various forms, according to the specific malady of the client. Whatever the form, it always served to interrupt the sense of pulsation, a core vitality that he termed the Life Force.

Jung also worked with breathing, using it as a tool for relaxation and release of active imagination. Some Jungian analysts use a breath-awareness process, freeing the breathing very subtly and slowly, allowing unconscious images, thoughts, sensations, and experiences to emerge.

We believe it is important to utilize the wisdom of both Western and Eastern views of human development. The Western world has contributed a great deal toward understanding the role of neurophysiology in the functioning of individuals. We recognize that for an organism to exist and to survive, it needs a regulatory nervous system with two principal qualities: a basic stability and a capacity for flexibility, change, and adaptability.

Stability and flexibility have to exist in a dynamic balance with each other. By fluctuating within a range narrow enough to maintain homeostasis, they create a steady state that gives us the consistency to be able to function as human beings. Each level of increased self-regulatory functioning generates a new steady state, and this new pattern of stability provides the foundation for the next new level of flexibility, and so on.

Reich originally viewed therapy as a process of reducing, or breaking down, armor. We need to rethink what this actually means, since the reduction or dissolution of an individual's armor can disorganize a person's whole system of adaptation and coping. When we, as therapists, intervene to remove some of this defensive armor, it is essential that other more functional resources are found for the individual. This enables them to maintain the stability they need to remain functional in the world.

When Reich originally developed this de-armoring process in pre-World War II Germany, people's defenses were particularly strong—an important point in the current development of theory and practice. Now our intent should be to create more functionality and organization, and use this perspective when considering any new type of intervention in a person's psychophysiological functioning so that these resources can be accessed in an integratable manner over the long term.

For example, we can look at what happens when transforming energy is applied to the human organism. When it is introduced judiciously, the organism or system is able to reorder itself to a level of even higher stability, and increase its potential for future flexibility. However, if energy is introduced in large amounts, flooding the system beyond the organism's ability to maintain its containment boundaries, the system breaks down in chaotic disorganization.

Behavioral extremes coexist in many people today, and people can and do exhibit both excess rigidity and a tendency to be unfocused or scattered in their energies at the same time. A person who uses intense high energy breathing methods to expand consciousness may operate under the illusion that he or she is becoming more spiritual and evolved, when in fact they are primarily becoming more dissociated. They may pursue hyperventilation and experience some type of relief, or they may create further dissociation. As a general rule, when a system moves too far out of equilibrium, it will continue toward further destabilization without realizing it. This is why repetitively following a person's "process" will often reinforce the maladaptive pattern.

However, gradual interventions can allow the organism to maintain integrity, maximize the functional reorganization process, and develop the potential for greater flexibility—as long as that flexibility is bounded by a stable system and is incremental. The process of using small interventions, assessing the impact, and reassessing what to do next, is a process we term *titration*.

Through evolution, organisms have developed ways of coping with attempts at changing the status quo, and any attempts to alter this coping ability have to move slowly. The innate wisdom of the neurophysiology, and how it has come to deal with attempts to change its orientation in the world, must be respected: We cannot change overnight that which has evolved over millions of years. If it were possible to make substantial changes quickly and easily, we would not be flexible but rather would be unstable!

The sudden introduction of vast quantities of energy, as happens during intense hyperventilation and catharsis, can destabilize a person's "self" organization. If a person has been overly stable, it may feel good to have a sense of letting go. This may make them feel like, "Wow, I'm on the other side and I'm free. I'm floating with the cosmos." However, with that floating feeling may come a disordering of the self, in such a way that the person cannot retrace their path through small steps; they must push the breathing all the way, or not at all. It's a lot like taking a drug such as LSD. The drug destabilizes the physiochemistry and this destabilizes the functioning of the self. No one can say exactly what the effect is.

LSD can be useful in certain circumstances, and can open the doors of perception, but it also initiates a potentially disorganized process. In most cases, people don't know how to use the experience to make useful changes, and this can lead to very dysfunctional outcomes.

Working with the breath can also open up an awareness to other realities, and to other dimensions of consciousness. In this form of therapeutic intervention, the art is in knowing how to integrate these experiences into the whole personality, and to do this in a way that is developmentally and psychophysiologically sound. If breathwork is used without proper integration, it simply recreates the same old path of disorder with which the person was struggling originally. It does not address the creative process of disintegration and reordering, and it does not introduce new information or parallel stabilizing patterns to support a person's sense of integration and wholeness.

Experience needs to be properly integrated in a repetitive, incremental, and self-organizing process. This is what drives all our developmental and spiritual processes. We see this reflected in a child's experience. At each developmental stage, a child acquires new skills and then they pass into a new stage, such as the "terrible twos," and order disintegrates. However, each falling apart is followed by a significant new synthesis.

An infant cannot be made into an adolescent by giving them a drug; the drug would simply disorder their reality. An infant would not have the life experience to contain the gonadal energy of an adolescent appropriately, and they would be seriously disoriented. This is what happens when drugs and intense breathing methods are used to generate intense experiences. The person needs information, preparation, experience, and pacing through developmental layers before these experiences can be integrated as part of their developmental shift toward realizing their full potential.

Some individuals can become fixated around new pathways, such as the use of intense breathing, so that they can continue to have an intense experience. When this happens, it indicates an addiction to the process. A certain type of experience may need to be generated several times in order to resolve it without the person feeling a sense of loss or incompleteness. People who are prone to becoming fixated (addicted) to a certain type of experience may not be able to adjust successfully to the intensity of the intervention used and healthy defense mechanisms may break down, reducing the person's ability to function. This can result in generalized or specific anxiety, somatization, illness, psychosis, or depression.

Some of the new psychologies, including those utilizing hyperventilation methods, have focused on catharsis, on the expressive get it out theme, and there is much concern around this technique. In 1990, Gendlin expressed his concern about the dangers of cathartic work and analyzed the theories of Janoff, contrasting them with those of Levine and Grove.

Section 2: Breath, Anxiety, and Consciousness

Here we examine the relationship between breath, anxiety, and consciousness. We address the two different patterns of breathing and their effects on consciousness.

Patterns of Breathing

There are two primary patterns of breathing which can be useful to understand in the context of psychotherapy: hyperventilation (overbreathing) and hypoventilation (underbreathing). These patterns are two polarities in a continuum of breathing patterns that range from gasping to very shallow, limited breathing.

The use of the term hyperventilation can be misleading. Most people who are called hyperventilators are actually hypoventilators who exhibit periodic episodes of relative hyperventilation. True hyperventilators are aggressive, type A individuals who develop a sense of aliveness by pumping their breathing. These people are often seen puffing in gyms, and they thrive on constant charge and excitement in their lives. They need to be sensitized to their inner pulsatory capacity, and weaned from the pushing and tightening rhythms that they use to develop and perpetuate their type A energy patterns.

Hypo/hyperventilator types, by contrast, shrink from experiencing the energy surge or charge. In their predominant mode of hypoventilation, their feeble breathing pattern accumulates carbon dioxide in the blood. This shift toward blood acidity and incomplete metabolism, which produces increased serum lactate, irritates the core regulatory functions of the brain in the hypothalamus and brainstem, contributing to the many digestive, allergic, immunologic, and general low energy problems that frequently plague them.

Repeated hypoventilation predisposes the individual to a metabolic imbalance. This triggers compensatory mechanisms involving the secretory systems of the kidneys and lungs in an attempt to restore homeostasis. This stimulates a respiratory increase in the lungs, reducing blood acidity and increasing alkalinity. Unfortunately, this abrupt change in pH, with associated sympathetic activation from receptors in the intercostal muscles, produces a rush of excitation leading to further overbreathing, which leads in turn to anxiety and still more charging, creating a vicious, escalating circle; in other words, a panic attack.

Viewing this from another perspective, what is actually happening is that overbreathing generates a charging pattern that mobilizes anxiety so that a chronic, low-grade anxiety becomes acute. When hyperventilation is carried to extremes, it removes control of the cortex and allows the anxious effects to flood, moving the person through the anxiety state. However, the person then regresses back into hypoventilation, and anxiety builds up again. This typically results in a flip-flopping between hypo- (anxious) and hyperventilatory (dissociated) states.

People who have done a lot of intense breathwork will sometimes create this pattern. They will hypoventilate for a period of time, almost not breathing, and then switch to hyperventilating. Here the system is not regulating itself and it is not stable. Rather, the two modes are separated—split from each other and disconnected. Breathing becomes dysfunctional, and is not coordinated with the overall functioning of the organism.

Thus it is absolutely essential to help hypo/hypervertilatory individuals contain and regulate their charging mechanism, and lead them toward normalizing biological rhythms. This helps them to develop a more flexible, adaptive stability. Although it is true that techniques which encourage runaway hyperventilation can ultimately take the person through to panic release, this kind of flip-flopping eventually encourages an even greater widening of the pattern. This is rather like setting the house thermostat to turn the heat on at 50°F and off again at 100°F. Although the average room temperature is 75°F, inhabitants of the house will be first chilled and then nearly suffocated in the process. It is obviously much more desirable to have a thermostat that turns on at 73°F and off again at 77°F.

When hyperventilation breathing techniques are used repeatedly, the person is encouraged to split hypo- and hyperventilation patterns even more, rather than restoring respiratory balance. This cuts the person off from a dynamic repertory of experience, and they can lose the sense of the essential, core self. Experience is no longer continuous and coherent but becomes expressed in terms of these extremes.

Then the person's internal experience is oriented around either anxiety or flooding, around holding and not breathing, or overbreathing and flooding. This phenomenon can occur in the Primal Therapy approach, where the orientation around *having a feeling*, usually a regressive feeling, becomes a goal, a pathway believed to lead to the *real* sense of self.

If this pathway of generating intense experiences becomes a part of the person's life evolvement approach, he or she may end up without a sense of self-regulation, leading to a diminished sense of self. We believe that the essential self evolves from a sense of internal regulation, and thus learning how to regulate the self is critical in the development of a person's full human potential. This includes paying subtle attention to shifts in regulatory patterns, and then using appropriate interventions.

When we become aware of the wide range of subtly-flowing sensations and feelings which make up the overall process of self-regulation, orientation, responsiveness, approach, and withdrawal, we know that we are alive, connected, and human. All of these orienting responses become parts of the self-regulation of homeostasis as a person begins to experience his or her breathing automatically.

Practically, it can be useful to generate mild to moderate breathing in order to access various states of affect and consciousness. For example, when working with a client's anger, a therapist can have the client push firmly on the therapist's hand, and breathe out while pushing. This discharges the energy associated with the anger. The therapist does not, however, encourage or allow the client to dramatize the anger he or she feels. In this way, the therapist has helped to contain the expression of the client's emotional experience.

Section 3: Intent of Using Breathing Techniques

As mentioned previously, the healthy opposite of stability is not instability; rather, flexibility is the complement of stability.

Stability and Flexibility: System Dynamics

When using breathing interventions, a therapist needs to develop a way of assessing the systems and parameters of the client in order to design an intervention to generate optimal adaptive tendencies. This raises several questions: What are the adaptive tendencies of a person? What are the maladaptive tendencies? How can these be assessed? Where does one begin an intervention? A therapist needs to develop a balanced approach, based on the interventions appropriate for each individual client.

Appropriate Assessment

As mentioned above, the hypoventilator is characterized by a pattern of avoiding charge. The client has an underlying anxiety of which he/she is often unaware, but is unconsciously driven by it all the same. The hypoventilator is driven to avoid excitement, has a tendency to minimize intense contact, and exhibits avoidance behaviors. In addition, they are likely to have unresolved developmental issues, family-of-origin issues, and other concerns related to their particular character structure (as explained earlier in the text).

A person with a primarily mental character structure will tend to be a hypoventilator, while a person with a more emotional character structure will tend to alternate between hyper- and hypoventilation. The more mental person may be lost in a dream world, with a philosophical or spiritual orientation to life, connected through a philosophical or spiritual cause. An emotional type, on the other hand, may utilize hyperventilation to generate emotionally transcendent spiritual experiences. This, however, reinforces their inability to be in the world and to contain affect.

It is sometimes believed in body psychotherapy that the body has its own innate wisdom, and that this wisdom will guide a person to wholeness. Like most blanket statements, this theory can lead us astray. For example, the premise that encouraging a client to hyperventilate and go into catharsis will naturally bring them to an improved state of well-being is just not true.

Strategies with Different Breathing Styles

Hyperventilator intervention: When working with an energetic and expressive hyperventilator, a therapist can push the client slightly to increase their breathing and raise the activation level. This encourages the nervous system to become sympathetically dominant, leading to a parasympathetic discharge and release response. This gives the client the experience of a charging and discharging cycle, and familiarizes them with the subtlety of their own internal experience. The therapist should encourage the client to develop a fascination with the internal experience, and with a more internal orientation (in contrast to emotional explosion). Through this type of experience, the therapist is teaching the client that gradual increments can lead to positive experiences.

The client needs to be helped to move slowly as they will want to push right through, wanting greater charge, intensity, and experience, and overriding the building blocks necessary for the broadening and deepening of personal development. When left to their own devices, clients will often try to use breathing to satisfy an addictive pattern. The therapist's task is to encourage enjoyment of the more subtle experience. An important goal of therapy is to replace the drive to generate more intensity with a sense of facilitating the building and containing of charge, leading to a gentle release. The therapist can discuss with the client the awareness of changes. This includes questions such as: "What's going on now? How is it to be like that? How is that different? What do you want from this place? What do you feel in this area? What are your images from your body? What sensations are you experiencing? How are they different from before?"

Hypoventilator intervention: When a client's breathing pattern is closer to hypoventilation, the goal is to titrate the experience just enough to stimulate the breathing mildly, leading to a minimal activation. This will tend to normalize the respiratory pattern and support the client to develop their own capacity to contain more charge without fragmentation, leading to more central vitality without anxiety.

The intent here is to shift the homeostasis in a direction that can embrace more life. The client will want to disassociate as they approach anything close to a hyperventilation response.

The therapist needs to assist the client to stay present with the gradually increased excitation. As the client's breathing begins to approach a more normalized pattern, they will actually begin to associate. This may not be comfortable at first, and they may need additional encouragement to tolerate the experience. They may again move into slight disassociation, and the therapist will need to direct the client back toward what is being associated.

The process of bringing the client back into awareness of a higher level association, stimulating slightly and then reassociating when the client slightly disassociates, is the preferred approach when working with this pattern. The idea is to use breathing techniques to help them reach the point where they can associate, without going over to disassociation. If they disassociate during the process, the therapist needs to recognize it, ensure the disassociation is minimal, and bring the client back through to reassociation.

In body psychotherapy, it is important to work with body awareness and an awareness of muscle. For example, the therapist might physically support the lower back, and ask, "What does that back support feel like?" or "How does that affect respiration?" This type of intervention can lead to increased body awareness and, until the client has awareness of the muscular sensations and the embodied experience of the self, they will not be able to change old patterns. This approach requires a great deal of education and information in order for the client to understand the personal benefit of the work.

Section 4: Developing Spiritual Experience

When we speak of spiritual experience, it might be more accurate to think about the undeveloped parts of ourselves. Extension of these parts will then lead to unfolding of spiritual dimensions. It is important to look at this as developmental, not just as a psychological or spiritual experience. It is a developmental process in human development.

We believe that the role of a therapist is to encourage clients to live more comfortably within themselves, and support them to move beyond an addiction to transcendent and spiritual experiences. In order to do this, we need to assist them to develop the everyday richness of internal experience. Once that richness is discovered and incorporated as a part of their ongoing experience, their spiritual life will be generated quite naturally out of the richness of internal experience, and will not be a goal in itself. We need to encourage the notion that we are biological beings, rooted in flesh and in the animistic spirit of the flesh; that we are a part of the cosmos, and of all existence.

The approach to spiritual experience will be different for the hypo- and hyperventilator. The hyperventilator will want to push, and will tend to become focused on or addicted to whatever approach can generate the transcendent experience. The hypoventilator, on the other hand, will go into the spiritual as something disassociated from daily life. The therapist's task is to bring both types back into everyday development. Then, instead of habituating to spirituality outside of self, the person will learn to surrender to his or her own vegetative currents, and find their internal truth within their authentic and inner instinctual self.

Section 5: An Explanation of Character Structure and Bodynamic Model

Throughout this article, the terms *Character Structure* and *Bodynamic Model* are used. The following section is intended to provide definitions and frameworks to clarify these terms for those readers unfamiliar with them.

Character Structure

The following material on character structure, although originally developed by Reich, is drawn from the Bioenergetics model of Lowen.

Character is defined as a fixed pattern of behavior, the typical way an individual handles his striving for pleasure. It is structured in the body in the form of chronic and generally unconscious muscular tensions that block or limit impulses to reach out. Character is also a psychic attitude, buttressed by a system of denials, rationalizations, and projections, and geared to an ego ideal that affirms its value. The functional identity of psychic character and body structure or muscular attitude is the key to understanding personality, for it enables us to read the character from the body, and to explain a body attitude by its psychic representations, and vice versa.

In Bioenergetics, the different character structures are classified into five basic types. Each type has a special pattern of defense on both the psychological and the muscular levels that distinguishes it from the other types. It is important to note that this is a classification not of people but of defensive positions. It is recognized that no individual is a pure type, and that every person in our culture combines some or all of these defensive patterns within his personality. The personality of an individual, as distinct from his character structure, is determined by his vitality; that is, by the strength of his impulses and by the defenses he has erected to control these impulses.

No two individuals are alike in either their inherent vitality or in their patterns of defense arising from their life experience. Nevertheless, it is necessary to speak in terms of types for the sake of clarity in communication and understanding. The five types are termed *schizoid, oral, psychopathic, masochistic,* and *rigid*. These terms are used because they are known and accepted definitions of personality disorders in the psychiatric profession. Our classification does not violate established criteria.

The schizoid character structure: *Schizoid* describes a person whose sense of self is diminished, whose ego is weak, and whose contact with the body and its feelings is greatly reduced.

The oral character structure: We describe a personality as being *oral* when it contains many traits typical of infancy, the oral period of life. These traits are weakness in the sense of independence, a tendency to cling to others, a decreased aggressiveness, and an inner feeling of needing to be held, supported, and cared for.

The psychopathic character structure: The essence of the *psychopathic* attitude is the denial of feeling. There is in all psychopathic characters a great investment of energy in one's image. The other aspect of this personality is the drive for power, and the need to dominate and control.

The masochistic character structure: The *masochistic* individual is one who suffers and whines or complains, but remains submissive. Submissiveness is the dominant masochistic tendency. If the masochistic character shows a submissive attitude in his outward behavior, he is just the opposite inside. On a deeper emotional level, he has strong feelings of spite, negativity, hostility, and superiority.

The rigid character structure: The concept of rigidity derives from the tendency of these individuals to hold themselves stiff—with pride. Thus, the head is held fairly high, the backbone straight. These would be positive traits were it not for the fact that the pride is defensive, the rigidity unyielding. The rigid character is afraid to give in, equating this with submission and collapse. Rigidity becomes a defense against an underlying masochistic tendency.

The character structure defines the way an individual handles his need to love, his reaching out for intimacy and closeness, and his striving for pleasure. Seen in this light, the different character structures form a spectrum or hierarchy, at one end of which is the *schizoid* position, a withdrawal from intimacy and closeness because it is too threatening, and at the other emotional health, where there is no holding against the impulse to reach out openly for closeness and contact. The various character types fit into this spectrum or hierarchy according to the degree that they allow for intimacy and contact.

Bodynamic Model

Founded by Lisbeth Marcher, the Bodynamic theory is the work of a group of Danish therapists who have studied, worked, and developed together for over fifteen years. The theory combines the experience of many people working with a powerful system, continually finding and expanding its limits. The diverse personalities engaged in this project are reflected in the many aspects of the theory. One such aspect, Somatic Developmental Psychology, achieves its power through integrating new research on the psychomotor development of children with depth psychotherapy systems. This developmental approach allows for direct activation of undeveloped motor (body) skills and psychological (mind) resources.

Marcher was aware of the Reichian idea that if children are frustrated in an activity, they may tense their muscles to hold back this activity. She realized that when the frustration of a developmental activity is early or severe the child may become resigned, and the corresponding muscles will be flaccid (undertoned). If the response of the environment is appropriate, the muscles will have a neutral tone, and the child will tend to have a healthy response to future situations. Since each developmental stage is comprised of a specific set of developmental psychomotor tasks, and since these tasks all have associated muscles, there can be any of three overall outcomes for each stage: 1) *resigned* (early frustration), 2) *held back* or *rigid* (later frustration), and 3) *healthy* (appropriate response).

The seven developmental stages, listed in increasing age and by the structural issue dealt with, are: *existence, need, autonomy, will, love/sexuality, opinion,* and *solidarity/performance.* Each will be understood in terms of an early position, a late position, and a healthy position. Using the *will* stage (two to four years of age) as an example, its early position is characterized by self-sacrificing, its later position by judging, and its healthy position by assertiveness. Viewing clients' difficulties in these terms allows the therapist to phrase interventions in an appropriate manner. A schematic of the seven stages is included as Appendix A, outlining the different early, late, and healthy phases with the stages, as well as an approximate correlation to the Lowen's Bioenergetics model.

Having this specific information allows the therapist to pinpoint the undeveloped areas corresponding to a particular issue. The ability to work directly with somatic resignation transforms the nature of psychotherapy. Rather than focusing on resistance, understanding, or emotional release, clients learn to sense their body in a way that helps to awaken these undeveloped resources, ones that have been given up or never learned. The acquisition of these new resources, which are exactly the ones needed (but missing), greatly facilitates the resolution of developmental trauma. At the same time, it empowers clients to new actions in daily life, including developing the resources to reposition themselves within their family-of-origin and their social context.

One of the profound aspects of the Bodynamic approach is the Bodymap, an empirically developed diagnostic tool. The Bodymap is a color-coded mapping of the elasticity (hypo, hyper, or neutral) of over two hundred muscles. Bodynamic therapists are trained to make this map for each client. The testing is done manually and has a repeatability of over ninety percent. With the map, one can read the history of the client's character development. One can literally see which stages are characterized by developmental trauma. The test results can be analyzed functionally, in terms of a client's resources and abilities in areas like bonding, grounding, centering, boundaries, etc. Shock and birth trauma can also be read directly from the map.

The somatic developmental approach can also lead to exciting new ways of working with a wide range of issues, including family-of-origin, somatic boundaries, shock (such as physical and sexual abuse), issues related to birthing and womb experiences, and the use of somatic therapies with children.

With this introductory information on Character Structure and Bodynamics in mind, we now look at the practical applications of breathwork. Strategies for working with a particular client depend not only on their psychological make-up, but also on their present character structure. For example, a hyperventilator could be a person with a great deal of *will* structure who has endured through difficult life situations, or could be a later developmental structure, such as the *rigid opinion* or *solidarity/performance* structures.

There will be slightly different strategies for each of those related structures, but they do have commonality. If a *will* structure client is having trouble moving through a charge, he or she may become afraid of explosion, and get stuck while trying to go through the charge to discharge. On the other hand, a client with a *rigid* structure will try without success to push through, failing to achieve relaxation. Both clients will have a similar problem as they become caught in the charge and cannot get through.

When working with these clients, especially with the withholding *will* structure, a therapist needs to be both firm and gentle. The therapist may need to assist the client as they breathe, and free the breathing by using massage or supporting the back. The breathing may be used as an adjunct to massage, just as the client is preparing to let go. This will diminish the person's thinking activity, promoting a sense of ease and stillness, and allow them to let go.

The later character structures all have some issues around surrender. When surrender happens, and the client is responding parasympathetically, he or she is much more aware of the subtlety of sensations. Comparing the sympathetic to the parasympathetic state can be likened to the Weber Fechnen Law: If you have a hundred candles in a room and you put one candle out, you don't notice it, but if there are only four candles and you put one out, you notice the difference.

In the parasympathetic state, the client begins to notice and experience sensations besides pain, bracing, and tension, and starts to realize that there is another universe available to them.

They are now able to experience a whole range of sensations. Later, they can learn to access these sensations themselves, with or without the breathing. They become aware of more subtle, softer sensations, and of fluidity, aliveness, connection, yearning, and power. Each of these sensations will feel different for people with different personality structures, but whatever their make-up, each person begins to have a sense that there is something underneath the tension and the energy. People with a *will* structure pattern are likely to be most aware of the tension, while those with a *rigid/achiever* structure will be most aware of excitement, the ability to handle the energetic sensations, and the subsequent move into surrender.

Since *will* structure clients need to learn to move through the tension and experience the charge, the therapist must work with their tension and help to ease the musculature. On the other hand, if the client has a *rigid* structure, the therapist needs to help them achieve a free flow of sensation so that they can connect their different experiences. The therapist must keep the client from going into the same stuck patterns. Once the client begins to accept and feel comfortable with new sensations, and gain the confidence that comes with a successful experience, then they will be able either to release their patterns of tension or move through their patterns of holding intensity.

A client who hypoventilates generally embodies the earlier character structures. The first benefit the hypoventilator will experience from increasing respiration is having more oxygen, and this enables them to get more energy and hold more charge. The *oral* or *need* structure person, for example, will be able to sense some vitality, core feeling, and satisfaction. It is crucial for the hypoventilator to learn to develop self-support. (Note: This is not regressive work, it is wiser to avoid using breathing for regressive work, but breathing work could be useful to give some extra self-support).

If the client has a *mental-oriented existence* structure, it's important to give them a strong sense of security so that they will not feel they are flying apart when they experience some charge.

They need to learn to feel charge directly in the body, and then work at containing it. Their natural tendency will be to escape from the increased sensation, so it is necessary to build up the charge a little at a time, helping the client to stay with the experience.

This pattern of avoidance is found in both the *mental* and the *emotional existence* structures but is expressed in different ways. The *mental* type is more likely to squirm, itch, and scratch, whereas the *emotional* type is more likely to emote, become hysterical, or end up compelled to express some feeling. It is possible to assist the client to experience the sensation. The *emotional* type needs to learn to connect with their energetic nature, to their bodily truth, whereas the *mental* type needs to connect more with their body sensations so that they can handle, tolerate, and contain some of the increased charge.

It is important for the therapist to take care not to push the *mental* structure into disassociation, or the *emotional* into catharsis, as both are actually forms of disassociation. The therapist needs to work at the level where the client is able to contain and tolerate charge. In the earlier character structures (*existence, need, autonomy,* and *will*), breathing is not the best approach for uncovering unresolved developmental issues. In later structures (*love/sexuality, opinions,* and *solidarity/performance*), breathing is more useful. The client has the resources to integrate its impact, having developed more ego strength and autonomic stability at the earlier developmental stages.

Clients who hyperventilate, and are characteristically the later structures, can use breathing as a tool to discover more subtle levels of their experience. Here the therapist assists, teaching the client how to relax by paying attention to the nervous system. Relaxation happens when the client navigates the excitation or charge successfully, and is able to enter into different altered states. This kind of deep relaxation can support hyperamnesia and an ability to make more associations, just as alcohol and some mild drugs can loosen up the super ego, our sensor and critical judge. When a client yields to deep relaxation, he or she is able to access more core material, not necessarily just memories, but also how they see the self, how they feel, and how they experience the difference between the public and private self, the heart feelings and desires.

By contrast, hypoventilator structures need to be strongly encouraged, supported, and helped to breathe. This can be done with a little gentle work on the chest. If the therapist places a hand gently on the side of the client's chest, it encourages the client to use side breathing, which is usually more spontaneous. The client may need only two or three breaths before experiencing a noticeable sense of nervous system charge. By staying with that experience until the charge becomes fully associated as a sensation or feeling, the client can move toward integration. The therapist can do some movement or emotive work at this time. The client may become a little dizzy, or become slightly uneasy, and may need contact or support to move through to release. It is important for the client to titrate the experience gradually, rather than pushing past this point of dizziness or light-headedness.

At this point, the goal of therapy is to develop some sense of energy flow, and reinforce the ability of the client to handle the charge without fragmentation. This is a very important corrective experience because it reorganizes the client's basic belief in self, and their capacity to integrate increased sensation. For example, a *mental* structure type believes that they are going to fall apart or disintegrate in some way. There are variations of this, but it is an overall theme. When a client can experience shifts in reality without falling apart, they are moving toward a more functional way of being in the world.

Section 6: Strategies for Developmental and Traumatic Issues

Having examined different character structures and the particular breathing patterns associated with these structures, it is now possible to look at therapeutic strategies for both developmental and traumatic issues.

We begin by examining how to work with the incomplete developmental issues of hyperventilators. Usually these people do not have much expressed or experienced spirituality. They may go to a church or synagogue, but actual spiritual experience generally eludes them. Except for an emotional sensitivity, hyperventilators are either bound up, like the *will* structure, or do not believe in spiritual experience, like a *rigid* structure does ("It's not rational" or "I'm trying but can't seem to find it"). They will sometimes express disillusionment, since they have tried to meditate to change their reality and nothing happened.

In these cases, a therapist can work directly with breathing to build up some charge. Eventually, the person will start going into deeper discharge experiences, altered states of awareness, and suspended respiratory states. They will be beginning to "see" images, and experience subtle body sensations.

These people can be substantially present in their bodies without having the problems found in early structure individuals. When their experience begins to shift, they begin to develop an interest in spirituality and want to explore it. *Love/sexuality* structure individuals then start to open up sexually, experiencing love with sexuality together as a spiritual union. They become more able to connect to their feelings and desire a more complete relationship than they have had before. *Will* structure individuals who have been trying to break through their sexual tensions, or achievers who were trying to achieve orgasm, begin to yield. A sense of melting is a positive step forward in their spiritual development.

For people with a *mental* (*schizoid*) structure, spirituality tends to be enhanced or linked to images and thoughts. As the person opens up, feelings contained within the body become more grounded in spirituality, beginning with mutual connection. Working with the breathing is a good approach here, because these clients have real feeling for the first time and start to open up in their bodies, moving with the breathing and feeling pleasure.

This initially invites a positive transference, and supports them to develop a good therapeutic alliance. Occasional breathwork at this point is very useful. It can also help the client to develop the strength to resist being flooded by sensations and any spontaneous emotional material that may emerge. As they learn to control the charge and tolerate it, the experience becomes one of developing increased personal capacity and healthy boundaries.

When working with hypoventilators and developmental issues, a therapist needs to teach them how to contain increased sensation and charge, so that they experience the charge in their body while remaining grounded in sensation. Otherwise the energy will move up and centre in the head. In order to be grounded, the client needs to increase his/her energy and then move it down. It is essential for the therapist to know when the energy moves from one area of the body to another. When a group works with hyperventilation-type overbreathing, often there is no one attending to the movement of each person's energy who has the ability to recognize vegetative flow and shifts. This can be hazardous. Breathing is a powerful tool for moving energy, provided it is used appropriately and directed by skilled practitioners. Ethical guidelines and adequate training are necessary if approaches are to be used wisely and well (Macnaughton, Bentzen, and Jarlnaes).

Developmental issues are different from shock or trauma issues, and need to be approached differently. Breathing can be used in traumatic issues to help a client tune into the autonomic nervous system and develop a sense of resources that can be used to help. A therapist may choose to do this before working with the shock itself. It is helpful to work gently with respiratory patterns during the renegotiation of the trauma response, before using breathwork to enhance integration and a sense of wholeness.

Section 7: The Contraindications

Breathwork may be contraindicated, or a cause for concern, in the presence of certain medical conditions, and it is important that a therapist is aware of this potential. Such medical issues include diabetes, hypoglycemia, lupus, muscular sclerosis, heart problems, cancer, stomach ulcers, epilepsy, glandular problems, kidney disease, and liver disease.

Hyperventilation can cause the blood sugar to drop, and this can be significant for clients with diabetes and hypoglycemia. A number of people have reactivated their symptoms of lupus, muscular sclerosis, and other autoimmune disorders and chronic conditions through intense overbreathing. People whose symptoms had been in remission for years have had to be hospitalized because their symptoms returned. The increased stress of hyperventilation could precipitate a heart attack in those with heart problems, and could possibly increase the rate of spread of cancer within the body.

Therapists should not start breathwork with clients who have an active stomach ulcer. However, if the therapist can use the breathing in a very sensitive, judicious way, it is possible to help to clear up stomach and intestinal problems. One of the diagnostic tests for epilepsy is that a patient's brain will produce spiking waves when they hyperventilate, even if it is only for a few breaths. Lupus is an autoimmune disorder characterized by major breakdown and disorganization of the system, and thus any energy that is introduced must be of the very smallest titration, otherwise the system will become further disorganized.

Similarly, endocrine problems (such as hyperactive thyroid—Graves disease) are most likely a result of central nervous system disorganization: If too much energy is introduced through breathing, the therapist may not be able to control what is going to happen to some of the organs. For example, a client with kidney problems uses hyperventilation. This will force the kidneys to secrete additional biocarbonate ions, and put more stress on the kidneys themselves. This could cause the kidney to fail. If the organ under stress is the liver, it may not be able to cope with all the additional toxic material that is being moved around as a result of the increased breathing. These are not necessarily absolute contraindications, but they are serious concerns and caveats for a therapist to consider.

Section 8: Psychological Concerns, Dissociative Problems, and Sexual Abuse

Consider this scenario: As the therapist, you are working with a client's breathing pattern and he or she disassociates significantly on the third breath. If you are surprised, something has been missed in the assessment phase. Obviously, a therapist must know character structure and psychopathology enough to know when not to use breathwork at all. If you have a client who would typically be diagnosed as a borderline personality or a multiple personality, it is very difficult to know what meaning he or she is going to place on that altered state experience. The client may take a few breaths and become flooded with images, projecting that out to you. Such a client needs to connect much more slowly, in terms of transference, rather than have a rapid transference provoked by hyperventilation.

A further example of the perceptual problems altered states can create: A person goes to the dentist and uses nitrous oxide. This releases some sexual images, feelings, or fantasies. Since the person's boundaries are unclear when they are in this altered state, they become confused as to whether or not the dentist molested them.

Breathwork is very rarely appropriate in working directly with shock and trauma, although it can be helpful in some situations (mentioned earlier in this article) to develop resources and uncover previously unconscious material. This is more true for individuals with later character structures. As the therapist, you don't want to push them through prematurely.

Hysterical, Obsessive, or Explosive Personalities

Obsessive clients can habituate to breathwork. If it is done correctly, a therapist can use hyperventilation to help break the obsession, but this takes finesse and skill. The therapist must know how to take the breathing up to a point, poke and prod a little bit, have a good rapport, and be able to use some other interventions to loosen it up. If you are too forceful, it will merely reinforce the obsessive behavior. If a person is hysterical, the therapist should only unmask emotional issues gradually, otherwise they will tend to experience flooding. There are, at the least, caveats in working with explosive and violent personalities. Pushing these clients could generate violent behavior.

It is not appropriate to introduce breathing for clients who are dealing with unresolved birth and intrauterine situations. Rather, it is important for the breathing to start from the generation of deep biological rhythms, not those imposed by the therapist. The person may have been respirated at birth, which created a shock or similar reaction. If the therapist introduces a mechanical respiration pattern, the client will be locked even more into the shock pattern. However, if the client has worked through some of the birth and intrauterine shock, gentle belly breathing, then some light panting patterns can be used as a resource, to recapture some "womb bliss." It is important to realize that these steps must be put into the appropriate context. A therapist should not do a Rebirthing session if a client is still exhibiting birth shock or any shock relating to the neck; responses can be unpredictable if the client tries to push physically through that shock.

Summary

This article has discussed the implications of attending to the respiratory response of individuals in the psychotherapy process. The patterns or styles of breathing were placed on a continuum ranging from those individuals who over breathe (hyperventilators) to the other polarity of individuals who under breathe (hypoventilators). The relationship between respiration, breathing, anxiety, and consciousness was discussed in relationship to these polarities. The importance of employing attention to the breath, and interventions in breathing patterns, were explored. This led to a description of appropriate interventions with various breathing patterns and character structures. The need to include caution and flexibility in employing breath interventions was described. This led to an examination of types of medical conditions and psychological issues where breathing interventions would be contraindicated.

Conclusions

Attention to the pattern or type of breathing displayed by a client can provide useful information for the therapist in the practice of psychotherapy. Intervening in the client's breathing pattern can be useful in moving the client toward self-regulation and a sense of wholeness. These interventions must be utilized within a context of understanding the client's breathing pattern, its implications in their psychological, neurophysiological, and developmental (character structure) issues. In addition, particular cautions need to be kept in mind when there is any evidence of shock and trauma, medical conditions, or dissociative issues. The authors hope that this piece will provide some guidelines for the therapist wishing to employ attention to, and interventions in, a client's breathing in the service of increased psychological and spiritual well-being.

References

Campbell, R. *Fisherman's Guide to a Systems Approach to Creativity and Organization* (Boston: New Science Library/Shambala, 1985), xi.

Gendlin, E.T. "Emotions, Psychotherapy and Change," In J.D. Safran and Les Greenberg (Eds.) *On Emotion in Therapy* (New York: Academic Press, 1990).

Levine, P. (1990). "The Body as Healer: Revisioning of Trauma." *Somatics* 8(1).

Levine, Peter. "Transforming Trauma, Giving the Body Its Due." In Maxine Sheets-Johnstone (Ed.) *Giving the Body Its Due (Suny Series)* (New York: State University of New York Press, 1992).

Lowen, A. *Bioenergetics* (New York: Penguin Books, 1975).

Macnaughton, I. "The Wisdom of the Body." Unpublished manuscript, 1983.

Macnaughton, I. "Developing a design inquiry model by conducting a retrospective design analysis." Unpublished dissertation. (San Francisco: Saybrook Institute, 1989).

Macnaughton, I., M. Bentzen, & E. Jarlnaes. (1993). "Ethical guidelines for the use of somatic psychotherapy." *Energy & Character* 24(2):64.

Reich, W. *Character Analysis* (New York: Simon & Schuster Inc., 1945).

Russell, P. *The Global Brain* (Los Angeles: J.P. Tarcher, 1983).

Toffler, A. *Future Shock* (New York: Bantam, 1984).

Afterword

It is clear to me and many others that a key usefulness of psychotherapy is assisting the emergent qualities of a person's own uniqueness—his or her fundamental character. That task cannot be done quickly. If psychotherapy is to be most helpful, it must concern itself with more than pathology. It needs to address people's struggles and suffering in such ways as to assist in the manifestation of their own soul expressions—connecting themselves with their unique selves, their families, the world, and the sacred.

A fast-paced technological culture can crush all the juices from therapy, leaving it a dry affair—a means for limited repair work, another technical pseudo-solution. It is imperative that therapists not encourage the erosion of the mystery of life. Rather, we should nurture a proper sense of reverence toward it.

To embrace life, we must address the whole person. That implies not leaving out anything vital. Each of us has a mind and a body, complete with a nervous system, sensations, muscles, blood, felt experiences, and the like. But even Freud, who began with the body, gave up on it early, and most therapists have followed his example. Fortunately, this narrow, nearly inorganic view of the human being is gradually being corrected.

Where earlier psychotherapy focused only on the individual, now a knowledge of the family system permits a more inclusive approach to each person. Yet here again, we can lose this new advantage if we fail to see our clients as human beings—people who come to us for assistance, yes, but who bring inside them callings from spiritual depths. Like Virgil in Dante's *Inferno*, we must serve as guides to those profundities, but we cannot do so unless we have respected the depths of our own being and explored them conscientiously. Only then, can we bring the timing and personal presence which will help our patients emerge from darkness into the light that Dante so magnificently describes.

Indeed, I often wonder what dark night may yet descend on all of us if we continue on our present path toward reductionistic thinking. Here, I am speaking not only of therapists. We have all been reared and schooled in linear ways to believe that the world's richness is bound by geometric lines describing discrete entities with separate parts. Most of us are still largely unaware of the degree to which we still think and act as if we can understand whole by studying parts. Fortunately, there is growing awareness among thoughtful people that only a systemic perspective can help us effectively explore the complexity of our inner and outer worlds. The articles in this book are a beginning attempt to address some interrelated aspects of that complexity—body/ mind/spirit/family/society. I hope their collection here may generate some new insights to move us toward that better world for future generations, which we all seek.

About the Contributors

Marianne Bentzen graduated as a relaxation therapist in 1980, and held a private practice in body psychotherapy until 1985, when she co-founded the Bodynamic Institute. After thirteen years there, first as a trainer and then as training director, she is now working as a freelance trainer and professional consultant in Denmark, Sweden, the Netherlands, Russia, and North America. She is a member of the European Association for Body Psychotherapy and the Danish Psychotherapist Association. Bentzen focuses on establishing truth and peace in the field of consciousness. Her subjects include psychomotor development, neuropsychology, evolutionary psychology, trauma theory, and a spiritual framework for ego-formation.

Peter Bernhardt, MFT, is adjunct professor of psychology at John F. Kennedy University in Orinda, California. He is a former core faculty member of the Somatics Department at the California Institute for Integral Studies and past president of the U.S. Association of Body Psychotherapy. He holds a private practice in the Bay Area.

Merete Holm Brantbjerg is co-creator, trainer, supervisor, and therapist in the Bodynamic System. She is Director of Bodynamic trainings in Scandinavia and originally trained as a psychomotor therapist. Brantbjerg has specialized in teaching body and cognitive coping strategies in relation to stress and shock, and also as related to self-care in the helping professions.

David Freeman received his MSW and DSW degrees from the University of Southern California. As Professor Emeritus at the University of British Columbia School of Social Work, his specialty is in family theory and therapy. Freeman maintains a private practice and is a highly regarded consultant to and a trainer of family therapists in the United States and Canada.

Dr. Freeman has written and edited six texts on family theory and therapy. His most recent books, *Multi-Generational Family Therapy* and *Family Therapy with Couples: The Family of Origin Approach,* emphasize the importance of working with the family elders.

Erik Jarlnaes is Co-creator of the Bodynamic System, a Cognitive Somatic Psychotherapy, and Bodynamic International. He has been creative director since 1982, and is presently director of Bodynamic International. He teaches and trains internationally, coaching Olympic chess players, European competitive runners, and world-champion rowing teams. He maintains a private practice in Denmark, his native country. Jarlnaes specializes in working with the concept of "peak experience," the subject in which he has done extensive research on Olympic gold medal winners as well as those who have experienced traumatic events.

Steen Jørgensen is a founding member of Bodynamic Institute, Denmark. He has a M.Sc. of Psychology from University of Copenhagen, Denmark. He has Danish training as an examined relaxation and movement therapist, as well as training in the field of somatic psychotherapy. He is a certified therapist in Bioenergetic Analysis. His main interests include understanding body language, character structure, and the effects of shock traumatic experience on the personality, and he has contributed to various articles and books on the Bodynamic view on these topics.

Maggie Kline is a marriage and family therapist who maintains a private practice in Long Beach, California. She is also a school psychologist for Long Beach Unified School District. She graduated from the Somatic Experiencing Practitioner Program in 1998 and is a supervising therapist and faculty member for the Foundation of Human Enrichment. Kline holds a master's degree in Counseling Psychology from California State University, Long Beach. She has also trained in Bodynamics and is a graduate of the Body-Mind Institute for Postural Integration. She has been bringing Somatic Experiencing awareness into the public school system through parent workshops of special needs youngsters and has maintained a private practice for over fifteen years.

Peter A. Levine earned his Ph.D. in Medical and Biological Physics at the University of California, Berkeley, and his Ph.D. in Psychology at International University. He has spent the last thirty-five years studying stress and trauma and has contributed to a variety of scientific and medical publications. He authored the book, *Waking the Tiger, Healing Trauma* (North Atlantic Books, 1997), which has received international recognition. He teaches his approach, Somatic Experiencing, worldwide, including consulting with NASA during the development of the space shuttle. He has consulted at a number of hospitals and Mental Health Agencies.

Josette van Luytelaar is a photographer who likes to "freeze" people in different situations. As a psychologist, however, she specializes in "unfreezing." Her main interests are peak and trauma work, panic disorders, and sexual problems. She is a certified therapist/supervisor in Bioenergetic Analysis, a Bodynamic Practitioner, and a European Certified Psychotherapist. She is also teaching general practitioners, unfreezing their professional attitude, at the University Medical Center in Nijmegen, the Netherlands. E-mail: josettevan-luytelaar@hetnet.nl

Lisbeth Marcher is Creator of the Bodynamic System, a Cognitive Somatic Psychotherapy, and Bodynamic International.   Since 1984, she has been director of training. She is a teacher and trainer who presents internationally at universities and at conferences (bodypsychotherapy, cognitive, pre-perinatal). She maintains a private practice in Denmark, her native country. She specializes in working with children.

Erving Polster obtained his Ph.D. from Case Western Reserve University in 1950. He is Director of the Gestalt Training Center in San Diego. He is also Clinical Professor in the Department of Psychiatry, School of Medicine at the University of California, San Diego. Along with his late wife Miriam, Polster is the co-author of an important text in gestalt therapy, *Gestalt Therapy Integrated*. Together they have also written *From the Radical Center: The Heart of Gestalt Therapy*. Polster is the author of *Every Person's Life Is Worth a Novel, A Population of Selves*.

About the Editor

Ian Macnaughton, Ph.D. (Human Science), is a registered clinical counselor in Vancouver, British Columbia, Canada. He maintains a private practice working with individuals, families, and organizations. He is currently on the teaching faculty of the Bodynamics Institute Inc. (Canada) and the Pacific Coast Family Therapy Training Association. In addition, he has served as a consultant to a number of organizations in the area of design and organizational learning.

He is a past president of the British Columbia Association of Clinical Counselors and Pacific Coast Family Therapy Training Associates. Ian has also taught for the business schools of the University of British Columbia, Simon Fraser University, Langara College, and the British Columbia Institute of Technology.

Ian brings to organizational consulting an extensive background in business, having owned a number of businesses both in Canada and the U.S.A. He is a past director of the Notaries Society of British Columbia, and also a past president of the Real Estate Institute of British Columbia, the Fraser Valley Real Estate Board, and the Real Estate Association of British Columbia. He has also served on the Executive Committee of the Canadian Real Estate Board.

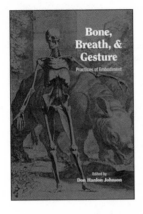

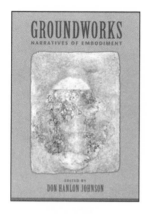

Groundworks
Narratives of Embodiment

Groundworks is the second in the series of Somatics texts edited by Don Hanlon Johnson. *Groundworks* gives accounts of the actual processes of working with individuals in six major schools of Somatics by either the creator of the method itself or a leading teacher of the method. The creators are Robert Hall of Lomi School, Bonnie Bainbridge Cohen of Body-Mind Centering, and Emilie Conrad Da'oud of Continuum. Leading teachers of methods include Michael Salveson on Rolfing, Elizabeth Beringer on Feldenkrais work, and Darcy Elman on F.M. Alexander Technique. Each therapist shows the complexity of working with somatic processes, as well as the reward, both for client and therapist.

• • •

Don Hanlon Johnson is Director of the Somatics graduate program at California Institute of Integral Studies and a former Rolf practitioner.

Edited by Don Hanlon Johnson

$14.95 paper, 1-55643-235-6, 138 pages, photos

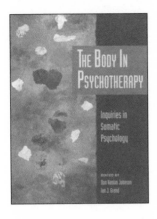